中医英译思考与实践

Thought and Practice of English Translation of Traditional Chinese Medicine

主　　编　陈可冀

编辑小组　陈可冀　刘　玥

　　　　　邱　禹　赵芳芳

北京大学医学出版社

ZHONGYI YINGYI SIKAO YU SHIJIAN

图书在版编目（CIP）数据

中医英译思考与实践/陈可冀主编．—北京：
北京大学医学出版社，2015.4
ISBN 978-7-5659-1063-0

Ⅰ.①中…　Ⅱ.①陈…　Ⅲ.①中国医药学-英语-翻
译-研究　Ⅳ.①R－092②H315.9

中国版本图书馆 CIP 数据核字（2015）第 055842 号

中医英译思考与实践

主　　编：陈可冀
出版发行：北京大学医学出版社
地　　址：（100191）北京市海淀区学院路 38 号　北京大学医学部院内
电　　话：发行部　010－82802230；图书邮购　010－82802495
网　　址：http：//www. pumpress. com. cn
E - mail：booksale@bjmu. edu. cn
印　　刷：中煤涿州制图印刷厂北京分厂
经　　销：新华书店
责任编辑：刘　燕　　**责任校对**：金彤文　　**责任印制**：李　啸
开　　本：710mm×1000mm　1/16　　**印张**：24.5　　**字数**：494 千字
版　　次：2015 年 4 月第 1 版　　2015 年 4 月第 1 次印刷
书　　号：978－7－5659－1063－0
定　　价：109.00 元

序

○○○

中医药名词术语的英译是中医药走向世界所必须逾越的沟坎。一般专业名词术语尚且在翻译上有困难，更何况一些寓意深刻的中医专业术语，例如“釜底抽薪”“扬汤止沸”“急下存阴”及“调理冲任”等中医治疗方法的描述，含义隐晦，不是三两个字就能够说明白的。要达到忠实原意并且说理通顺，实属不易。中外文化背景尚且不同，更何谈乎信达以外之雅也。中医词汇术语的翻译失当，不仅时常影响中外中医药学术交流，更可能引起医药沟通和医疗上的误解或曲解。

《中国中西医结合杂志》一向重视国内中医药名词术语的英译动向。1992年在当时常务副主编陈维养的倡议努力下，杂志设立了“中医英译”栏目，旨在通过在这个平台的讨论、交流，为中医药名词术语等的英译取得较为一致的意见，为以后的中医药名词术语标准化提供参考意见。20余年来，杂志刊登了数以百计的相关文章，虽未达到初衷，尚在路上，但在推动中医英译的心得经验交流、提高英译水平及表达合理化建议方面，还是起了一定的作用。这里面有老专家的大力支持与关注，有全国相关作者的踊跃参与，也有编辑部同仁的辛勤耕耘。

今经中国中医科学院心血管病研究所刘玥医师及《中国中西医结合杂志》编辑部赵芳芳医师、邱禹医师等合作，整理了20余年来在本杂志发表的有关中医英译文章并汇编成册，以提供大家参考，希望能在这方面起到抛砖引玉的作用，推进中医英译工作的发展。本书的出版得到了广州医药集团总工程师刘菊妍博士及广州娇兰佳人集团董事长蔡丙国先生的协助和支持，谨致谢忱。是以为序。

陈可冀

2014年隆冬

于北京西郊

目　录

上篇　总论　中医英译思考

谈中医名词术语的英译名问题…………………………………………………………… 3
关于中医生理学术语英译的意见………………………………………………………… 4
中医术语英译问题的商讨………………………………………………………………… 5
关于中医名词术语英译的讨论 ………………………………………………………… 12
浅谈中医翻译 …………………………………………………………………………… 19
Terminology Standardization in Chinese Medicine：The Perspective from
UCLA Center for East-West Medicine(Ⅰ) ………………………………………… 21
Terminology Standardization in Chinese Medicine：The Perspective from
UCLA Center for East-West Medicine(Ⅱ) ………………………………………… 27
中医基本理论名词术语英译探讨 ……………………………………………………… 35
中医药术语英译的探讨 ………………………………………………………………… 37
关于中医名词术语英译标准化的思考 ………………………………………………… 39
借鉴国外翻译经验和理念，促进国内中医英译事业发展 …………………………… 41
中医英译中的音译现象与翻译的等值理论 …………………………………………… 45
中医术语英译原则探讨 ………………………………………………………………… 48
中医文献英译的异化和归化 …………………………………………………………… 52
中医英译规范化中的译者素养问题探讨 ……………………………………………… 57
中医英译的多元文化系统视角探微 …………………………………………………… 60
中医名词术语英译中的信息密度与翻译策略和方法 ………………………………… 63
音译法在中医英译中的应用原则与策略 ……………………………………………… 67
浅议连字符在中医术语英译中的使用 ………………………………………………… 77
中医名词术语英译标准化应用之因“地”制宜 ………………………………………… 82
不同翻译手段在中医文献翻译中的辨证施用 ………………………………………… 85
中医名词术语翻译层面观及其译语特点 ……………………………………………… 88
论名词化在中医文本英译中的运用 …………………………………………………… 92

“东方情调化翻译”在两套中医名词术语英译标准化方案中的体现………… 98
中医英译的语言学思考…………………………………………………… 102
中医术语英译标准化讨论………………………………………………… 107
中医文献英译的文化对等………………………………………………… 110
从接受理论浅谈中医翻译中的文化传达………………………………… 113

中篇　分论　中医英译实践

第一节　中医基础理论英译实践……………………………………… 119
试论中医基础理论名词术语英译的标准………………………………… 119
中医因果关系病名的特征及其翻译……………………………………… 122
试析中医“证”的几个常见英译名……………………………………… 125
中医学疾病的概念………………………………………………………… 129
中医病症名称的英译方法………………………………………………… 132
中医病因学常用名词术语英译…………………………………………… 136
中医“证”及其相关术语的英译………………………………………… 140
也谈中医术语“六淫”的英译…………………………………………… 141
关于“风、寒、暑、湿、燥、火”中医术语英译的商榷………………… 143
谈中医病因学说有关术语的英译………………………………………… 145
中医“神明”的英语翻译………………………………………………… 147
谈“脏象”与“脏腑”术语的英译……………………………………… 150
谈中医名词术语“辨证论治”的英译…………………………………… 152
“证”的新译 ……………………………………………………………… 154
试论“证”及其相关词语的英译………………………………………… 156
有关中医五行学说术语的英译…………………………………………… 158
谈中医术语“气”的英译………………………………………………… 159
谈谈中医学中“虚实”的翻译…………………………………………… 161
中医诊断学中常用辨证证名英译探讨…………………………………… 163
谈谈中医“实”和“虚”的英译………………………………………… 166
“整体观念”翻译之浅见 ………………………………………………… 168
中医反治法英译评析……………………………………………………… 170
浅析活血化瘀的英译……………………………………………………… 174
中医脉象翻译的原则和方法……………………………………………… 176
基于隐喻认知的脉象术语英译研究……………………………………… 179
论中医脉象术语的翻译…………………………………………………… 187

《黄帝内经》英译中美学价值的损失与补偿 …… 194
《黄帝内经》常用文化负载词英译 …… 202
《黄帝内经·素问》英译事业的描写性研究 …… 208
论《黄帝内经·素问》篇名的英译…… 224
《黄帝内经素问》书名英译探讨 …… 230
关于《黄帝内经》书名英译的商榷…… 235
当代翻译理论在《黄帝内经》英译研究中的应用…… 237
“Huangdi”还是“Huang Di”? …… 245

第二节　中药方剂英译实践…… 247
中药方剂名的英译技巧与原则…… 247
谈中药药性理论有关术语的英译…… 251
中药名词英译标准化的探讨…… 253
中药商品名称的美学特征与英语名称的翻译…… 261
论中药七情的英文翻译…… 265
中成药说明书“功能与主治”的文体特点与翻译…… 271
中医方剂名称英译的归化与异化…… 275
“Zhibai Dihuang”还是“Zhibo Dihuang”? …… 279
方剂学“君、臣、佐、使”英译的探讨…… 281
浅谈中医英译中方剂名称的翻译…… 284
试论方剂学“君、臣、佐、使”的英译…… 286
中成药名的常见英译结构…… 291
方剂名称英译…… 293
中医方剂名英译问题探讨…… 295

第三节　针灸经络英译实践…… 298
浅谈“络穴”的英译…… 298
中医针灸学论文标题的英译…… 300
经络学说术语的英译…… 303
腧穴本义与英译…… 304
奇经八脉英译当议…… 306
关于针灸学中“寸”的英文译名…… 307
经络和穴位名称的翻译…… 309
也谈针灸穴位名称的翻译…… 312
针灸穴位翻译与中医文化传承…… 315

下篇　书评及其他

为谢竹藩教授英译中专著 *On the Standard Nomenclature of Traditional Chinese Medicine* 写的序言 …… 321
评杨谦志著《中药与方剂手册》(*Handbook of Chinese Herbs and Formulas*) …… 323
评魏迺杰先生的《实用英文中医辞典》 …… 327
评《英汉·汉英中医词典》出版 …… 338
《补注洗冤录集证》第一个英译本简评 …… 344
中医翻译要追本求源和衷中参西 …… 349
对《中医药常用名词术语英译》的一些意见 …… 355
关于《汉英医学大辞典》中某些中医药词条的商榷 …… 362
评《中医药学名词》中的对应英文名词 …… 366
中医对外英语交流的经验与体会 …… 373
英译《中医妇科学》的几点体会 …… 376
中医药期刊的刊名英译 …… 378

上篇　总论　中医英译思考

谈中医名词术语的英译名问题

周金黄

近来在阅读国内中医药期刊时，我感到中医名词术语的英译名问题值得讨论。例如，有下列译名："气"为 functional activities，"阴"为 vital essence，"阳"为 vital function，"补气药"为 drugs for replenishing the vital energy，"补血药"为 blood tonics，"补益药"（补养药）为 tonics，"理气药"为 drugs for regulating the flow of vital energy 等。中医名词术语的优点是字少而意深，其英译名似应仿此，但不要与西医常用专门名词混淆。有的可音译，如阴、阳，现在世界上均通用 Yin、Yang。但"气"则未见通用外文译名，译法也不一致。有人用译音 Qi，似乎只有标音的用途，但不能作为译意的名词。"气"在中医理论中是一个最基本的概念，是构成宇宙和人最本质的元素（basic element）。为了突出这一特点，是否可以创造一个新的派生字"energen"（原意为"能"，从 energy 派生），字尾加"gen"，有类似氧（oxygen）、氢（hydrogen）、氮（nitrogen）等元素的字尾。"气"就具有中医理论"能动元素"这一概念。"补气药"则为 energenic drugs 或 energenics，"理气药"则为 energen modulating drugs 或 energen-modulators，"气虚"则为 energen-deficiency，"气不足"则为 energen-insufficiency 等，均属同源派生字，原外文字根为 energein、energos 等。

提出英译新名词的设想，是为了请有关专家考虑这个问题，而不是以为把"气"译为 energen 就一定可取，仅以此作为抛砖引玉之一线。

中医的"证"译成 syndrome，也是一个值得推敲的词。要使译名突出中医"证"的概念，似乎也应创造一个新译名词，从而既能体现中医的学术思想，又便于现代科学的理解。

总之，希望在中西医结合工作中，逐步使中医名词术语有标准英译名，供国内外学者采用。北京医学院编的《汉英常用中医药词汇》可供参考，有其优点，可以更进一步修改、充实，使之更加完善。本刊可以为探讨中医药名词术语标准英译名草案开辟一个不定期专栏，以在这方面提出建议。

[原载《中国中西医结合杂志》，1984，1（1）：9.]

关于中医生理学术语英译的意见

季钟朴　谢仁敷　沈雪勇　孔海云

中医生理学术语英译需要规范化，这是毫无疑问的。国际上日益重视中医学，国际医学界迫切希望了解中医药学。中医药学若要走向世界为全人类做贡献，首先是要求中医药学翻译名词术语的规范化。

我国已经有一批西医学中的中西医结合的专家。他们对中医学、西医学以及英语均有较深的修养和较高的素质。其中部分专家还在国外讲授过中医学，写过英译中医药学的文章，编写翻译过有关中医学的英译教材，还出版了若干种中医英译的名词术语辞书。所以中医学名词术语英译规范化是完全有条件办到的事。

建议中国中西医结合学会负责组织专家进行这件大事，成立中医药学术语英译规范化小组，协同有关方面分工编写出版一部比较权威的中医药学英译名词术语词典。

中医生理学名词术语英译对中医学各科影响广泛而深远，现提出几点粗浅意见供参考：

1. 凡是中医学的名词概念内涵比较复杂，各家对它的理解也不尽相同，难以确切英译成西医学中对应的名词的，则采取用中医学名词的汉语拼音，如 Qi（气）、Yin-Yang（阴-阳）等以保留原貌，以便深入探讨、研究。汉语拼音第一个字母要大写。

2. 凡是中西医名词概念内涵明确、一致，所指器官的结构与功能统一的，可完全采用中西医学名词直接对应意译，中外学者均不会产生误解，如胃（stomach）、肠（intestine）、膀胱（bladder）、胞宫（uterus）等。

3. 凡是中西医名词所指器官的结构与功能不完全统一，宏观概念与微观概念不一致的，如心、肝、脾、肾等脏象，中西医名词不能对应意译时，可采取兼顾处理，例如中医学的心、肝、脾、肾，分别英译为 Heart（Xin）、Liver（Gan）、Spleen（Pi）、Kidney（Shen）等。中医学的“心”是宏观的，故英译时应将英文首字母改为大写并附汉语拼音。

4. 生理解剖术语虽也有拉丁文，但与中草药名词用拉丁文不同，中草药用拉丁文较易被接受，而生理名词术语用普通英语加第一字母大写并附汉语拼音，具有音译、意译兼顾并有中医学特色。以上建议不成熟，供参考。

[原载《中国中西医结合杂志》，1993，13（10）：626.]

中医术语英译问题的商讨

侯　灿

编辑部让我参加关于中医术语英译问题的讨论。这方面我经验不多，但有几个不成熟的想法，提出来和同道商讨，希望对中医英译有所裨益。

1. 中医术语概念的规范化理解问题

众所周知，翻译应做到“信、达、雅”（清・严复语）。对英译中医术语（包括名词在内的专门用语）来说，首先要求“信”和“达”，要求译出来的词语能准确（信）反映（达）原中医术语所含概念的内涵，特别是中医特有的有别于西医的思想内容。为此，英译中医术语首先必须对各术语所含概念有明确、统一、规范化的理解。而当前有些特别具有中医特色的术语，古今中外人士对其所含概念内涵的理解却很不规范，这就给英译造成很大的困难。

以公认最具中医特色的“辨证论治”的“证”来说，它首见于《素问・至真要大论》，“证有中外，治有轻重”，对此王冰注“病证有表里，药用有轻重”，将“证”等同于“病证”；而吴昆注“证候有中外，药用有轻重”，将“证”等同于“证候”。对于《伤寒论》中“平脉辨证”的“证”，现代肖氏认为是“症候”，认为“结胸证”的“证”是“病症”。以上各家给“证”下定义的四个定义项（病证、证候、症候、病症）是否含有同一概念，很不明确。若按《辞海》（中华书局，1965年）所认为：医学名词的“证”与“症”同义，可以通用，则上述“证”的定义都犯了同语反复（即定义项“病症”“证候”都直接包括被定义项“证”字）的逻辑错误。由于上述“证”的定义不明确、不规范，就无法从英语中去寻找对等词或对应词，也无法创造英语新词。

另外，新中国成立以来对“证”的理解，有认为是“医者赖以作出诊断和治疗的各种证据”者；有认为是“整个外观病象的总和，现代术语叫症候群”者；有认为是“中医通过四诊所得到的患病机体即病后的全部临床表现”者；有认为是“中医的诊断总称”者；有将显然属于症状的“小便多”“小便失禁”等定义为“证名”者。若按第一种理解来翻译，“证据”可译为 evidence，但西医诊治疾病同样需要证据，“症状”就是西医认识病情或疾病的功能性“证据”（美国《道兰图解医学词典》给症状“symptom”下的定义是：“any functional evidence of disease or of a patient's condition”），因此，这种理解及其相应英译法不能准确反映中医特色。若按第二种理解来翻译，“症候群”即英文 syndrome，但“症候群”是现代西医有特定含义的术语（指构成某种病理情况而其特征尚未完全确定、其原因不明或原因多种多样的症状和体征的集合）。而依照赵金铎主编《中医证候鉴别诊断学》（人民卫生出版社，1987 年）给“证”下的定义：“证”是“证候”的简括总称，既不是症状，也不是病名，而是“集中地反映疾病的原因、性状、部位、范围、动态等病理要素的综合性诊断概念”。或依照冷方南主编《中医证候辨治规范》（人民卫生出版社，1991 年）的定义，即疾病某一具体阶段的本质反应和病理概括，则将“证”译为 syndrome 显然不准确，而且抹杀了中医“证”的上述特色。若按第三种理解，“临床表现”有现成的英文对等词 clinical manifestation，但即使加上“中医通过四诊得到的……”这个定语从句，也未能反映“证”的上述特色，因为四诊是通过医者感官掌握患者的临床表现，而西医同样要通过感官了解患者的临床表现。若按第四种理解，“诊断总称”可直译为 overall diagnosis，但西医的诊断指将一种疾病（disease）与其他疾病区别开来的艺术，或对疾病性质的确定（《道兰图解医学词典》），因此，将“证”译为 overall diagnosis 也不能准确表达“证”不同于西医“疾病实体”（disease entity）的中医特色。

外国学者对“证”的理解也不一致。如 Porkert 在其所著德文《中医诊断学教科书》的有关八纲辨证章节中将“辨证”译为 differenzierung der Krankheitszeichen（英译为 differentiation of symptoms and signs，即症状与体征的鉴别），相当于把“证”理解为“证候”（我国有学者认为“证候”就是“症状与体征”）；但在具体讲到表证与里证时却将其译为 species-symptome 及 intima-symptome（英译为 outer-symptom 及 inner-symptom），即将“证”等同于“症状”；而有的地方又把表证和里证分别译为 aubenseit eer krankung 和 innerseit eer krankung（英译分别为 outer-disease 和 inner-disease），即将“证”等同于“疾病”。20 世纪 30 年代 Morse 在其所著《中医学》中也将“证”等同于“疾病”，如将“表证”译为 superficial disease。而 Kaptchuk 在其专著中则将“证”理解为“类型”（pattern），认为“八纲辨证”是通过症状和体征认识身体失衡状态的八种类型，因而将“八纲辨证”译为 eight principal patterns。新近魏迺杰等在其《中医术语规范化建议》一文中使用了 Kaptchuk 的“类型”一词，但却将“八纲辨证”译为 eight parameters of disease-pattern identification，即不将“辨证”理解为“身体失衡状态类型的确认”，而将其理解为“疾病类型（disease-pattern）的确认”，也就是将“证”理解为“疾病”（disease）。

由上可见，仅“证”一个术语就有如此不同的理解，多么需要加以规范。当然这要靠学术研究来逐步解决。

2. 英译中医术语的规范化问题

即使若干中医术语概念理解规范化问题得到解决，其英译词本身也存在规范化问题。英译词规范化同样要以信、达、雅为准绳，具体说就是用词的准确性（所用英译词的词义与中医术语所含概念的符合程度）、合理性（表达中医术语思想内容的能力）和可接受性（被人们认可、赞同而乐意加以使用的程度）。下面我们试分析现有的一些英译中医术语不规范和（或）不符合上述准绳的情况。

加拿大术语学权威 Dubuc 在其专著《应用术语学》中提出，术语的规范化决定可由权威机构用法令或表态方式规定或建议人们使用某种术语。按此观点，英译中医术语的权威机构在我国应是《汉英医学大词典》（人民卫生出版社，1987 年，下简称《医典》）的编委会及《中医药主题词表》（北京科技出版社，1987 年，下简称《词表》）的主编单位。但在他们所编的上述两部工具书中，有些中医术语英译词就不够准确、合理，因而难以接受，影响了其权威性。

例如，《医典》将“证”等同于“证候”，英译为 syndrome、symptom complex。将“证”译为“症候群”或“综合征”的不妥之处，已如前述。又如以上两书均将“辨证”英译为 differentiation of symptoms and signs，将“证”等同于“症状和体征”。由于西医诊断疾病同样需要对症状与体征进行鉴别，因此，这种译法同样不能准确表达中医“辨证”的思想内容，不能反映中医特色。再如《医典》将“辨证论治”译成 187 个印刷符号的英文，内容可反映中医特色（因文中指出是以中医基础理论为基础的鉴别诊断），但这是对“辨证论治”的“释义”而不是英译“术语”。而《词表》则将其译为 treatment according to differentiation（按照鉴别进行治疗），由于“鉴别”（differentiation）后面没有加上与“证”相应的介词短语，人们将不明白用“什么”来进行治疗，因此，这种译法也难以接受。欧明主编的《汉英中医辞典》（广东科技出版社，1986 年）将“辨证论治”译为 selection of treatment based on the differential diagnosis，同样缺少 diagnosis 后面的介词短语而没能反映出“证”的中医特色。

在规模庞大的编委会的指导下由张恩勤主编的《英汉对照实用中医文库》也应被视为权威著作，但其中某些提法和译法也不尽如人意。例如其《中医诊断学》分册（上海中医学院出版社，1990 年）中给“证”下了一个疾病的“病理概括”的定义，而将其译为 pathological generalization of a disease。generalization 在西医术语中有“局部病变扩散为全身性疾病”的意思（To convert from a local to a general disease.）（《道兰图解医学词典》）英语读者可能接受不了或被误导。另外，该书汉语部分给“辨证”下了个定义，即“辨证是……辨明其为何证的过程”，这又是一个定义项直接包括被定义项的同义语反复定义，而其英译为 differentiation of syndrome…to determine the type of a disease（症候群的鉴别……以确定疾病的类型)，即将原汉语部分的“辨证”译为“症候群的鉴别”，然后又将“辨明其为何证”译为“确定疾病的类型”（将“证”等同于“疾病”)。这种译法看来也不符合上述三性的要求，特别是未能准确体现中医辨证的特色。

外国学者英译中医术语也存在不规范和（或）不符合三性要求的情况。除了本文前面提及的“证”和“辨证”外，还可举出其他例子。

例如八纲中的“虚”与“实”。据称最早由美国 Bensky 分别译成 deficiency 和 excess，以后 Kaptchuk 加以沿用，但 ILza Veith 在翻译《素问·通评虚实论》时却将其分别译为 emptiness 和 fullness。从岐伯所下定义“邪气盛则实，精气夺则虚”看，Veith 在该场合的这种译法显然不准确。英国著名汉学家李约瑟（JTM. Needham）分别译为 asthenic 和 plerotic。前者源于希腊语 asthenikos，表示虚弱、没力气（weak，lack or loss of strength)，用于八纲虚证较准确、合理，而且可以接受，但后者来源于拉丁语 pleroticus，表示填满、装满（filling up)，用于八纲实证显然不妥，因实证的症状和体征是机能亢进（邪气盛)，而不是什么“填满”。不过 emptiness 和 fullness plertoic 用于另一场合如《素问·五脏别论》“水谷入口则胃实而肠虚”中的虚实或脉的虚实看来就很合适。对用于八纲的“实”，欧明主编《汉英中医辞典》译为 sthenia 看来较准确、合理，因该词源于希腊语 sthenos，意为 strength、force（有力气，与“邪气盛则实”和实证的症状与体征相吻合)。而 Porkert 将“八纲虚实”中的“虚”“实”分别译为拉丁语 inanitas（emptiness，空虚）及 repletio（fullness，充满)，魏迺杰将其分别译为 vacuity（空虚）及 repletion（充满）都存在同样的问题。

再如脏腑。Veith 将五脏六腑译为 the five viscera and the six bowels。viscera（拉丁语）指所有三个体腔内的器官，已包括 bowel（源于古法语，指肠道)，而且这两个词仍特指西医解剖单位，未能反映中医脏腑作为一种现代系统论中的“概念单元”（conceptual unity）的特色。Porkert 强调脏腑是一种充满能量的功能集合体，而不单纯是解剖单位，因而将其译为 energetic sphere，即一种与大宇宙有关的小天体“orb”［源自拉丁语 orbis，《韦氏英语大字典》对此词也有 collective whole（即“集合的整体”）的释义］，然后依照中医理论将“脏”译为拉丁语 orbishorreal（horreal 派生自拉丁语 horream，即英语 storehouse，指藏东西的仓库，与张景岳“脏，藏也……犹言库藏之藏，所以藏物者”相吻合)，将“腑”译为拉丁语 orbis aulici（aulici 派生自 aulicus，指大庭院、宫廷，蕴含“中空”——空腔器官之意，与《素问·金匮真言论》“胆、胃、大肠、小肠、膀胱、三焦、六腑……”相吻合)，并将“脏象”译为 orbis-iconography（icon 为图像，iconography 即用图画描述某种东西的形象)，有其准确性和合理性，可惜可接受性差。就作者所知，至今仅有个别人采用这种译法。欧明等将“脏”译为 solid organ（实质性器官如心、肝、肾等)，“腑”译为 hollow organ（空腔性器官，如胃肠、胆、膀胱等），更符合中医对内脏解剖学的粗浅认识，但在功能上特别是病理生理上则与中医脏腑概念相去甚远。

还可举出其他事例，不过以上例子已足以说明英译中医术语本身也存在规范化问题有待解决。

3. 中医术语英译的方法学问题

按双语术语学的一般研究方法，要将一种语言的术语译成另一种语言的术语，首先要弄清前者的概念特性和使用范围，再从后者寻找前者的对等词（equivalent word，指在同一专业领域中所含词义内容几乎完全一致的词）或对应词（correspondent word，指一种语言的术语只包含另一语言术语中的部分词义内容），或创造后者中的新词。据此，相当一部分中医术语，特别是那些可直接感知其现象如症状和体征的术语或可通过症状和体征等临床表现加以判定的病名，其所含概念及使用范围与英语原有的医学术语几乎完全相同，因而可从后者中找到对等词。例如：下利（diarrhea）、中脘痛（epigastric pain）、日晡发热（afternoon fever）、不更衣（constipation）、小便短小（oliguria）、小便难（dysuria）、消谷善饥（polyorexia）、崩漏（metrorrhagia & metrostaxis）、鼻齆（anosmia）、皶（rhinophyma）等。

但另一部分中医术语不能从英语中找到对等词而只能找出对应词（相当于一种意译）。下面是魏迺杰关于英译某些中医特有术语规范译法的建议，似可看成是一些对应词，可供参考和商榷：五行（five phases）、八纲（eight parameters）、脾胃虚（splenogastric vacuity）、伤寒（cold damage）、导（abduct）、疏（course）、肃（depurate）、利（disinhibit）、散（dissipate）、发（effuse）、渗（percolate）、宣（perfuse）、升（upbearing）、降（downbearing）、滞（stagnation）、瘀（stasis）、郁（depression）、闭（block）、痹（obturation）、结（bind）、积（accumulation）、聚（gathering）、停（collection）、壅（congestion）、补（supplementation）、育（fostering）、滋（enriching）、养（nourishing）、柔（emolliating）、强（strengthening）、生（engendering）、健（fortification）、益（reinforce）、活血（blood quickening）、破血（blood breaking）、熄风（extinguishing wind）、祛风（dispelling wind）、壮阳（invigorating Yang）、救阳（salvaging Yang）、回阳（restoring Yang）、助阳（reinforcing Yang）、通阳（freeing Yang）、宣阳（perfusing Yang）等。

寻求中医术语在英语中的对应词时还应注意该术语在不同场合的不同含义（一词多义），即注意它的上下文，同时要注意英语词类搭配习惯。例如上述魏迺杰对中医治疗学术语“宣”字的英译建议使用 perfuse。按《韦氏英语大词典》，perfuse 意为“to cause to flow or spread”（致使流动或散布），则 perfuse 用于以温热通阳方药治疗因寒湿阻遏、痰凝瘀阻所致阳气不通（即“宣通阳气”，perfusing Yang）较合适，用于治疗邪阻心窍（“宣窍”）或“宣毒”的场合就不合适。另外，“宣可去壅”，魏迺杰将“壅”译成 congestion，但按英语搭配习惯，congestion 不能与 perfuse 搭配，因此，在此场合“宣”似可译为 relieve（减轻、解除）或 reduce（减轻），或 disperse（to cause to vanish，使逐渐消除或消散）。

Porkert 认为中医术语的翻译方法可有三种，即直译、根据上下文灵活翻译（flexible translation adapted to the context）和规范化翻译（normative translation）。他曾直译“太极”为 supreme pole，直译“命门”为 gate of destiny（另一些外国学者认为译为 gate of life 较符合中医“生命之门户”的原意），但更主张采用“规范化”译法。例如他强调用拉丁语创造新词，并希望大家都加以使用从而使其规范化。可惜他的这种译法可接受性差。如他将“脏”译为拉丁语 orbis 或相应英语 orb。除了在他出版有关专著的次年有瑞典学者 Agren 采用外，至今尚未见有人采用。当然我们不能因此否定他这种主张和努力的合理性。

众所周知，中医理论体系及其术语对西方国家及其语言来说大都是外来的东西，因此，我们在英语中找不到相应对等词或对应词时可以采用各国外来词的构词方法，为英语构造一些新的外来词。由于英语越来越取代了世界语的功能，加上英语语法简单，因此，为汲取其他语言敞开了大门。如 Mawson 在其编撰的英语《外来词词典》的前言中指出，英语的外来词来自 50 种以上的外语，可见将中医术语特别是独具中医特色的术语变成英语外来词的可能性和潜力是很大的。

外来词是“一种语言从其他语言里吸收过来的词语”，一般多使用音译、音译加表意成分、半音译半意译以及直接借用等方法。例如“休克”是英语 shock 的音译，“阿米巴原虫”是 ameba 的音译加表意成分，“单克隆”是 monoclone 的半意译半音译；有的则直接借用自日语，如：血栓、流感等。日本的医学外来词绝大部分用片假名音译英语医学术语，而对中医术语则大都直接借用汉语。采用拉丁字母拼音的英语与采用笔画表意的汉语不同，它可以直接借用拉丁语医学术语（如 abdomen“腹”，cancer“癌”等），而不能像日语那样直接借用汉语中医术语，因此，只能使用其他几种外来词构词法。例如“阴阳”音译为 Yin and Yang（这种翻译方式已被载入权威的《韦氏英语大词典》），“脏”音译加表意成分为 Zang organ，“正气”半音译半意译为 normal Qi，“湿热痢”calor-humidus-dysenteria 为希-拉构词法。

在本刊“中医英译”专栏讨论中，有同志认为音译法即用汉语拼音英译中医术语应是“最后一种选择”，主要理由是害怕外国读者无法或不容易接受。我不同意这种看法。相反，我认为对中医独有而在现有英语词汇中找不到适当对等词或对应词，或无法用英语惯用希-拉词素构词法构造恰当新词的情况下，用汉语拼音加以音译［当然开始时应同时加注 1867 年英国人威妥玛（Thomas F.

Wade）设计的用以在英文中拼写汉字的拼音法，而且在正文中首次出现时可加注汉字］是唯一可行的出路。对本文第一节提到的尚未能加以规范化理解的中医术语（例如“证”）更是如此，因为这种音译而成的英语外来词就是中医术语本身，可以最准确、合理地反映该术语所含概念的思想内容和使用范围，而不受意译或希-拉构词法可能产生的曲解或歧义的影响。

人们最担心的是英语读者的可接受性问题。我认为这种担心不必要，关键是国人要有信心和决心。

信心从何而来？首先，像陈可冀同志在讨论中指出的，“汉字拼音已被联合国承认，是合法的”。其次，汉字拼音法与威妥玛式汉字拼音法虽有不同，但有规律可循，主要是14个声母（辅音）的写法和发音略有不同（以汉语拼音在前，威妥玛式拼音在后，其对照如下：b→p，c→ts′，ch→ch′，d→t，g→k，j→ch，k→k′，p→p′，q→ch′，r→j，t→t′，x→hs，z→ts，zh→ch。如“八纲”bagang-pa kang，“气”Qi-ch′，“证”zheng-cheng等），这两种拼法的韵母（元音）基本相同。掌握这一简单规律，英语读者就可很快学会音译中医术语的正确发音。再次，也是很重要的一点是，音译另一种语言的医学术语，在已出版的用英语介绍不同民族传统医学的若干医学专著中已有不少先例。如Heyn 1990年介绍印度传统医学的专著时，其书名“Ayurveda”就是古印度天城体梵文的拉丁字母转写形式 āyurveda 的音译（汉语音译为“阿由吠陀”，半音半意译为“长寿吠陀”）。书中的很多术语如Tridosha、Vata、Pitta、Kapha等都是在第一次出现时从梵文的拉丁字母转写形式音译加注释，以后重新出现时就不再注释，当成英语外来词使用。Svoboda 1989年介绍了长寿吠陀体质学说的专著，其书名“Prakruti”也是梵文的音译。书中关于三种基本体质类型——Vata型、Pitta型和Kapha型等也都是音译，也是开头加注释后就不再注释。Rechung 1976年在介绍西藏医学的专著中大部分术语也都采用类似的方法。上述三本书有一个共同点，就是在书末附有一个词汇表（glossary），将音译术语按字母顺序排列并逐一加以简要说明，这就大大提高了这种译法的可接受性，而且十分有利于学术交流。

语言是约定俗成的产物。音译中医术语能否被英语读者接受，还要看我们有无决心发挥主观能动性去施加影响。在以汉语为母语的中国，外国人学习中医时要学会汉语拼音，就像我们学习西医时要学会英语一样，是理所当然的事。1985年我访美期间参加过一个印度长寿吠陀医学短训班，白人教师和学员在课堂上用音译梵文医学术语熟练地讲授和讨论，给我留下很深的印象。难道咱们中医就不能这样做吗？

［原载《中国中西医结合杂志》，1994，14（1）：46－49.］

关于中医名词术语英译的讨论

谢竹藩

自1992年《中国中西医结合杂志》开辟了"中医英译"专栏以来，已刊登文章70余篇，其中有很多宝贵的意见值得我们翻译中医书籍、文章时参考。另外，这些文章中也存在着不少分歧。综合所讨论的内容，这些分歧大致可归纳为下列几个方面。

1. 中医名词术语英译标准化的指导思想

专栏的编者按指出，开辟此专栏的目的是"就国内目前中医药名词术语英译中存在的不同意见及难点加以探讨，希望取得较为一致的看法，为将来翻译的标准化提供参考意见"。要达到此目的，首先须对英译标准化的基本原则或指导思想有一个统一的看法。这里所说的不是单纯指"信、达、雅"或"准确、简洁、实用"等标准，而是指如何来判断是否达到这些标准。一开始建立"中医英译"时专栏就有人提出，"我们搞中医术语英译的对象不是中国人，而是外国人，目的是为了扩大中医学在世界上的影响，所以一切要以外国读者的接受性为主要尺度来衡量，哪一种方式最容易被接受，就应采用哪一种，……当然要能基本正确表达原意。"[1]在以后的讨论中也不断有人强调这一点，例如"在将源语转化为目标语时需要考虑目标语读者的承受能力"[2]。但也有人持相反的看法。例如，有人认为中医药英译的主动权应掌握在中国学者手中[3]。还有人提出"要建立一个有权威性的国际化的中医语言学，必须以自身语言为本……，至于西方人在学习新的中医语言时怎么去强化理解和方便记忆，这是他们的事。……用我们的语言去教育他人，而不是用我们的语言去适应他人"[3]。在这样对立的思想指导下出现种种争论当然就不足为奇了。

2. 音译问题

对中医名词术语音译问题争论的焦点有二：一是音译术语的数量，二是汉语拼音的使用。对于数量，没有人主张全用音译，但如"肾阴虚"这样的术语也须音译[3]，恐怕就没有多少中医术语不该音译的了。较多的意见是音译在万不得已时才使用，应尽量控制其数量，只适宜用于确实难以用其他译法表达其概念的术语[4]。这一点显然是合理的，因为汉语用的是单音象形文字，同音异义字很多。音译多了，出现同音字词时就会造成混乱。

关于用汉语拼音"音译"，争论很多，但忽略了音译的定义和汉语拼音的功用这两个最根本问题。在《辞海》《辞源》等辞典中未能找到关于音译的定义，但无论是汉英字典还是英汉字典，音译与 transliteration 是对应的。Transliterate的定义很明确，是指"把一个字或词用另一种语言的同音字母来表达"（to represent, as a word, by the alphabetic characters of another language having the same sound,《韦氏国际英语词典》，1996 年)。这里说明音译须有两个条件，一是翻成另一种语言，否则不能叫做"译"；二是必须同音，不然就不是音译。从理论上讲，汉语拼音只是用拉丁字母拼出来的汉语，根本不是音译的英语。从实际情况来看，汉语拼音虽然也用 26 个拉丁字母，但是连字母的读音都与英语字母的读音有很多差别，拼出来的字词更不可能全都符合英语音译的要求。当然，有时也有符合英语拼音的，如阴 Yin，阳 Yang。但这两个音译与汉语拼音无关，早在汉语拼音问世之前，"阴""阳"作为中国古代哲学概念就已被音译为 Yin 和 Yang 了。《韦氏国际英语词典》中还收载了不少由汉语音译的字，都不是根据汉语拼音音译，而是根据英语本身的发音规律和习惯音译（顺便提一下，也非完全根据威妥玛拼音法。后者同样只能形成拼音的汉语，不一定能成为音译的英语）。

汉语的拼音有多种方案，现行的方案是 1958 年由我国第一届全国人民代表大会第五次会议批准推行的。制定此方案的目的是帮助识字，统一读音，改进学校语言教学，推广普通话，并为创制汉语拼音文字准备条件。总之，用汉语拼音是解决汉语的语音问题。世界卫生组织在针灸国际标准命名法建议中确实采用了汉语拼音，而且还加注了声调，但明确指出"汉字代表经脉和穴位的全名和原名……，由于汉字的发音各地不同，故根据中国的标准语音加注拼音名以助发音"[5]。该命名法在"十四经"项下列出了四种名称。以肺经为例，依次排列如下：英文为 lung meridian，拼音为 shǒutàiyīn fèijīng，汉字为"手太阴肺经"，字母编码为 LU。至于穴位名称，由于英译困难，故把字母编码放在第一位，如中府是 LU1。西方人士一般都用字母编码。

英语中的确有很多外来词，有的音译成英语，这些词能按英语的规律用前缀、后缀或词尾变化来改变其意义和词性。有的直接把其他语言的字词或短语一成不变地用到文章里，原来是什么语还是什么语，即使是拉丁文也不例外。这些词语不是音译的英语，更不能按英语的规律来添加词缀或改变词性。用汉语拼音属于后一种情况，所以国外作者在编写英文中医书籍时对一些汉语拼音文字常作如下的交代：由于这些字词翻译困难，故未译。有的作者还给汉语拼音加英语注音。说"未译"是合情合理、实事求是的。

音译并不是那么简单的。汉语中由外语音译来的词，很多都是几经改动才得到公认的。音译不仅要考虑语音规律和习惯，还要有一个约定俗成的过程。举例来说，"艾滋病"是个音译过来的汉语名词，意译是"获得性免疫缺陷综合征"

acquired immunodeficiency syndrome，AIDS)，这个词太长，按缩写“AIDS”音译，严格地说应该是“诶滋”，但听起来不大顺耳，于是译成“艾滋”，还加了个“病”字。现在“艾滋病”这个词叫开了，约定俗成，成了公认的译法。如果写文章时直截了当用 AIDS，这没有什么不可以，但不会有人认为这是音译的汉语。在中医的英译中用几个汉语拼音的名词术语，与汉语中加几个英文语词没有什么区别，全都与“译”无关，因此，还是应把精力放在名词术语的真正翻译上，直译也罢，意译也罢，如果实在没有合适的译法，那么只能暂用汉语拼音，待日后再解决。这种汉语日后能不能以及如何成为音译的英语，这只能由以英语为母语的人来进行约定俗成。

3. 创造新词

这里所说的词是指 word，在中文常称为“字”。有不少人提出种种方法来创造英文新词以适应中医术语英译的需要，例如借用拉丁文和希腊语的词根、前缀或后缀构成新词，甚至有人认为中文的汉语拼音就是英文新词，而且在此基础上还可以进一步发展[6]。但这些意见遭到了很多人的反对[3,6~8]。Manfred Porkert 在 20 多年前就曾用拉丁文创建了一套中医名词术语，结果无人采用，只好将之束之高阁。至于创造新的英文字词，回顾一下西医中译的历史可能对解决这个问题有所帮助。在 19 世纪末 20 世纪初西医传入中国时就遇到了西医名词中译的问题。1886 年，西方的传教士医生在上海成立中国教会医学联合会，在中文的西医名词方面做了许多工作，还编造了一些新字。对于这些新字，中国人根本未予接受[9]。不以英语为母语的人要当英文的仓颉，这大概是同样难以被接受的。即使是以英语为母语的人，在这个问题上也是采取十分谨慎的态度。例如英国学者魏迺杰在其编著的收载了 1 万多词条的《英汉汉英中医辞典》中只造了屈指可数的几个新词，而且是“根据自己的母语直觉（native speaker intuition)，西方读者应该会觉得这些新造词在语境里面传达中医概念的表达力很高，甚至很可能根本不会想到它们是新造的词”[10]。实际情况也确实如此，把“胁”译为 ribside，把气逆的“逆”译为 counter-flow，一眼便能了解字义，不会想到是新造的英文词。但是这样的词能否被公认，也还有待时间的考验。只有大家都愿意用，才能成为公认的词。

4. 语法结构

一般来说英译的语法结构最好与中文相符。有人在中医术语的分类中着重讨论了从语法角度的分类，认为只有根据分类才能对中医术语进行准确的翻译[11]。这种意见很有参考价值。有些中医术语英译的混乱确实是因为难以确定其语法结构所致。例如在讨论中有几篇文章都涉及“活血化瘀”的英译，认为目前有多种译法，亟须统一[12-14]。问题的关键在于如何分析“活血化瘀”这四个字的语法关系。中医术语来源于古汉语，言简意赅，又常常将虚字省略，以至于对其语法可做多种解释。这类由两组动宾短语组成的术语在中医学中十分常见，这两组短语可以并列，可以是同义重叠，也可以是动宾状关系。不同的语法关系必然带来不同的含义，明确中医术语的汉语语法结构，这固然是翻译者的任务，更是中医专家所义不容辞的责任。

5. 具体名词术语

讨论最多的是五脏的英译，按心、肝、脾、肺、肾等汉字直接用对应的英语，容易与西医概念混淆。为了避免混淆，在讨论中提出了许多办法，如在对应的英语后加注汉语拼音[15-16]，加 system[17]，加“-SO”（“-SO”为 storing organ 的缩写，表示是中医的“脏”）[18]等。但也有人持反对意见，认为越加注释，误解越多[19]。其实，这个问题在世界卫生组织的针灸国际标准命名法建议（1991）中已经解决。十二经的英文名称中都带有脏腑名称，全都被直译为相应的英语（“三焦”则译为 triple energizer），还把以前几稿中的大写字母开头一律改为小写。

“证”和“辨证论治”是中医学中极为重要的术语。一般认为以前把“证”译为 syndrome 无大问题[1]，因为 syndrome 并非任意一组症状和体征，而是代表某种异常状态。但国内有人对这种译法不满意，认为没有显示中医的特点。国外也受到这种意见的影响，将 syndrome 改为 pattern，且已相当流行。后者的问题是 pattern（式样、模式）根本没有病态或异常的含义，所以在实际运用时有时还得加字，例如 disease pattern[20]。讨论中未能提出更好的译法，看来目前只能把这两种译法并用。也许在一篇纯中医的文章中，译为 syndrome 好些；在西医病名下讨论有关的各种证时，用 pattern 比较适宜。

对于“辨证论治”的译法，在讨论中虽有不少倡议[21,14,22-23]，但都嫌冗长，不像术语，而像解释，真正应用起来很难得心应手。有人介绍在国外教学中用 TCM differentiation and treatment 来表达，简洁实用，容易被接受[19]。有些国内外出版的英文中医教材就是采用这种译法的，例如《中国针灸学》（英文版，外文出版社出版，1997 年）和 Giovanni Maciocia 的《中医妇科学》（英文版，Churchill Livingstone 出版社出版，1998 年），因为是中医书，连 TCM 也删去了。

另一个讨论较多的是“中医（学）”。对于 traditional Chinese medicine（TCM）的译法有人有异议，提倡用 Chinese medicine 或 China's medicine[22-24]。但后两种译法无法除外“中国的西医学”和“中西医结合医学”。有人根据对国内外近百种中医和中西医结合医学期刊的英文名称及其题录或摘要的查阅结果，提出 TCM 的译法已达到“约定俗成”的地步[25]。虽然如此，这个问题并未真正解决，尤其在国外 traditional Chinese medicine 和 Chinese medicine 两个名称都在应用。以美国为例，美国国立卫生研究院（National Institutes of Health，NIH）的补充和替代医疗办公室（Office of Alternative Medicine，OAM）（国家卫生院另种医学处）的官方出版物称中医为 traditional Chinese medicine，而一些学者编写的有影响力的书籍大多称中医为 Chinese medicine，看来这两种译法大概会长期共存。

对“虚”“实”的英译也有一些讨论。有人比较了各种现有的译法，都不能令人满意[25]。翻译这两个词之所以困难，主要是因为主语的改变。“邪气盛则实，精气夺则虚”，在英语中想要找到这样一对词，它们本身是反义的，又须针对两个相反的主体，确实困难。目前一般只能沿用多数人的译法，即 deficiency 和 excess[20]，但用作形容词时有可能需要考虑其他译法。在讨论中还对其他许多名词术语的译法提出了建议，限于篇幅，不再一一赘述。

综上所述，《中国中西医结合杂志》开展中医英译的讨论确实取得了很大成绩，理应继续进行下去，但讨论的重点宜有所转移。

第一，宜更多讨论国外中医英译的情况。中医西译不是从 20 世纪 70 年代我国实行改革开放政策后才开始的。早在 1682 年就出版了 Andreas Cleyer 翻译的拉丁文版《脉诀》，其后陆续有中医典籍被译为法文和德文。20 世纪 40 年代美国加州大学的 Ilza Veith 翻译了《黄帝内经·素问》的前 34 篇，并由 Williams & Wilkins Co. 出版（1949）。其后有一些欧美人士专门从事中医研究和翻译，如 Nanthan Sivin、Paul U. Unschuld、Manfred Porkert 等。我国在 20 世纪 80 年代早期出版的中医名词术语英译有不少就是参考了这些译文的。近年的情况更有所发展，例如 Giovanni Maciocia 编写了不少英文中医著作，其中《中医舌诊》（*Tongue Diagnosis in Chinese Medicine*，1987 年）、《中医学基础》（*The Foundations of Chinese Medicine*，1989 年）、《中医临床》（*The Practice of Chinese Medicine*，1994 年）和《中医妇科学》（*Obstetrics and Gynecology in Chinese Medicine*，1998 年）已成为海外英语国家的重要中医教材。魏迺杰于 1990 年出版了其编著的《英汉汉英中医词典》，1996 年又出版了修订版，该词典收载的词条达 1 万余条。多了解一些国外学者的译法，有助于我们对中医英译的讨论。

第二，宜争取以英语为母语的外国人参加讨论。过去参加本栏目讨论的各位专家尽管英语水平很高，但除个别人外，均不以英语为母语。很多中医术语来自日常生活的用语，完全根据英语语法和科学词汇不易解决，有时甚至会造成误解。例如，“吐舌”“弄舌”“吐弄舌”在几本汉英词典中都译为 wagging tongue 或 wagging of the tongue。wagging 这个词确有“动来动去”的意思，但常与尾巴（tail）搭配，与舌头（tongue）搭配在一起，首先令人想到的是喋喋不休的饶舌。此外，还有语感问题。如前文所举的“艾滋病”，如译为“诶滋”，就难以被人接受。汉语讲究语感，英语也一样，而只有以英语为母语的人才最能体会英语的语感。为了便于外国学者参加讨论，建议有关文章可在本刊的中文版和英文版同时登载。

第三，宜争取中医界的支持和帮助。除词条的一般注释外，有些问题如术语中所用汉字的字源学出处、字义学依据以及术语的汉语语法结构等，只有中医专家的意见才具有权威性。例如，前述有关“活血化瘀”英译的争论，归根结底是汉语语法上的分歧。又如“真气”的“真”字，如能明确该字作“本原”解，相当于“返璞归真”的“真”，而不是“真假”的“真”，就不会把“真气”译为 true Qi 了。“一夫法”的“夫”字是怎样成为针灸学中的度量单位的，如讲明其来龙去脉，翻译起来当然就会有较大把握。

总之，中医是中国的医学，名词术语如何解释，译文是否符合中医原意，中国的学者最有发言权。同时，英语是英美人士的母语，英译是否通顺、规范，应多听听他们的意见。只有中外学者密切合作、共同努力，中医名词术语英译的标准化问题才能较好地解决。

参考文献

[1] 刘干中，吕维柏，谢竹藩，等．中医基本理论名词术语英译探讨（一）．中国中西医结合杂志，1992，12（6）：327－329.

[2] 任斌，王晓平，季俊虬．中医术语翻译技巧初探．中国中西医结合杂志，1998，18（1）：53.

[3] 黄欣贤，樊蓥，金科奇，等．中医基本理论名词术语英译探讨（四）．中国中西医结合杂志，1993，13（4）：240－242.

[4] 戴莲仪．浅谈中医术语英译体会．中国中西医结合杂志，1998，18（1）：52－53.

[5] 吕少平，钟靖．中医英译的一点看法．中国中西医结合杂志，1992，12（12）：752－753.

[6] 佟彤．中医英译不等于医学英译．中国中西医结合杂志，1998，18（7）：398.

[7] 倪明．中医英译几个问题的思考．中国中西医结合杂志，1999，19（9）：560－561.

[8] 张大庆．早期医学名词统一：博医会的努力和影响．中华医史杂志，1994，24（1）：15－19.

[9] 王一方，魏迺杰，陈可冀．《英汉汉英中医词典》．中国中西医结合杂志，1996，16（2）：122－124.

[10] 王朝辉，林岩，陈淑芬，等．中医名词术语的分类及其英译的标准化．中国中西医结合杂志，1997，17（2）：107－108.

[11] 梁俊雄．中医术语的文体和风格．中国中西医结合杂志，1996，16（4）：250.

[12] 赵瑞安．浅析活血化瘀的英译．中国中西医结合杂志，1996，16（4）：250－251.

[13] 王得奎．谈中医名词术语“辨证论治”的英译．中国中西医结合杂志，1996，16（4）：250 .

[14] 欧明，李衍文，张家庆，等．中医基本理论名词术语英译探讨（二）．中国中西医结合杂志，1992，12（7）：433－435.

[15] 季种朴，谢仁敷，沈雪勇，等．中医基本理论名词术语英译探讨（六）．中国中西医结合杂志，1993，13（10）：626－628.

[16] 邓宇，朱栓立，徐彭，等．藏象分形五系统的新英译．中国中西医结合杂志，1999，19（9）：562.
[17] 陈道纯．有关中医英译的几点浅见．中国中西医结合杂志，1997，17（6）：371－372.
[18] 周杰．关于中医英译作品内容的思考．中国中西医结合杂志，1996，16（1）：55.
[19] 杨伊凡．中医术语英译浅见．中国中西医结合杂志，1999，19（9）：559－560.
[20] 成肇智．试论“证”及其相关词语的英译．中国中西医结合杂志，1999，19（9）：561－562.
[21] 樊蓥．中医药名词术语及论文英译若干问题再议．中国中西医结合杂志，1996，16（7）：441－442.
[22] 陈家旭．对中医英译的几点看法．中国中西医结合杂志，1996，16（7）：442.
[23] 吴振斗．应该重视中医药对外翻译的研究．中国中西医结合杂志，1996，16（1）：57.
[24] 张庆荣．中医及相关学科名词的英译．中国中西医结合杂志，1998，18（1）：51－52.
[25] 卢文超．谈谈中医“实”和“虚”的英译．中国中西医结合杂志，1999，19（6）：366.

[原载《中国中西医结合杂志》，2000，20（9）：706－709.]

浅谈中医翻译

陈可冀

关于中医翻译问题，报纸和杂志中有过很多讨论，但看来恐怕远远不够。继续讨论并逐渐深化认识，仍属必要。

中医英译是中英双语在中医药学专业方面的语言转换活动，有专业知识层面的问题，也有语言表达水平的问题，更有中、英语使用者文化素养方面的问题，所以要做到译得丝丝入扣、不失原意，而且又能为使用英语者所乐于和易于接受，即所谓两相接轨、水到渠成，实非易事。以“三焦”一词而言，有 triple warmers、triple heaters、triple energizer、tripyrogens 及 Sanjiao 等种种译法，各有千秋，何时方能得到共识？又如“辨证论治”的“证”，有诸如以下译法：symptom-complex、pattern、symptoms and signs 及 syndrome 等。由于时代的更替、科学的发展，对中医学认识的深化，何况当前更有宏观与微观结合辨证的“证”，则似乎 syndrome 较 symptom-complex 更适宜。“辨证”则也以 syndrome differentiation 更为恰当了。

现在中医药走向世界，实现中医药现代化的呼声甚高，中医英译正处于生机勃勃发展之时，我相信会日有所进。首先还应当强调准确性，要真正转达中医药学术中的真正信息。中外概念相似的可以直译，也可移植。例如，中医学中气血的“血”并不等于现代医学中的血，但译为 blood，大概大家意见不大。又如，“弦脉”译为 taut pulse，“舌苔”译为 tongue coating（fur），都是八九不离十的。

语言是科学文化的载体，译文中求同易，统异难。由于中医学术语歧义性或模糊性词条较多，翻译时难免难于用一词而以求表达多意，真正做到准确是有困难的，这就要求在专业范围内多多思索并推理。中医学词条中的“脉三五不调”讲的是心律失常，“釜底抽薪”讲的是一种治法，如同我们日常讲“三天打鱼，两天晒网”。意思知道了，翻译得简明易懂则不易。英语里“writing a sugar report”意谓写一封情书，若要说写一份糖业的情况报告，则谬以千里了。其他如“银河”应是 milky way，翻译成“牛奶路”就不对了。clearing hospital 的意思是“野战医院”，若译成“平静的医院”就错了。

中医英译词条中最使国外西医“丈二和尚摸不着脑袋”的是脏象（state of viscera 或 visceral manifestation）的各个词条，如心、肝、脾、肺、肾等，现代一般都分别直译为西医的 heart、liver、spleen、lung、kidney。但根据我个人在国外参加学术交流的体会，由于多数国外学者并不了解中医药学，此种词条一出，并且其概念与当代西医知识迥异，他们就不想听了，甚至认为你在胡说什么。我想有人建议音译为 Xin、Gan、Pi、Fei 和 Shen 也未尝不可，再加一个注脚说明。又如中医学中的“痰”，其概念和现代医学的痰也不同，译为 phlegm 或 sputum 都有不甚了了的情况，需加注脚，不像“湿”字译为 dampness 较易被接受。

我对中医英译素养不够，不该侈谈，谨以浅谈应约，以促进大家共同切磋、共同进步。

[原载《上海中医药杂志》，2002，22（3）：7－8.]

Terminology Standardization in Chinese Medicine: The Perspective from UCLA Center for East-West Medicine(Ⅰ)

Ka-Kit Hui and Sonya Pritzker

1. Introduction (Ka-kit Hui, M. D.)*

Because we recognize the clinical, educational, and cultural importance of translation and terminology in Chinese medicine, we feel that it is imperative to understand the perspectives of all concerned parties. This article thus addresses the issue of terminology standardization in English language Chinese medical publications from the point of view of multiple stakeholders in this field at the UCLA Center for East-West Medicine. A great deal of discussion about the issue has arisen among faculty and staff at the Center, prompted especially by my invitation by the World Health Organization (WHO) Western Pacific Region to review the draft document of English terminology standards in Chinese medicine. As the discussion within the Center reflects the wider debates within the field, we would like to address the topic by inviting seven Center staff and faculty, all of whom have been trained as clinicians and teachers rather than translators or linguistic scholars, to formally provide their insights into the matter. Sonya Pritzker, M. S. , M. A. , L. Ac. ** will first offer a brief background derived from her presentation at the original Grand Rounds at the Center upon which the current article is based. Staff and faculty from the Center then offer their contributions to the discussion, after which I discuss participants' views and conclude by suggesting that a biomedical interface system[1] in combination with a system of open standards[2] offers a possible solution to the several divergent views brought up by the terminology debates.

Note: * Ka Kit Hui, M. D. , Wallis Annenberg Chair in Integrative East-West Medicine, Founder & Director of the Center for East-West Medicine at UCLA, is a fellow of the American College of Physician, clinical pharmacologist and an expert on Chinese medicine and Integrative medicine. He is fluent in both Chinese and English.

** Sonya Pritzker, M. S. (Oriental Medicine), M. A. (Anthropology) is a practicing acupuncturist and practitioner of Chinese herbal medicine in Santa Monica, CA, and has been involved with the terminology debates for over five years. She is currently a part time staff research assistant at the center and is in her third year of graduate studies in medical and linguistic anthropology at UCLA, where she is researching the role of language in Chinese medical education for her doctoral dissertation.

2. Background (Sonya Pritzker, M. S. , M. A. , L. Ac.)

In the field of Chinese medicine, the issue of term standardization for English language Chinese medical publications constitutes a matter of intense debate. With many prominent authors involved, including Nigel Wiseman, Bob Flaws, Marnae Ergil, Dan Bensky, and Xie Zhufan, among others, the terminology debates have also received attention from the China-based World Federation of Chinese Medical Societies (WFCMS) and the Western Pacific Region of the World Health Organization (WHO). Both organizations have hosted several international meetings in order to develop English language Chinese medical term standards. While the WFCMS is interested in developing these standards in order to enhance communication across the wide variety of traditional, biomedical, and integrated professional organizations that it interacts with, the WHO is invested in the standard terms so that they may be included in a section on Chinese medicine in the traditional medical portion of the upcoming ICD-11. This project requires standardized terminology especially because the terms will be linked to computerized international health information systems[3].

Attendees at the WFCMS and WHO meeting shave included both Chinese and Western experts, and debates have consisted of discussions focusing on specific terms as well as general themes, especially the question of whether to use biomedical terminology or more traditional terminology to translate Chinese medical terms. This argument, made public most recently in a series of Chinese Journal of Integrated Medicine articles by Xie Zhufan and Nigel Wiseman[4-6], Wiseman 2006, revolves around the issue of what type of language most accurately represents Chinese medicine. Xie and colleagues, for instance, argue that standard English terminology for the translation of Chinese medical material should be based on modern biomedical/Western medical concepts so as to accurately represent Chinese medicine as a viable medical system appropriate for use in international contexts[4,5,7]. Not only does the use of biomedical terms to represent Chinese medical concepts help in making Chinese medicine feel more familiar and accessible to Western audiences, facilitating a broader bridging of the gap between the two systems, Xie and colleagues argue that translating using biomedical terms also effectively brings Chinese medicine into the current age, saving it from being considered a cultural relic in the modern world[4,5,7]. Wiseman and others who support a more traditional approach to translation, argue that the use of biomedical terms to translate Chinese medicine "destroys the integrity and independence of Chinese medical concepts"[6]. They suggest, for example, that when the Chinese medical term feng huo yan, or 'windfire eye', is translated as 'acute conjunctivitis', the fact that 'wind-fire eye' is rooted in a Chinese medical conception of the body distinct from biomedicine is ignored. Instead, the biomedical understanding of the body implied by the term 'acute conjunctivitis' is linguistically mapped onto the traditional body of Chinese medicine, thereby negating it[8]. Standard terms that preserve the original Chinese medical conceptualization of illness, these scholars argue, are needed to prevent such degradation.

Outside of the WFCMS and WHO meetings, other Chinese medical scholars suggest that any form of standardization betrays the multiple meanings inherent in most Chinese medical terms, a plurality that has developed over 2,000 years of use by different scholars in different contexts[9-12]. In addition to arguing that more than one English term for a single Chinese medical word "does not necessarily obscure its meaning", these scholars suggest that "the rigid application of the principle of one to one correspondence in translating Chinese terms into English easily oversimplifies Chinese medical ideas"[10]. In American Chinese medicine in particular, these scholars have engaged in a heated debate with proponents of standardization, who counter that multiple and un-standardized English terminology leads to a loss of critical knowledge. Citing cases where multiple Chinese words for a type of symptom or illness pattern, such as pain or diarrhea, are translated into a single English term that doesn't differentiate between the multiple concepts originally represented in Chinese, supporters of standardization argue that lack of term standards leads to a decline in clinical efficacy[1,2,8,13,14]. They also point out that when different authors use different terms, cross-referencing books and relating them back to the original Chinese becomes impossible.

The American debates have continued for several years, carried out in journals, informal meetings, and internet discussion groups, and recently culminated in a day-long conference on nomenclature in Chinese medicine, hosted by the American Association of Oriental Medicine (AAOM). The discussion at the conference, as elsewhere, revolved around several main issues arising out of the principal debate about whether or not standards are necessary. Firstly, the discussion around the notion of translatability is especially animated. Many scholars thus feel that, as a result of the cultural and linguistic divide between China and the West, completely accurate translation is impossible[9-12,15]. Alterations are thus bound to occur, and should in fact be welcomed as American authors adapt Chinese medicine to meet the needs of their English speaking audience. For those that support standardization, on the other hand, it is clear that when the original concept is altered via inaccurate or multiple translations, new ideas emerge and the fundamental concept changes. This translates into an essential adaptation of Chinese medicine that abandons the original, traditional knowledge that Americans are supposedly seeking to represent. For these scholars, the true meanings of original terms are translatable, i. e. they can be accurately represented in English, but only using a standardized, coherent set of translation strategies[8,13-167].

Secondly, the issue of whether or not Chinese medical language in English should be comprised of specialized and standardized technical terms has also been debated. Those seeking standardization feel that the translation of Chinese medical language is a technical language that "differs from other forms of translation chiefly in that technical writing is characterized by technical terms that must be given equivalents in the target language if the concepts they represent are to be upheld in the transmission process"[17]. This argument thus classifies Chinese medical language as a "Language for Special Purposes" (LSP) that qualifies for a formal, standardized terminology. The notion that Chinese medical language is an LSP, however, is contested. Because the words that are used to make up Chinese language Chinese medical terminology are often the same words used in common Chinese language, some argue, we do not need a highly specialized terminology in English[9].

Finally, the issue of deciding upon the best way to teach Chinese medicine to clinical students is a prominent theme of American debates. Some scholars thus suggest that a multiplicity of terms creates a "terminological chaos" that actually benefits students as they learn to negotiate the depths of Chinese medical concepts[10]. Others argue that terminological precision is necessary for instructing students who will eventually become experts in the field of Chinese medicine[14].

The salient themes in both the international and American debates can thus be separated into two major themes:

1. Single standards versus plural terms (Involves issues of clinical accuracy, historical diversity, translatability, and technical language)

2. The basis for standards (Biomedical or traditional knowledge/terminology)

As this brief introduction alludes to, perspectives on all of the issues contained within these two categories are very different and often incompatible. Participants' viewpoints on standardization differ greatly in both degree and orientation, and reflect a widely variant set of priorities, goals, and philosophical biases.

References

[1] Brand E. Unpublished conference report. World Federation of Chinese Medical Societies meeting to develop terminology standards in Chinese medicine. 2006, April.

[2] Felt R. The role of standards in the transmission of Chinese medical information. Am Acupunct, 2006, 37: 18-20.

[3] Kang J. Perspective on the Asian medical nomenclature debates. Presentation given at the American Association of Oriental Medicine Annual Expo, Phoenix, AZ. 2006.

[4] Xie ZF, White P. Comments on Nigel Wiseman's "A Practical Dictionary of Chinese Medicine" (I)—On the "word-for-word" literal approach to translation. Chin J Integr Med, 2005, 12 (4): 305-308.

[5] Xie ZF, White P. Comments on Nigel Wiseman's "A Practical Dictionary of Chinese Medicine" (II)—On the use of Western medical terms to express the concepts of traditional Chinese medicine. Chin J Integr Med, 2006, 13 (1): 61-65.

[6] Wiseman N. English translation of Chinese medicine: Concerning the use of Western medical terms to represent traditional Chinese medical concepts (answer to Prof. Xie and his colleagues). Chin J Integr Med, 2006, 12 (3): 225-228.

[7] Xie ZF. On the standard nomenclature of traditional Chinese medicine. Beijing: Foreign Langua-

ges Press，2003.

[8] Wiseman N. Translation of Chinese medical terms：a source-oriented approach (unpublished doctoral thesis) . University of Exeter，2000.

[9] Beinfield H，Korngold E. Centralism vs. pluralism：language，authority，and freedom in Chinese medicine. Clin Acupunct Oriental Med，2001，2：145-154.

[10] Bensky D，Blalack J，Chace C，et al. Toward a working methodology for translating Chinese medicine. Am Acupunct，2006，37：14-15.

[11] Fratkin J. Asian medical nomenclature debates. Am Acupunct，2006，37：22-23.

[12] Shima M. Asian medical nomenclature debates. Am Acupunct，2006，37：8-11.

[13] Ergil M. Considerations for the translation of traditional Chinese medicine into English. Available：http：//www. paradigm-pubs. com/refs/Translation. html. 2001.

[14] Ergil M，Ergil K. Issues surrounding the translation of Chinese medical texts into English. Am Acupunct，2006，37：24-25.

[15] Shen XT. An extra thought about nomenclature. Am Acupunct，2006，37：12-13.

[16] Wiseman N. Why the fuss about terminology? Available (restricted access)：F：\ Papers \ Dossier \ 3CHA2Fuss. doc. 2002

[17] Wiseman N. The extra linguistic aspects of English translation of Chinese medical terminology. Available：http：//www. paradigm-pubs. com/paradigm/refs/wiseman/Extralinguistics. pdf. 2001

[原载 *Chinese Journal of Integrative Medicine*，2007，13 (1)：64 - 67.]

Terminology Standardization in Chinese Medicine: The Perspective from UCLA Center for East-West Medicine(Ⅱ)

Ka-Kit Hui and Sonya Pritzker

1. The View From Ucla Center for East-West Medicine (Ka-kit Hui, M. D., and Sonya Pritzker, M. S., M. A., L. Ac)*

Center staff and faculty below provide their commentary and perspective on the two major issues (single standards versus plural terms and the basis for standards) comprising the terminology standardization debate as outlined by Sonya Pritzker above. Where most or all members of the discussion agree, that perspective is summarized. Members with distinct or outstanding positions on an issue are offered the opportunity to describe their viewpoint in their own words.

1.1 Single Standards Versus Plural Terms

All but one of the members of the discussion agreed that some form of standardization should be developed in Chinese medicine. Reasons included increased ease of communication with other practitioners and providers and increased clarity in terms of conducting clinical trials and other medical research. Only one discussant, Marc Brodsky, M. D. *, felt that any standardization of terminology in the field would be inherently limiting. He explained that the use of different terms by different authors facilitates the student's ability to use more than one resource to get the full meaning of the term. Multiplicity and plurality, he noted, help build conceptual clarity in the same sense as when a member of the public gathers an impression of the situation in the Middle East from various media sources. Rather than focusing on exact words, Marc argued, efforts should be directed towards helping English speakers grasp the essence of the concept, a feature that is often best expressed in multiple terms that reflect the change in meaning over its 2000 years of use in China. Marc Brodsky also pointed out that one-to-one translation of Chinese medical terms is difficult to impossible because of the changes that the meanings of the Chinese words have undergone over the course of their 2000 years of use in China.

Note: * Marc Brodsky is a board certified family practice physician who has been associated with the Center as a clinician for four and half years. His interest in Chinese medicine was sparked by experience as a family practice physician in the U. S. Navy, when he was exposed to many forms of Asian medicine in Japan and other Asian countries. In addition to several courses in acupuncture and Chinese medicine offered by faculty at the Center, he has completed the 300 h course in medical acupuncture at UCLA Extension and finished a 2-year fellowship in Integrative East-West medicine at the Center. His formal title is Assistant Clinical Professor of Medicine at UCLA. He speaks no Chinese.

Although they agreed on the need for standardized terminology, many discussants' feelings about the usefulness of standardization were tempered by various limitations they felt to arise from the nature of language. Lawrence Taw, M. D. ** expressed the opinion that, while standardized language is useful and necessary in texts, it is not necessarily a requirement for accurate communication in a clinical context. "In dialoguing with people," he said, "you can still convey or communicate what you're trying to say." Dr. Taw emphasized that the importance of standard terms for teaching clinicians does not necessarily translate into the need to use standard terms when expressing the concept in order to help a patient. Because this is his overall goal, he maintained that the usefulness of standardization would be limited to an academic context only. Furthermore, he felt the standardization of specific words to be less important than the standardization of general concepts.

Note: ** Lawrence Taw, M. D., is a board certified internist and Center clinician who is currently completing his final year of a Masters in Traditional Oriental Medicine at Emperor's College of Oriental Medicine. His original exposure to Chinese medicine was as a fourth year medical student at UCLA, when he attended the 2-week elective course in East-West medicine held at the Center. He has been associated with the Center on and off for four years, the last of which he has spent as a fellow in Integrative East-West medicine. He speaks minimal to no Chinese.

Lawrence Taw also expressed the opinion that standardized terminology should not be formulated using overly technical language. Instead, he argued, common language that common people can understand should be used to translate Chinese medicine and formulate standardized terms. This view stems from his goal of wanting to be able to more clearly communicate with patients. Because he believes that common terms are sufficient in this context, he argues that they are also sufficient for standardized Chinese medical terms.

Malcom Taw, * M. D. * also pointed out the limitations of standardized language in terms of helping students and patients understand Chinese medical concepts. Stressing the importance of experience in learning the meaning of concepts like qi, he noted that many Chinese medical concepts require direct experience before one is able to fully appreciate their meaning, regardless of the word. He thus expressed the opinion that for many Chinese medical technical terms and/or concepts, one-to- one translations are often impossible. The meanings of such concepts, such as Qi, cannot be captured in language alone. Instead, they require both experience and discussion within an educational context, especially because the concepts are so foreign to a Western audience.

* Malcolm Taw, M. D., is also a board certified internist and Center clinician who is currently completing his final year of a Masters in Traditional Oriental Medicine at Emperor's College of Oriental Medicine. His original exposure to Chinese medicine was as a fourth year medical student at UCLA, when he attended the 2-week elective course in East-West medicine held at the Center. Having just completed the 2 year integrated medicine fellowship at the Center, he has been associated with the Center for 6 years. He has studied Chinese for two years.

In relation to the issue of whether or not Chinese medical terminology is a technical language, Malcolm Taw suggested that while common terms are often useful in a clinical context, more technical terms are appropriate in professional and educational contexts. This view led Malcolm to point out that part of the reason standardization is so difficult has to do with the different backgrounds of people consuming Chinese medical language. What a biomedical practitioner will understand is thus vastly different from what a student of Chinese medicine or patient will understand a fact which makes any single standard difficult to decide upon, especially from the perspective of integrated East-West medicine.

1.2 The Basis for Standards

Two discussion participants, Marc Brodsky and Xiuling Ma, O. M. D. (China), Ph. D. **, strongly expressed the belief that biomedical terminology can and should be used to explain and translate Chinese medical concepts other than those that are unique to Chinese medicine, such as Qi, Yin, or Yang. In

Marc's view, the knowledge that biomedicine has of the body, such as how the different systems are interrelated and how and why it breaks down, should be utilized in describing and translating Chinese medicine to a Western audience. For Dr. Ma, Chinese medical concepts and disease categories, such as stroke, are often no different than the corresponding biomedical concepts. The use of different terminology is therefore unnecessary. These ties into her view that a single, correct translation is possible for most Chinese medical technical terms.

** Xiuling Ma, O. M. D. (China), Ph. D. earned her doctorate in Chinese medicine and acupuncture over 12 years of formal study at Beijing University of Chinese Medicine in Beijing, China. She is currently the Director for Chinese Medical (TCM) Education at the Center, where she has worked for 4 years. Her duties at the Center include teaching the fellows, residents, and medical students, in addition to helping compile their curriculum. Dr. Ma is fluent in both Chinese and English.

Ryan Abbott, M. T. O. M., L. Ac. *** and Ed Hui, M. D. **** disagreed, arguing that translating Chinese medical concepts directly into biomedical terms comes at the expense of true integration. Emphasizing that Chinese medicine and biomedicine are distinct systems, Ryan Abbott explained that integrating terminology sends the incorrect message that they share a similar set of core beliefs. Because of the different way in which the two medical systems fundamentally approach health and disease, he stresses, the terminology is not equivalent.

*** Ryan Abbott, M. T. O. M., L. Ac. is a licensed acupuncturist as well as a second year medical student at the University of California at San Diego. He first became involved with the Center 4 years ago, when as a UCLA undergraduate he embarked on a major in "Integrative Medical Theory". Concurrently carrying out his B. S. and Masters. in Traditional Oriental Medicine (MTOM) at Emperor's College of Oriental Medicine, Ryan also worked at the Center, where he served as principal investigator of a randomized controlled trial of Tai Chi for tension headaches. He has had 2 years of formal training in Chinese language.

**** Ed Hui, M. D. is a board certified internist and geriatrician currently on the faculty practicing general internal medicine at UCLA. He has been associated with the Center for 13 years since its inception and is currently seeing patients part time at the Center clinic and as a teacher. He has completed a limited fellowship in Integrative East-West medicine at the Center while completing his fellowship in Geriatrics at UCLA. He speaks some Chinese, but is not fl uent in terms of medical language.

2. Conclusion (Ka-kit Hui, M. D.*)

From my perspective, it is crucial to consider all of the diverse opinions on terminology in Chinese medicine expressed by East-West Center discussants, as well as in the broader debates.

In considering opinions on the matter of whether or not to standardize terminology in Chinese medicine, for example, it is important to note that when we look closely at the details of their opinions on the issue of single standards versus plural terms, there is no clear black and white separation between those who support standardization and those who don't. Marc Brodsky's doubts about the translatability of Chinese medical terms are thus echoed in Malcom Taw's point that finding an exact term for many Chinese medical concepts is next to impossible. Even though Dr. Brodsky does not support standardization and Dr. Taw does, their points are actually quite similar and reflect the positions of those in the U. S. who argue for a plurality of terms[9-12,14]. Like these scholars, both of these physicians also brought up the issue of how best to teach the complexity of Chinese medical concepts and the need for students to be introduced to multiple ways of thinking about terms. Finally, while they agreed that standards are necessary, both Lawrence and Malcolm Taw agreed that some variability in terminology is necessary depending on the audience being addressed (patients, biomedical students, Chinese medical professionals, insurance companies).

All of these points are critical to consider when approaching the terminology standardization issue. Given the developments at the WFCMS in China and the WHO, however, it is clear that we no longer can debate about whether or not there should be standards. Standard terminology is an imminent occurrence at this point, and is going to need to be developed for its inclusion in the new ICD, as well as for communication across international organizations. Along with most of the discussants in the present conference, I agree that such standards are necessary for the smooth integration of Chinese medicine to mainstream medical culture through clinical trials and patient care. Similarly, as many supporters of standardization point out, standards ensure the preservation of critical clinical details as well as they allow a reader to cross-reference different authors terms[2,8,13-15]. Our contribution to the discussion at this point can therefore most appropriately consist of suggestions as to how these standards can be built to represent Chinese medicine in the best possible way, and to do so with the utmost respect, diplomacy, and understanding for the views of all concerned parties.

Despite the many divergent views raised by the issues, I believe that it is possible to arrive at an acceptable solution to many of the problems. Firstly, in terms of peoples' reservations about the ultimate translatability of Chinese medical concepts into single English words, a system of open standards[2] encourages plurality in teaching, speaking, and clinical use, at the same time allowing for different texts, ideas, and systems to be linked via a single standard. In this system, standard technical terms can continue to be discussed and debated at the same time they are acknowledged as standards. As Robert Felt explains, "A term standard is not a list of words you must use, but a method for linking your words to those of others"[2]. It is therefore comparable to the ICD-9 or the DSM-Ⅳ, where standard definitions are constantly contested and revisions made to each new edition[18]. Furthermore, like these biomedical standards, open standards in Chinese medicine need not dictate the behavior or thinking of teachers, students, or clinicians, who can use common terms or other technical terms when talking to patients or teaching students. In fact, it is certainly true that Chinese medical terms often indicate multiple and variant realities. As long as they are linked to a single technical standard, I am thus in agreement with Marc Brodsky, Malcolm Taw, Lawrence Taw, as well as supporters of terminological plurality, that all of these must be discussed and taught via both text and experience in the context of Chinese medical education in order to convey the full depth of Chinese medicine to future practitioners. An open system of standards allows for this diversity in teaching at the same time as it makes communication across contexts possible.

Secondly, in terms of the disagreement around whether biomedical or traditional knowledge and terminology should be used to translate Chinese medicine, the possibility of a biomedical interface system, which has been suggested by several experts involved in the debates at the WHO and the World Federation of Chinese Medical Societies (WFCMS) in Beijing[1], creates a flexibility wherein a standard traditional or literal translation is paired with a standard biomedical translation only when a precise equivalent exists. Both terms are acknowledged as official, and the translator or author can variably draw upon these terms depending on the audience that he or she is writing for. This solution fashions a bridge between the views of Xiuling Ma and Marc Brodsky (as well as Xie Zhu-fan and colleagues), who argue for the use of biomedical terminology in the translation of Chinese medical texts, and Ryan Abbott and Ed Hui (as well as Nigel Wiseman and colleagues), who support a more traditional approach. Chinese medical concepts are thus not forced into biomedical categories, but a conceptual and linguistic connection between the two medical systems is established. Furthermore, this system solves the problem of needing to use different terms for different audiences, brought up by Malcolm Taw in the present discussion.

By way of conclusion, I therefore suggest that a system of open standards in combination with a biomedical interface system is an ideal solution to the terminology standardization problem. In addition to allowing for the continued debate about specific terms, it also makes clear communication between experts within the field and in the broader international medical context possible. In short, it generates a responsible flexibility that incorporates both theoretical and clinical concerns and ultimately helps facilitate the ethical treatment of patients and the accurate transmission of Chinese medicine to the contemporary Western world.

Acknowledgements

The authors gratefully acknowledge financial support for this project from the Gerald Oppenheimer Family Foundation, the Annenberg Foundation, the David Chu Bequest, the Sirpuhe & John Conte Foundation, the Stephen Philibosian Foundation, and the Stanley Dashew Trust.

References

[1] Brand E. Unpublished Conference Report. World Federation of Chinese Medical Societies meeting to develop terminology standards in Chinese medicine. 2006, April.

[2] Felt R. The role of standards in the transmission of Chinese medical information. Am Acupunct, 2006, 37: 18-20.

[3] Kang J. Perspective on the Asian medical nomenclature debates. Presentation given at the American Association of Orienta Medicine Annual Expo, Phoenix, AZ. 2006.

[4] Xie ZF, White P. Comments on Nigel Wiseman's "A Practical Dictionary of Chinese Medicine" (Ⅰ)—On the "Word-for-word" literal approach to translation. Chin J Integr Med, 2005, 12

(4): 305-308.

[5] Xie ZF, White P. Comments on Nigel Wiseman's "A Practical Dictionary of Chinese Medicine" (Ⅱ)—On the use of Western medical terms to express the concepts of traditional Chinese medicine. Chin J Integr Med, 2006, 13 (1): 61-65.

[6] Wiseman N. English translation of Chinese medicine: concerning the use of Western medical terms to represent traditional Chinese medical concepts (answer to Prof. Xie and his colleagues). Chin J Integr Med, 2006, 12 (3): 225-228.

[7] Xie ZF. On the standard nomenclature of traditional Chinese medicine. Beijing: Foreign Languages Press, 2003.

[8] Wiseman N. Translation of Chinese medical terms: a source-oriented approach (unpublished doctoral thesis). University of Exeter, 2000.

[9] Beinfi eld H, Korngold E. Centralism vs. pluralism: language, authority, and freedom in Chinese medicine. Clin Acupunct Oriental Med, 2001, 2: 145-154.

[10] Bensky D, Blalack J, Chace C. Toward a working methodology for translating Chinese medicine. Am Acupunct, 2006, 37: 14-15.

[11] Fratkin J. Asian medical nomenclature debates. Am Acupunct, 2006, 37: 22-23.

[12] Shima M. Asian medical nomenclature debates. Am Acupunct, 2006, 37: 8-11.

[13] Ergil M. Considerations for the translation of traditional Chinese medicine into English. Available: http: //www. paradigm-pubs. com/refs/Translation. html. 2001.

[14] Ergil M, Ergil K. Issues surrounding the translation of Chinese medical texts into English. Am Acupunct, 2006, 37: 24-25.

[15] Shen XT. An extra thought about nomenclature. Am Acupunct, 2006, 37: 12-13.

[16] Wiseman N. Why the fuss about terminology? Available (restricted access): F: \ Papers \ Dossier \ 3CHA2Fuss. doc. 2002

[17] Wiseman N. The extralinguistic aspects of English translation of Chinese medical terminology. Available: http: //www. paradigm-pubs. com/paradigm/refs/wiseman/Extralinguistics. pdf. 2001.

[18] Bowker FC, Star SL. Sorting things out: Classification and its consequences. Cambridge: MIT Press, 2002.

[原载 *Chinese Journal of Integrative Medicine*, 2007, 13 (2): 152-155.]

中医基本理论名词术语英译探讨

欧明　李衍文　张家庆　蔡景峰　陈可冀

“八纲”是中医辨证的基本纲领，即阴阳、表里、寒热、虚实。

对“阴阳”的英译，过去曾有 negative-positive、feminine-musculine、ebb-wax 及其他译法，均只反映阴阳概念的一个方面，显然是不理想的。近年来，在中外的中医书刊中均已通过 Yin 和 Yang 的音译法，这两个词也已收入《韦氏国际英语词典》中，其定义如下：“Yin is the feminine and negative principle (as of passivity, depth, darkness, cold, wetness) in nature that according to traditional Chinese cosmology combines with its opposite Yang to produce all that comes to be. Yang is the musculine and positive principle (as of activity, beight, light, heat, or dryness) in nature according to traditional Chinese cosmology combines and interacts with its opposite Yin to produce everything that comes into existence.”上述定义是着眼于中国古代的宇宙观，虽未能与中医的阴阳概念完全吻合，但中医学的阴阳亦源出于中国古代哲学，出现于中医著作则可代表中医的特定概念，因而，Yin 和 Yang 的音译法已为中外学者广泛接受。

八纲中的表里是辨别病位的深浅，代表空间的相对性。“表”可译为 superficies (the purely external aspects, features, or characteristics of a thing) 和 exterior (an outside of outside surface; outward appearance)。“里”作为其反义词，应分别译为 deepness (the state of being deep, in all its sense) 和 interior (the inner part of a thing; the inner nature of a person or thing)。但 deepness 的词义较广，其与 superficies 的对应不如 interior 与 exterior 那么严谨明确，故现多采用后者。《汉英医学大辞典》亦采用这样的译法。

寒热是辨疾病的性质，较通行的英译是 cold 与 heat。事实上，从《韦氏国际英语词典》的解释中，亦有一个明确表达古代生物科学的概念，即：“Cold is naturally without heat-used in ancient and medieval sciences to describe one of the qualities of the four elements. Heat is one of the fundamental qualties of bodies elements, or humors recognized in medieval physiology.”因此，借用这两个词来表达中医八纲辨证中的寒热是较为合理的。

至于虚实，则是辨正邪的盛衰。“虚”一般翻译为 deficiency (a shortage of substances necessary to health) 或 asthenia (lack or loss of bodily strength; deficient vitality)。“实”作为其反义词，应分别译为 excess (the state of exceeding that which is normal, sufficient, or needed）和 sthenia（health：strength；virility；specifically，in medicine，unusual vigor）。sthenia 一词一般用于描述精力充沛的健康状态，这显然不适用于反映中医的实证，但从其释义当中，特别指出在医学上代表“unusual vigor”的异常状态。从中医辨证纲领、机体整体反应的角度来考虑，以 sthenia 表达八纲中的“实”也未尝不可，但对其出现于具体的病证与病理，则应作别论。

[原载《中国中西医结合杂志》，1992，12（7）：433－435.）

中医药术语英译的探讨

钱自奋

中医药学文献英译的历史已很悠久，随着国际上中医药热的掀起，中医药文献英译工作显得更加迫切。目前虽已有许多中医药术语英译辞典及英文中医药著作出版，但对中医药术语的翻译仍欠规范和统一。《中国中西医结合杂志》发起的中医药术语英译的探讨很有必要，非常及时，我也想借此园地谈一些个人不成熟的意见。

1. 明确读者对象

中医药文献英译的主要读者应是熟悉英语的医务工作者，因此，翻译应以通顺、规范的英语为主，尽量少用其他文字，如拉丁语、汉语拼音等。因为这些读者对这些文字并不熟悉。他们遇到汉语拼音时往往用英语方式来发音，听起来很别扭。据我所知，对中医药感兴趣的外国学者往往对中文也有兴趣，许多人或多或少学过一些中文。如果在中医药专门术语英译的后面加上中文，无疑会有利于他们进一步查阅有关辞书，来弥补译文的不足。这种方式在将外文译成中文时也常常被采用。

2. 翻译应简明

中医药术语的翻译与中医药术语解释的翻译是不同的，术语的翻译应简洁明了。例如，有人把“辨证论治”译作 diagnosis and treatment based on overall analysis of symptoms and signs，the cause，nature and location of the illness and the patient’s physical condition according to the basic theories of traditional Chinese medicine. 另有人译为 planning treatment according to diagnosis。显然，前者属于术语解释的翻译，后者是术语本身的翻译。个人认为可把“辨证论治”简单译成 Diagnosis and Treatment。因为中医的“辨证论治”与西医的诊断和治疗虽然在内容与方法上有所不同，但其基本含义是十分相近的。为了显示两者的区别，故英译时“D”与“T”均改为大写并附中文。再如，有人把“脾统血”译成 Spleen participates in regulating hemopoiesis and keeps the blood flowing normally in the vessels。另有人译为 The spleen governs the blood。很明显前者是“脾统血”含义的翻译，后者是忠于原文的译法。这两种译法哪一种好呢？我认为如果自己写文章，这两种译法皆可用；如果翻译他人文章，则以后者为优。因为翻译应忠于原文，不能随便发挥，而且对“脾统血”的含义可有不同的理解。传统的、狭义的脾统血仅指脾能使血液在脉管内正常运行，并不包括造血的功能。脾确有造血的功能，因为中医早有“脾胃为气血生化之源”之说，但这属于脾主运化功能的范畴。

建议中国中医药学会与中国中西医结合学会协作，首先编写一本规范的、权威性的中医药术语解释辞典，然后再组织权威专家将其译成规范化的英语。

3. 中药名称翻译以英语为主

据我所知，一般中外医务工作者精通拉丁语的不多，而且拉丁语辞典也甚少，因此，用拉丁语翻译中药名称会给这些读者带来很大困难。大多数中药名称均有相对应的英语可以翻译；对少数无适当英语可译的中药，可用拉丁语翻译，但应注明中文。如果国家明文规定中药名称非用拉丁语不可，最好在其后注明中文，以为多数中外读者提供方便。另外，如果在国外行医时开中医处方，不论用英文或拉丁文，最好都注明繁体的中文，因为国外绝大多数中药店是华人开设的。

［原载《中国中西医结合杂志》，1995，15（8）：499.］

关于中医名词术语英译标准化的思考

李照国

关于中医名词术语英译标准化的理论问题，笔者曾在“中医翻译标准化的概念、原则与方法”[1]及“中医名词术语英译的标准化”[2]两篇文章中作了较为深入的探讨。本文拟就标准化过程中涉及的其他问题进行概要的分析。

1. 技术问题

所谓技术问题，是指对标准化的方法与程序的研究有较大影响的问题。这些问题包括以下几个方面。

1.1 名词术语的界定

首先要明确名词术语的定义。《朗文当代英语词典》将“名词术语”定义为“使用于特定学科、职业或运动的一套专门词汇或用语系统”。《汉语主题词表》在选词原则中更明确提出，所选定的主题词“必须是名词和名词性的词汇”。在中医翻译中，许多译者往往把名词术语与疑难语句混为一谈。对于名词术语，我们强调要译语一致，但对于句子，翻译上就不能强求一致了。这是原则问题。

1.2 名词术语的分类

中医名词术语的构成方式各不相同，如果用同一方法来翻译不同类型的术语，必然会使一些译语词不达意。为了使标准化的研究有的放矢，很有必要对其进行分类。笔者在以往的研究中根据语义的明晰度及实在性将其分为5类[3]，这种分法是否恰当，尚需进一步研究。

1.3 翻译单位的确立

翻译单位指源语在译语中具备对应物的最小单位。目前尚未确立中医翻译单位，但大多数译者实际上都将词看作翻译单位。词虽然在有些情况下可以充当翻译单位，但并不总是最小的语言单位。根据我们的研究，我们认为将中医翻译单位确立在“词素”层面上比较恰当（详见《中医翻译学导论》）。

2. 学界问题

学界问题是指在中医翻译及中医名词术语翻译标准化的研究中，中医翻译界与有关学科的关系问题。这些关系包括以下几个方面。

2.1 与中医界的关系

为了使标准化的研究具有客观实在性，中医翻译界应与中医界建立密切的联系并接受后者的指导。

2.2　与语言翻译界的关系

为了使中医翻译摆脱“各家学说”的混乱状态，中医翻译界应与语言翻译界建立联系并接受其指导与帮助。

2.3　与医学外语界的关系

为了使中医走向世界，还有赖于医学外语界的协助。

3. 行政问题

所谓行政问题，是指国家有关部门对中医翻译及标准化研究的统一领导和有效干预。目前，有关方面对中医翻译基本上采取的是一种放任自流的政策，这只能导致更大的混乱。

4. 国际问题

中医翻译并不只限于中国，实际上大量工作是在海外进行的，因此，在标准化的过程中，我们必须注意研究国际方面的发展。

5. 结束语

在此，笔者愿以朱自清先生《译名》一文的结尾作为本文的结束语：“争名只在名初出现时剧烈，终究总应该定于一，才便利，这固然靠着名自身的价值，也有人为的力量”。我认为这种人为的力量有四种，就是：①政府审定；②学会审定；③学者鼓吹的力量；④多数意志的选择。这四种力量是并行不悖的，一种也不可少，由此最终所得的译名才可适当，并被大多数人所接受。

参考文献

[1] 李照国．中医翻译标准化的概念、原则与方法．中国翻译，1991，12（4）：27－31．
[2] 李照国．中医名词术语英译的标准化．西安：西安医科大学出版社，1992．
[3] 李照国．中医翻译学导论．西安：西北大学出版社，1993：143－147．

［原载《中国中西医结合杂志》，1994，14（3）：144.］

借鉴国外翻译经验和理念，促进国内中医英译事业发展

——从几个中医术语的英译想起的

兰凤利

目前，中医英译可以说是百花齐放、百家争鸣。20 世纪 80 年代，世界卫生组织（World Health Orgnization，WHO）就曾专门组织专家、学者对针灸学方面的术语的英译进行规范化，这在一定程度上促进了针灸学的国际交流和对外教学，但也存在不少明显的误译。比如，以 meridian 对译“经脉”。实际上，用 channel 来翻译“经脉”要比 meridian 好得多。“经脉”可以运行气血，显然是三维的。meridian 的本义是指地图上的子午线、经线（“an imaginary line drawn from the top point of the Earth to the bottom over the surface of the Earth，one of several used on maps to show position”[1]），是二维的，而 channel 指三维的、可以容纳某种物质的管道（“suggesting a three-dimensional conduit that contains some kind of substance”[2]），在含义上更接近中文。而 triple energizer［三焦，energizer（energize，v. give energy to[1]）］这一译语至今未能得到大多数人的认同，triple burner 倒是相当流行。

下面我们看几个常见的中医学术语的英译。

1. 五行学说

目前国内几乎都将“五行学说”译成 the theory of five elements。笔者认为，这一译法或许是受了 Greek system of the four elements 的启发而来。五行学说虽然起源于“五材”说，但是“五行”就是“五材”吗？第 5 版《中医基础理论》教材是这样解释的：“五行，即是木、火、土、金、水五种物质的运动。”[3]商务印书馆出版的《古汉语常用字字典》中“行”字条的第三个释义是“运动，运行”，并在其后举“五行”为例加以说明[4]。此外，从内容来看，五行学说并非孤立地论述五种物质的特性，可“进一步引申为世界上的一切事物都是由木、火、土、金、水五种基本物质之间的运动变化而生成的”[3]，“同时，还以五行之间的生、克关系来阐释事物之间的相互关系”[3]。令人汗颜的是，西方学者，比如英国的魏迺杰[5]、美国的 Ted J. Kaptchuk 等却都能对“五行”作出正确的理解，将之译成 Five Phases。请看 Ted J. Kaptchuk 的一段论述：“The Five Phases are not in any way ultimate constituents of matter. This misconception has long been embodied in the common mistranslation ‘Five Elements’ and exemplifies the problems that arise from looking at things Chinese with a Western frame of reference. The Chinese term that we translate as 'Five Phases' is Wu Xing. Wu is the number five, and Xing means 'walk' or 'move', and, perhaps most pertinently, it implies a process. The Wu Xing, therefore, are five kinds of processes; hence the Five Phases, and not the Five Elements. The theory of Phases is a system of correspondences and patterns that subsume events and things, especially in relationship to their dynamics"[2]。鉴于"五行，即是木、火、土、金、水五种物质的运动"[3]，笔者建议国内采用西方公认的译法，将"五行"译为 Five Phases，将"五行学说"译为 the theory of Five Phases。

2. 辨证

自从吕维柏教授建议用 syndrome differentiation 来翻译"辨证"以来，这一术语便成了国内中医翻译界达成共识的为数不多的中医术语之一。用西方人容易理解的 syndrome 来翻译"证"这样一个中医独有的概念合适吗？试想，我们如何对 climacteric syndrome（更年期综合征，中医病名为"绝经前后诸证"）再进行 differentiating syndrome（辨证），然后将患者再辨为肝肾阴虚证（syndrome）或阴虚火旺证（syndrome）？Ted J. Kaptchuk 认为："From a modern Western perspective, it is tempting to translate the Chinese words as 'differentiating syndromes', but that rendering would distort the uniqueness and potential validity of the Chinese idea. 'Syndrome' is a purely descriptive term, suggesting an arbitrary grouping of signs and symptoms that is meaningless without an underlying cause. 'Syndrome' implies that something is missing."[2] 他把"辨证"译为 distinguishing patterns。如果联想到八纲辨证的表、里、寒、热、虚、实、阴、阳证的话，用 pattern 来翻译中医的"证"显然比 syndrome 更妥。著名英国中医翻译家魏迺杰将"辨证"译成 pattern identification 和 identify patterns[5]。实际上，英美国家出版的中医药学教材几乎都采用这一术语，如 *Fundamentals of Chinese Medicine*[6]、*The Foundations of Chinese Medicine*[7]。

3. 通因通用

通因通用是反治法中的一种，"是以通治通，即用通利的药物治疗具有实性通泄症状的病症。适用于食积腹痛，泻下不畅，热结旁流；瘀血所致的崩漏；膀胱湿热所致的尿频、尿急、尿痛等病症"[3]。目前国内对这个术语的翻译主要是 treating diarrhea with cathartics[8]（cathartics refers to medicine which causes a bowel movement）等，即"以泻法或导泻药治疗泄泻"，是很明显的误译。魏迺杰将这一术语译为 using flow to treat flow[6]，从信息密度、回译性以及"信"的角度，这一译语都很值得采纳。

4. 下法

下法，是“运用泻下、攻逐、润下的药物以通导大便、消除积滞、荡涤实热、攻逐水饮的治法”[8]。国内一般都将这一术语译为 purgation[8-9]或 purgative therapy[9]。《朗文当代高级英语辞典》将 purgation 释义为“清除、清洗；净化；消除不良影响；通便”[1]。《英汉双解医学词典》将 purgation 释义为“noun，using a drug to make a bowel movement；催泻”，将 purgative 释义为“noun & adjective，laxative；（medicine）which causes evacuation of the bowels；催泻的，催泻剂”，将 purge 释义为“verb，to induce evacuation of a patient's bowels”[10]。可见，purgation 或 purgative therapy 只具有“通导大便”的含义。从上面的“下法”定义，我们可以看出，不管是“下”大便、“下”积滞、“下”实热，或者是“下”水饮，“下”的意义是“使……下”。魏迺杰认为，“‘下’，其字面上意指‘使……降下’，但是一般使用的英文自然对应词 purgation，其字面上的含义却是 clean（清洁）。由于中医四种基本动态形式（出、入、升、降）的观念十分重要，因此，‘下’应当以符合中医原词字面含义的译文译出”[5]。他将之译为 precipitation[5]，意为“使……突然下降，猛然投下”。同样，这一术语也很值得国内同行借鉴。

翻译既是语言之间的转换，更是文化之间的交流。中医翻译与中医文化密切相关。国内中医翻译工作者总是采用“归化”的方法，试图以西方医学或文化中固有的概念来诠释中医学独特的术语。著名学者文树德先生说，“过于频繁地滥用现代西医学专业术语来意译中医书籍，已经混淆了中医学思想的独立性”[5]，而这主要是由于中国译者造成的。

中医学和西医学是根植于两种不同文化的医疗体系。100 多年来，国内外很多中西医学专家都努力在中医学与西医学之间搭起桥梁，然而这绝非翻译工作者的职责所在。国内的中医翻译工作者应该虚心借鉴国外的翻译经验和理念，在理解、把握中医术语的含义后，采用“异化”译法，还中医以本来面目。

笔者认为，为了适应中医医学与文化交流的客观要求，对中医英译中的医学文化空缺现象的处理应本着文化平等的态度，尽量运用“异化”译法，将医学文化空缺术语译成“中国式英语”。著名的英国中医翻译家魏迺杰先生说：“在西传的过程中，中医并不能为了配合西方人的需求而有所改变。而西方意欲学习中医的人也绝对无法经由一种‘以其本身较为熟悉的知识系统将中医学重新过滤’的学习方式获得成功，他们必须真正地进入中医的世界。总之，只有当翻译者遵循中医原来被接受的传统方式去看待中医学并将中医忠实地翻译出来，才得以为西方真正想学习中医的人士开启一条迈入中医的大道”[5]。

参考文献

[1] 艾迪生·维斯理. 朗文出版公司辞典部编. 朗文当代高级英语辞典. 北京：商务印书馆，1998：948，487，1219.
[2] Kaptchuk TJ. Chinese medicine：the web that has no weaver. London：Rider，2000：132，217.
[3] 印会河，张伯讷. 中医基础理论. 上海：上海科学技术出版社，1988：18，133.
[4]《古汉语常用字字典》编写组. 古汉语常用字字典. 北京：商务印书馆，1998：319.
[5] 魏迺杰. 英汉·汉英中医词典. 长沙：湖南科学技术出版社，1996：685，407，21，689，3，35.
[6] Wiseman N，Ellis A. Fundamentals of Chinese medicine. Paradigm Publications，1996：127，250.
[7] Maciocia G. The foundations of Chinese medicine. London：Churchill Livingstone，1989：175.
[8] 欧明. 汉英中医辞典. 广东科技出版社三联书店（香港）有限公司，1993：425，11-12.
[9] 汉英、汉法、汉德、汉日、汉俄医学大词典编纂委员会. 汉英医学大词典. 北京：人民卫生出版社，1995：1779.
[10] Collin PH. 英汉双解医学词典. 北京：外语教学与研究出版社，2001：477.

[原载《中国中西医结合杂志》，2003，23（8）：627-628.]

中医英译中的音译现象与翻译的等值理论

蒋建勇

中医英译难，要在英译中实现翻译等值更是难上加难。问题的关键是翻译的等值理论在中医英译实践中的再现，即如何既要准确地传递原文，又要将中医作为中国传统文化中一个不可分割的部分全面地在译文中准确地表达出来，努力使译文有一个坚实的理论基础，一个具有中国特色的鲜明导向性特征，一个能被英语母语使用者接受的流畅篇章。

Theo-Hermans 在《翻译的再现》中认为，“译本绝不可能是原作内容的翻版，因为译本所使用的文字不同，语言和文化体系既不对称也不同形”。李照国博士也在最近的讲座中提出：“翻译是由一种语言转化成另一种语言的过程，如同一个冰山，无论如何翻译，落实于文字的只是冰山的一角，而关键的是冰山在海平面以下的部分却无法准确地再现出来。我们所能做到的永远只是达到相似而已”。上述思想应该看作对等值理论的深化，因为追求译文与原文的近似等值，始终应该作为一名诚实译者必须信奉的准则，只有这样，译者及其译作才有存在的价值。

那么在具有典型中国文化特征的中医英译实践中，尤其是翻译如《黄帝内经》等古典医籍及特有的中医术语时如何努力使译文与原文更为相似、更能趋近于信、达、雅的翻译标准就值得我们深究了。徐象才先生在《谈中医术语的错误英译》一文中痛陈了 20 多年来中医英译的错误和弊端，并将矛头直指“解释翻译法”和“比照西医翻译法”。遗憾的是文中没有提及解决的办法。要根本解决上述问题，可能要如李照国先生在《中医英语》所指出的：“要使中医学特有概念在英语译语中保持特有的内涵，音译恐怕是唯一可行之路”。但许多译者在音译的使用上却是顾虑重重，或是因为害怕音译难以有效传递原文，甚至认为音译没有充足的理论依据。表现在译文、论文中是就点谈点，不敢涉及或回避面的问题、体系的问题。如鞋匠一般修修补补，乍看上去似修好了一些，实际上却是一片斑驳。对于前后文不统一、无总体性译则可言的英译文章，试问谁能相信？如果前怕狼后怕虎，结果非但无济于事，反而会祸害无穷！

北京大学的孟华在探讨西学东译过程后认为，“在中西文化交流中，翻译具有传递‘相异性’的功能，即‘它可在一国的文化传统中，亦即在一个民族的身份认同中植入相异性因素’”。实际上不仅汉语的吸收表明了这一点，它的输出也是有案可查的。从 Kowtow，到 Beijing，从 tea 到 Mandarin，一直到中医的 Qi、

Yin、Yang。中国文化在与其迥然不同的西方文化中植入了许多相异性因素。稍稍研究前面提到的已经融入现代英语的词汇中具有鲜明中国文化特色的词，可以发现一个重要特征就是音译，这是译者们在目标语文化对原作的改造中，无法找到既与原文对应且为读者理解的词语来进行置换造成的，也是他们所能将这类词语较为全面地表达出来的方式，这已经成为人们在翻译专有名词时的通常做法。例如我们完全不会极端地将 Mr. Black Smith 译为“铁匠先生”，将某某灵先生译为“Mr… Cleverness”。

据《翻译名义集序》记载，唐朝大翻译家玄奘早已提出采用音译的五种情况——“五不翻”，即秘密故、含多义故、此无故、顺古故、生善故，尤其是含多义故、此无故、顺古故。这种翻译理念对中医英译有着极其重要的帮助。中医中一词多义的现象普遍存在，如“气”，在中医中有功能之气、物质之气、先天之气、后天之气，还有元气、卫气、营气、宗气之分，如果用 vital energy、nourishment、vital-Qi 等来分别指代，恐怕会引起极大的混淆，也会使读者对译作的忠实度产生怀疑。就此而论，音译在某种程度上就理应成为中医译者的宠儿。但中医英译是绝不能搞一刀切，全用音译或只用音译。前者是因为许多中医术语还是能在英语中找到对应语的，如“带下医”就是今天的妇科医生，直接译为 gynecologist 就行了。对于后者我们必须认识到现代医学与中医从理论体系到临床实践是大相径庭的，若仅是音译，只是达到形式等值，实质并不等值。不客气地说，若该音译尚未约定俗成的话，这不叫翻译。因为读者将得不到充足的有效信息，这大概就是严复先生所批评的“译而不译”了。这样我们就得对音译作一点技术补充，即采用加注释的办法。在注释中就可以对这些音译术语进行解释，读者在上下文所创造的语域中参看注释，相信是不难理解译文的，而注释本身无疑会传递该术语所承载的中国传统文化等文内含义。这种方法分别被萧乾和金隄在《尤利西斯》的译本中成功应用。西方在《圣经》的翻译中也大量采用了这一方法。而部分术语采用了以拼音为手段的音译法，避免了歧义产生，也使之烙上了鲜明的中国特色，最大限度地使中医术语英译实现了名从主人原则，符合语言国情学的要求。这样的中医英译从理论上最接近原文，即再现其内涵和外延，又体现了其民族特征，还最大限度地传递了中医作为中国传统文化中一个不可分割的部分的深刻文化内涵，从形式到实质都实现了最大的近似等值。

另外，提倡音译也不能不分场合。中医英语的实际运用分为：中医诊疗基础理论、中药方剂和临床带教，故应根据其具体特征对音译的实践策略进行变化。基础理论部分的音译术语在文中首次出现时，可用注释、括号方式给出具体语境解释，直至新义出现再予新解。如，“天人相应”可译为 Tian Ren Xiang Ying (correspondence between man and nature)；中药音译术语的使用因用药的准确性要求，可于首次出现时用附注形式标示拉丁文，显示用药部位，如：大黄 Da

Huang（Radixet Rhizoma Rehi）。临床带教中由于医疗实体和语境的存在，音译是应该不会对医疗实践造成混乱的。

音译在中医英译中正逐渐地显现出其巨大魅力，它是处于传统与现代、西方与东方的种种张力间的译者的被动选择，也是他们试图将一种文化的特异性因素传递给另一种文化，实现最大限度等值转移的探索。但如果使用音译泛滥又将可能导致对音译的极端全面否定，这又成为一个棘手的问题。

[原载《中国中西医结合杂志》，2004，24（8）：750－751.]

中医术语英译原则探讨

王锦方　毛　红　杨守忠

中医学是灿烂的中华文化宝库中的一朵奇葩，现在已经绽放在世界上各个角落。然而，我们发现在中医术语的英译中，存在着不可忽视的误译、漏译甚至乱译现象，这种现象不利于中外的交流，不利于中医的进一步推广。本文旨在探讨中医术语英译中几个最基本的最亟需明确的原则，这些原则不求涵盖整个中医翻译理论，但希望能对中医术语翻译的科学化、规范化有所裨益。

1. 切忌滥用汉语拼音

中医术语言简意赅，内涵丰富。某些术语基于古老的东方哲学，概念独特，在任何其他民族的语言中没有相同甚至于近似的表达方式。例如："气"是中医的基本概念，它涉及中医的生理学、病理学、症候学等许多方面。它可能指人体及脏器组织的功能，有人译成 vital energy，还有人译成 immunity system；它可能指"水谷之气"，有人译成 refined nutritive substance；它还可能指空气、呼吸、致病因素、话语、宇宙生成等，这时有人会译成 air、breath、pathogen、voice、ether 等。这种意译把"气"这个概念肢解了，其哲学积淀荡然无存。而且仅就"气"的某一特定含意来讲，比如与血相对的人体基本生理功能之"气"，其含义也不是 vital energy 等词汇所能真正揭示的。这些术语除了采用音译的办法外别无选择：气即 Qi，采用音译是不得已而为之，它只能被训练有素的专业人员理解，对于外行来说可能就是天书。不过许多专业术语都是如此，比如多普勒、胃镜、过磷酸钙这些很普通的医学名词，可是普通中国人恐怕都不知其所以然。然而，西方人接受中医时需要在头脑里建立全新的观念，其困难可想而知。如果译文里充斥着大量的音译，无疑令学习者坠入云里雾中，因此，限制音译数量已成翻译界的共识。现在的问题是，许多术语本来已经有了约定俗成的好译法，音译依旧大行其道。比如脏腑，有人直接译成 Zang-Fu，这就很值得商榷。既然五脏六腑可以意译成 heart、lung、kidney 等，且已得到公认，脏腑却采用音译，岂不圆凿方枘？在一些译著或辞书里，我们经常会看到不当音译诸如 Couli（腠理）、Fenrou（分肉）等。更有甚者，连上膊、下膊有人也竟采用音译 upper Bo、lower Bo！使用 arm 多么简便而贴切。国内外公认只能音译的中医术语屈指可数，译者只要稍微下点儿工夫就不会出现如此低级的误译。这里需要指出，针灸学里的经络名称等在国际上流行意译（个别采用音译），但穴位名称普遍采用音译，这已经得到联合国卫生组织的认可。但有人也对穴位名称进行意译，目的是令学习者理解穴位名称的含意。

2. 借用西医术语，力求英汉内涵和外延的对等

将中医与西医比照，我们不难发现中医术语阐述的是功能概念，而西医术语阐述的是解剖学上的概念，其差异显而易见。如前面提到的“心、肝、脾、肺、肾”等，中医的概念与西医的概念含义不同，但相同之处也甚多，因此，译为 heart、liver、spleen、lung、kidney 为好。在翻译过程中，经常需要借助英语的基本词来表达中医学特有的概念。比如“肝血”译成 liver blood，“血虚”译成 blood deficiency，“活血化瘀”译成 activating blood to resolve stagnation 等，非常方便。对“心”之类的中医名词曾经也有人主张音译，他们认为译成 heart 等会造成误解，会令人以为中医的“心”等就是西医所说的 heart。并由此断言，这种译法会影响中医在世界上的发展。一种语言里的词汇和另一种语言里的现有词汇完全对等的情况极少。有人会说，汉语的“淋巴”和英语的 lymph 概念就完全一致。但“淋巴”并非汉语里固有词汇，而是源自英语的音译。

我们现在研究一下西医传入中国时的早期情况，当时就是采用音译、直译或意译并行的办法，然而这并未引起西医与中医的混乱，并未影响西医在中国的传播，因此，担心把“心”等中医术语译成 heart 等会造成误解是多余的。术语的翻译应该是统一的，即如前面所说，“气”不能此处译作 nutritive substance，彼处译作 vital energy。但是，也不能走极端，即不能硬性规定汉语的一个字无论何处都必须译成英语里的某个词。汉语和英语都是典型的多音词语言。一个字（词）很可能有若干不同的解释，因此，在翻译过程中，在注意统一性的同时，要准确把握中医术语的内涵和外延。例如“精”字，在“肾藏精，精舍志”中指“精气”，可译成 essence；在“精伤则骨痠厥，精时自下”，第一个“精”是指“肾精”，译成 essence，第二个指“精液”，则该译成 seminal；在“脉理精微，其体难辨”中，“精”指的是“精深”，对应译文为 profound。中医术语高度凝练，内涵丰富。如果英译也如此短小精悍，往往不能涵盖要传递的全部信息；如果要准确全面地揭示这些信息，英译则需要长长的短语，那么这就不像术语了。很多情况下折中的办法也行不通，译者因此而常常陷入两难境地。

不过，有时出现的两难是由于我们过分强调毫无遗漏地揭示中医术语的全部内涵，而忘记了术语的本质。比如“虚胀”，有人明知道译得不像术语却偏偏要译成 flatulence due to Yang-deficiency of the spleen and kidney，声称直译成 deficiency flatulence 会导致概念不清。我们则觉得后者很好。外行人会觉得一头雾水，可对内行人来说则一目了然。其实，任何语言里的专业术语都是如此。专著翻译不是科普写作，面对的不是普通读者（外国的普通读者也不会涉猎中医）。

有人以“辨证论治”为例，说明翻译如何才能做到忠实地揭示其内涵。推荐的译文是 diagnosis and treatment based on the overall analysis of symptoms and signs，这种翻译很直白，但是无论如何也算不上术语了。我们认为有人斥之为不当的翻译反倒更为可取：treatment based on syndrome differentiation。不过，对这种翻译还可以补充几种供参考：planning treatment according to diagnosis、determining treatment by patterns identified、identifying patterns and administering treatment...

3. 忠实、忠实、忠实

中医是科学，翻译过程中不允许艺术加工。译者的任务就是再现原作，要尽最大可能地保存原作的语言风格、韵味、历史和文化的特征。中国的翻译工作者都明了“信”字当头的翻译准则，对此翻译界没有任何分歧。然而，问题是什么样的翻译才是忠实的。有一个关于《黄帝内经》译法的例子，我们认为是极可笑的，但该文作者是郑重其事提出来的。该文称与秦始皇不一样，黄帝非帝也，因此，凡使用了 emperor 字眼的都不忠实。又云，“经”指长存之义理、法则、原则，非《圣经》或《金刚经》之经，故而凡使用 classic、canon 等字眼的，均非忠实的翻译。忠实的翻译是什么呢？人类的词汇随着历史的发展会发生变化，比如内涵与外延可能扩展或收缩，但是大多数基本词汇的变化往往都有承续性。三皇五帝的确和后来的帝王在地位、权利等诸多方面有很大的不同。但“皇”与“帝”表示的是最高统治者这一基本概念并没有改变，这正是秦始皇所以取“皇帝”而称之的原因。使用（yellow）emperor 有何不妥呢？如果照该文标准，忠实的译文看来只有一种：把全书全部改写成拼音！

我们在一篇文章中曾说，直译或鲁迅先生所说的硬译是保证翻译忠实的最主要的原则。直译就是源语怎么说的就怎么译。比如关于症状的术语，中医是根据症而治，因此，对症状的描述细致入微。对于这类术语，生套西医往往有悖于中医的本义。我们应该仔细揣摩它们描述的情景，然后再用恰当的英语表达出来。“不思饮食”译成 no thought of food and drink 就比译成 poor appetite 更忠于原文；同样，wind clenched jaw（风口噤）比 lockjaw 更可取；arched back rigidity 就比 opisthotonos 更符合中医本义。然而，和任何原则一样，不能走极端。比如“大便秘结”的翻译。既然直译不允许添加也不允许减少任何东西，那好，就译成 constipation of stool。constipation 就是便秘，再加上 of stool 岂不是画蛇添足？中医学的形成与发展深受中国传统文化的影响，因此，它的许多术语具有中国语言文化的特色。比如大量结构严谨、蕴涵丰富、音调和谐的四字结构的存在就说明了这个问题。在翻译时，即使是直译，也不能逐字（词）翻译。忠实要求抓住主旨，不能过分拘泥于汉语的词汇结构形式。

做到翻译的忠实很不容易。我们在一篇论文中曾举“虚夹寒”作为例子，提出较妥当的译法之一是 vacuity sandwiching cold。这在近现代的中医作品中使用还是可以的。然而，sandwich 这个词在英语里是从 18 世纪出现的，因此，用于较古老的中医典籍翻译则不忠实了，不忠于历史。在翻译中医术语时要想做到忠实，译者必须涉猎一些汉语的训诂、文字学，英语的修辞学、词源学，当然还要认认真真地学一学中医。

综上所述，中医术语的翻译在综合运用音译、直译、意译等方法的同时，还要严格限制音译词的数量；比照西医翻译时，要注意中医术语的内涵和外延；要科学忠实地再现原文。尽管中医术语的使用还存在模糊、歧义、笼统的缺点，相信通过广大译者从科学的原则出发，一定能使译文得到中外医学界的认可，为中医走向世界并开展对外学术交流更好地发挥桥梁作用。

［原载《中国中西医结合杂志》，2005，25（12）：1129－1130.］

中医文献英译的异化和归化

梁俊雄　王冠军

在翻译中存在着异化（alienation）和归化（adaptation）两种彼此对立的方法。异化是以源语为归宿的语际转换，主张保留原文中的异国情调，使读者可以充分欣赏借鉴其他文化的异质成分，以丰富本国的文化，但同时加重了读者对译文的陌生感；归化是以译语为归宿的语际转换，把源语中的异质成分转化为译语中人们所熟知的内容，从而降低读者接受的难度，但往往会丢失源语中负载的文化信息。例如，英语中有这样的说法，“Never offer to teach fish to swim”，译成“永远别想教鱼游泳”就是异化的方法，准确地传递了源语文化的信息；译成汉语中对应的成语“班门弄斧”，就是归化的方法，准确地再现了译语文化的信息。这两种翻译方法各有利弊，在中医文献的英译中如何恰当地运用异化和归化的方法就是我们面临的一个问题。

随着世界各国人民的经济文化交往日益频繁，语言文化的交融成为可能，各民族语言就会越来越多地吸收外来营养，丰富本民族的语言，因此，翻译中的异化现象就变得更常见了。汉语在不断地发展自身、拓宽语言内涵的同时，也越来越多地从其他语言特别是英语中广泛地吸收有益的成分，例如超级市场（supermarket）、因特网（internet）、信息高速公路（information highway）等。英语民族由于其自身开放性的心理特点，善于从其他语言中吸收外来语，因此，表达方式就极其丰富。近年来，随着中国国际地位的提高，对世界经济和文化的影响越来越大，有更多的汉语表达方式进入了英语词汇。例如，随着神舟五号和神舟六号载人飞船的成功发射，英语中就出现了一个汉化的词汇——“Taikonaut”来表达中国航天员，这就是英语中典型的异化。

事实上，随着各国人民文化交流的逐渐深入，异化的表达往往会加深对异族文化的理解，促进各民族文化的融合。异化的翻译方法可以将一种文化语言中陌生的现象介绍给其他文化的人们，并逐渐让人们了解、熟悉，从而人为地拉近了不同文化间的距离。在将英语翻译成汉语的过程中，我们可以感受到，一些英语成语、谚语和习语的翻译如以接受外来文化为翻译的出发点，采用异化的方法，往往会带来异国情调。如“Never offer to teach fish to swim”译成“永远别想教鱼游泳”，能给我们更多异族文化的联想，如译成“班门弄斧”，很明显我们将失去很多原汁原味。而且，从幽默和诙谐的角度来看，我们也很难把汉语“班门弄斧”和“Never offer to teach fish to swim”的确切内涵等同起来。同样的，

"Spend money like water"译为"花钱如流水"，而不用"挥金如土"；"Among wolves one must howl"直接译为"在狼群中你就得嗥"，而不用归化为"入乡随俗"。

诞生于东方的中医学与中国的人文地理条件及主导的传统文化有着相互依存的关系。在中医文献中，许多术语言简意丰，经历了历史文化的积淀，反映了汉民族的社会状况、宗教信仰、价值观念等，蕴含着丰富的文化含义，往往难以在英语中找到同等的表达法。遵循文化对等的原则，应使用各种翻译方法以最大限度地传递源语中的文化意蕴，因此，就翻译的内容而言，就应更多地考虑异化的方法。

音译的方法是一种常用的异化法，它能够最忠实地传递原文的文化意蕴。在各民族之间的文化交流中，对外来文化中的独特的现象、概念，如在本民族语言中难以找到对应的词汇翻译，采用音译的方法不失为一种明智的选择，因此，很多中医词汇用音译法作为外来词进入英语已不成问题了。事实上，一些中医词汇如阴阳（Ying，Yang），脏腑（Zang Fu），寸关尺（Cun，Guan，Chi），三焦（Tri-jiao），卫气营血（Wei，Qi，Ying，Xue）已进入英语词汇。

直译的方法也属于异化的范畴，可以直接传递语言中蕴藏的文化信息。"百闻不如一见"的英译"To hear hundred times cannot be compared with seeing once"，虽不完全符合英语的思维习惯，却直观生动地传达了鲜明的中国特色。我们中国人常说的"丢脸"和"船小好掉头"分别被译为"to lose face"和"A small boat turns easily"，也成了英语的有机成分。总之，在翻译过程中尽量传达源语中的民族形象和文化特点，有利于帮助人们接受异域文化和智慧，输入新鲜血液，促进本族语言与文化的发展。

如"东施效颦"这一汉成语典故，可直接译为"Tungshih imitates Hisshih"。但对不甚了解中国历史文化的西方人来说不知所云。为了让西方读者了解这一成语的内涵，可以在后面加注（Shishih was a famous beauty in the ancient Kingdom of Yueh，Tungshih was an ugly girl who tried to imitate her way.）[1]。这样译会使西方读者一目了然。很多中医术语都可以用直译的方法，例如，中医的"提壶揭盖"是一种治疗方法，指通过宣通上焦的气机而使下焦腑气畅通，进而达到排出大小便的目的。这个术语形象生动，有着很浓厚的中国文化特色。如果直译为"lifting the lid to pour off water in the pot"，保留了源语文化的情调，使读者感到新鲜生动，扩大了读者的知识视野。当然，如果在该术语首次出现的时候用括号加上解释（opening the lung Qi to treat constipation or dysuria），这样读者就容易明白了。

在对中医文献英译的时候，我们自然地会考虑异化的方法，以期更多地传递当中蕴含的文化信息。在音译法和直译法都不能解决问题的时候，就要求助于意译法了。意译法属于归化的范畴，它摆脱了原文表面结构形式的约束进行翻译，追求的不是两种语言在词义、句子结构、思维方式上的表面对应或一致，而是译文与原文在实质内容上的相近或相同。例如，中医的“转筋”（俗称抽筋）和“转胞”（指胎儿压迫孕妇的膀胱所致的小便不通），运用异化方法的音译或直译处理是不太恰当的。用意译的方法就分别译成 spasm 和 dysuria due to the pressure of the fetus，这是“重神似而不重形似”[2]。

同时，我们还必须注意到另外一个问题，就是思维方式对语言结构的影响。每个民族都有自己独特的思维方式，在观察事物与思维方式上都存在着一定的差异，这样就产生了不同的语言表达方式，有不同的语言结构[3]。例如，英语民族习惯直截了当地把要点放在句首说出来，然后再把各种标志一一补进，而汉语民族习惯于从侧面说明，阐述外围环境，最后点出话语的信息中心。将“胆者，中正之官，决断出焉”翻译成“The gallbladder seems to be an upright officer who is in charge of making a decision”，译文句法结构就反映了汉语的特点，不如译成“The gallbladder is in charge of making a decision，which seems to be an upright officer”更能迎合英语民族的思维特点。

受传统哲学“天人合一”的世界观影响，汉语民族习惯于从总体方面认识事物，把世界看成本质上是一个不可分割的有机体，这就形成了整体思维模式。重悟性、讲含蓄的哲学思想对汉语民族思维方式有很大的影响。汉语民族的这种思维方式就会体现在汉语句子结构上。汉语句式重意会，以意统形，是一个形散意合的系统，表意手段十分灵活丰富，往往不受严格的形态规则的制约。汉语句子往往按逻辑事物或时间先后顺序排列，是典型的流水结构[4]。例如，《黄帝内经》中有如下表述，“阴阳者，天地之道也，万物之纲纪，变化之父母，生杀之本始，神明之府也，治病必求于本。”这句话中每个小句都可独立成句，基本没有主次关系，典型地反映出汉语句子注重内在关系、隐含关系、模糊关系的语言结构特点，只是依靠意义上的连贯意合，其间很少用逻辑连接词；而英语民族往往把自己看作独立存在的个体，人与自然相互对立，人处在支配和改造自然的位置，天人相分，两者对立，认为世界上万物都是对立的。这种天人相分的思想使英语民族在处理问题时，常常把具体问题从总体中分离出来，将极复杂的问题划分为比较简单的形式和部分去研究，从而形成了与汉语民族思维模式截然相反的个体思维模式。这种思维模式反映到语言结构上，就是句子要受严格的形态规则的制约，其实际含义只能根据句中词汇的逻辑顺序来推理和归纳，是典型的树状结构[4]。如：Young men who have reasons to fear that they will be killed in battle may justifiably feel bitter in the thought that they have been cheated of the best things that life has to offer。该句的基本结构是：Young men…may justifiably feel bitter in the thought，跟在 Young men 后面的 who have reasons to fear that they will be killed in battle 是 Young men 的修饰语。在这个定语从句中，that they will be killed in battle 又是该句的宾语从句。另外，thought 后面还跟了一个同位语从句，在这个从句中又有一个定语从句 that life has to offer 修饰 the best things。这是一个典型的英语句子，句中有许多修饰和限制成分，但逻辑严密，语义关系一目了然。

对前述《黄帝内经》的原文如译为：Yin and Yang serve as the Dao（law）of the heaven and the earth，the fundamental principle of all things，the parent of change，the beginning of birth and death and the storehouse of Shengming. The treatment of disease must follow this law. 这样的翻译照搬了汉语结构，汉语味十足，可能不为英文读者所乐道。过分强调源语的语言结构必然给译文读者的理解造成很大的困难，因此，翻译在语言结构上应以归化为主。笔者尝试将该段原文译为：The treatment of disease must follow the principle of Yin and Yang for they serve as the Dao（law）of the heaven and the earth，by which all things must abide，from which change originates，to which birth and death can be traced back，in which Shengming is stored. 读者最关心的是阴阳在中医的应用，所以就以“The treatment…must follow the principle of Yin and Yang”为主句，突出治病求本，然后跟着以“for”引导的原因状语从句，说明要治病求本是因为阴阳是天地之道，世间一切事物的变化都必须遵从阴阳的运动，后面再跟着三个以介词＋which 引导的定语从句修饰 Dao（law），以说明阴阳在其他方面的应用。这样的翻译在句法结构上把汉语原文蕴含的逻辑语义关系按照英语的语言结构重新展开，符合英语的树状结构。汉语民族重视形象思维，惯于用具体形象的词语来表达虚的概念；而英语民族重视抽象思维，常常使用大量指称笼统的抽象词汇来表达复杂的理性概念。汉语原文中的“纲纪”“父母”“本始”“之府”“本”等都是很形象的名词，翻译时我们就用了比较抽象的动词短语来处理，这样就符合英语的思维习惯，这些都是归化的方法。当然在翻译中我们也采用了异化的方法，例如“道”“神明”分别用音译的方法处理，以期能传递其中蕴含的文化信息。

异化法和归化法作为翻译中的两种原则和方法，都具有其存在和应用的价值。在中医文献英译时，就语言的内容而言，应更多地应用异化法，以期忠实地传递其中蕴含的文化信息，当然在不得已的情况下可采用归化的意译法。由于汉语和英语的思维模式不同，汉英语言结构呈现出极大的差异。译者一方面要忠实于原文，另一方面又要使译文流畅，符合英语读者的思维习惯，因此，在翻译时，必须进行语言结构上的转换以适应英语读者的思维模式，就语言结构而言，应遵从归化的原则。总之，异化与归化两种方法应相辅相成，共同使翻译起到跨越不同文化的桥梁作用。

参考文献

[1] 陶明星．翻译教学中的文化导入．湖南社会科学，2005，(3)：122－124.
[2] 怒安．傅雷谈翻译．沈阳：辽宁教育出版社，2005：12.
[3] 张小曼，胡作友．英汉思维差异与翻译策略运用．合肥工业大学学报（社会科学版），2005，19（2）：108－112.
[4] 司显柱．论英汉民族思维模式、语言结构及其翻译．外语学刊，1999，(2)：78－86.

［原载《中国中西医结合杂志》，2006，26（10）：950－952.］

中医英译规范化中的译者素养问题探讨

何 阳

中医翻译作为一门新兴的特殊学科，既不同于一般的文学翻译，也不同于一般的工程技术翻译。而且，随着对外交流的日趋增多，中医翻译规范化也逐渐凸显其举足轻重的地位，这无疑给译者提出了更多的要求。

1. 提升中医英译者的知识结构是规范中医翻译的基础

中国传统医学已有几千年的发展历史，它不仅有独特的中医学理论体系，而且还有丰富的临床经验。以《黄帝内经》和《伤寒杂病论》为标志的中医学理论体系以整体观念为主导思想，以脏腑、经络的生理病理为基础，以辨证论治为诊疗特点，因此，中医学科本身的特点就要求译者在翻译实践中，首先具备一定的基础中医学知识，既要关注其丰富的古代朴素自然辩证法思想，更要学习其古奥精炼的学术术语并理解其概念的丰富内涵，否则，必然会影响到译文的质量。在处理像"怒伤肝"（anger impairs the liver）、"喜伤心"（overjoy impairs the heart）、"思伤脾"（anxiety impairs the spleen）、"悲伤肺"（melancholy impairs the lung ）、"恐伤肾"（fear impairs the kidney）这样的中英互译时，很难达到医文并举、用词精确、行文立说、文采熠熠、百诵不厌、回味无穷的效果。

此外，由于学科的日渐融和，中医的临床与科研大量借鉴了西医的检测方法与实验技术，并已成为中医药学发展的新趋势，这无疑给译者又带来了新的困难。要想做一名高水平的中医翻译人员，还应学习一些诸如生理学、解剖学、免疫学、药理学、病理学和生物化学等西医学科的基础理论知识，学会使用专业地道的医学语言，阐释传统的中医学特点，以达到交流之目的。例如：中医中的"血瘀"（blood stasis）指的就是西医血液流变学（blood-rheology）中的异常变化，并通常可以用血液黏稠度（blood viscosity）、血液循环（blood circulation）的异常改变来解释其发病机制。还有，中医学常说的"蛇串疮""缠腰火丹"，即是西医的带状疱疹（herpes zoster），若译成"the snakey beaded sore"，势必是会引起歧义的。

2. 关注中医药文献中的文化因素是规范中医翻译的首要策略

英语界知名前辈王佐良先生在《翻译中的文化比较》中提出译者"处理的是个别词，而面对的则是两大片文化"，并要求每位译者做"一个真正意义上的文化人”[1]。中医学在几千年的发展过程中，深受历朝各代政治、经济、科技和文化的影响，那些富含深奥哲理的医籍文献还蕴涵着厚重的古代文化知识，因此，关注中医药文献中的文化因素是规范中医翻译程中译者理应采取的首要策略。比如，《黄帝内经》就是一本包罗万象的大百科全书，它不仅深入探讨了有关医学的基本问题，还对中国古代文化，如天文历法、地理气象、名物典制、数术音律、天干地支、官制避讳和心理等知识均有所运用。阴阳、五行、气、形、神既是中国古代的哲学范畴，又是中医学理论的基本概念。《黄帝内经》中形气转化、形神统一、天人感应、辨证求因、四诊合参、异法方宜、五运六气、精气学说等理论均是传统哲学思想在中医学理论上应用的典范，无不渗透着华夏文化的精髓。作为传播中医文化的中国译者，在规范中医翻译的任务中，如何做到信、达、雅，忠实而有效地再现中国传统医学的博大精深？除了一些常用的古医籍的翻译策略，如比喻借代、互文对举、稽古引经、倒装省略等修辞策略的运用外，关注并有效地传达中医药文献中的文化因素，乃是高水平译者理应采用的首要翻译策略，同时它能确保中医翻译的精确与规范。比如，在中药配伍的理论中有君（monarch）、臣（official）、佐（adjuvant）、使（guide）之说，这和中国古代等级制度是相似的，因此，在翻译的过程中，如采用取类比象的保存其文化精华的策略，可以很好地处理如下的英汉互译：“心者，君主之官”（the heart is supposed to be the monarch），“肺者，相傅之官”（the lung acts as a prime minister），“肝者，将军之官”（the liver acts as a general），“膀胱者，周都之官”（the bladder serves as a reservoir）。此外，为了迎合翻译学科发展的新趋势，译者还必须学习一些西方较成熟的翻译理论，借鉴一些语言学研究的成果。因为无论东方还是西方，在翻译理论方面都是相似的，这也直接决定了译者翻译策略的运用。

3. 译者参与制定中医药翻译工具书的标准是规范中医翻译的必然趋势

在具体的翻译实践中，译者通常以一些中医英译的专著作为参考，兼以一些出版的中医翻译的各类工具书作为选词的指导，如《中医名词术语选释》《简明中医辞典》《中医大辞典》《中药大辞典》《针灸大辞典》《中国医学百科全书》（中医学各分卷）《中国大百科全书·中国传统医学》《中医药学主题词表》《汉英双解中医大辞典》等。但是，这些书目的翻译是否标准规范？至于中医药名词术语的英译，更是众说迭出，莫衷一是。如“针灸”，蔡宗健先生列举了10多种辞典的译名或释义，有译 acupuncture、acupuncture therapy needling、stylostixis 为“针刺疗法”“针术”“针灸”，有译 acupuncture、acupuncture and moxibustion 等为“针灸”，有译 moxibustion 为“艾灸术”。有趣的是 moxibustion 一词，它是由“moxa”（艾）和“combustion”二词合成的。而“艾”字之所以用“moxa”，是因为“艾”字的日语发音为“きぐぉ”，音译使然[2]。该如何进行类似中医名词术语标准的制定及翻译方法的规范呢？这一问题势必会随着中医学对外交流及中医英译规模的不断扩大成为一个突出的问题，亟待解决。而作为中医英译主体的译者，参与制定中医药翻译工具书的标准更是规范中医翻译的必然趋势。令人可喜的是，近年来有关中医药名词术语规范化的研究以及在制定相关行业标准和国家标准上已经取得了一定的成就，如《中华人民共和国药典》《中医诊断疗效标准》《经穴部位》《耳穴名称与部位》《中医病证分类与代码》《中医临床诊疗术语》等相继问世，这些工作以及所取得的成就为译者在中医英译规范化中发挥更实际的作用打下了较好的基础，因此，中医英译规范化中的译者素养问题，既是中医药现代化、国际化的基础性工作，也是一项迫切而艰巨的任务，更是需要有关方面参与、支持的一项系统工程。

参考文献

[1] 王佐良. 思考与试笔. 北京：外语教学与研究出版社，1989：35－50.
[2] 蔡宗健. 国际文化交流与术语标准化. 自然科学术语研究，1992，(1)：46－47.

[原载《中国中西医结合杂志》，2007，27（7）：667－668.]

中医英译的多元文化系统视角探微

张玉红

多元文化系统理论阐述了翻译文学在译入语文化系统中的不同地位会影响译者翻译策略的选择。本文拟从多元文化系统视角来探讨中医文化（中医英译文本）在西方医学文化中的地位及其对译者选择翻译策略的影响。

1. 多元文化系统翻译理论

多元文化系统翻译理论是由以色列著名学者 Even-Zohar[1] 在 20 世纪 70 年代提出来的。他认为，任何一种文化都是由不同等级而又相互转化的子文化系统所构成的一个动态发展的集合。从历史的角度来看，翻译文学可能会作为弱势文化在某个特定的译入语文化系统之中占据次要地位，也可能会作为强势文化在其中占主导地位。翻译文学在译入语文化系统中的不同地位不仅会影响到译者翻译策略的选择，而且在很大程度上也会影响译入语文化，使其语言、文学范式等随之发生变化。

当翻译文学在译入语文化系统中处于弱势时，它位于译入语文化系统的边缘[2]。这时，它不会对译入语文化的主流范式产生重大影响，因此，译者在翻译过程中会自觉遵循译入语文化原有的文化结构和文学范式，沿用译入语文化中现有的语言表达形式，而不会把源语文化中的异质性成分和语言表达方式输入到译入语来。

当翻译文学从译入语文化系统的边缘逐渐转入中心，它就由原来的弱势文化上升为强势。此时，它积极参与建构译入语文化的新的文学范式，为译入语输入一些异质性文化成分和新的表达方式，进而丰富译入语文化的内容。

2. 从多元文化系统视角看中医英译

中医的英译文本最初在西方医学文化中是作为一种弱势文化而存在的。当时西方还不太了解中医的价值，了解中医的目的无非就是想找“替代疗法”。要想让中医在西医强势文化中找到生存空间，让外国人了解并接受中医，译者只得向译入语文化妥协，遵循西医文化固有的规范，采用“尽可能使原作接近读者”[3]的“归化”译法，以迎合英语读者固有的接受水平，中医的推广和传承也因此受到西医主流文化的冲击和排斥，许多中医术语的英译只能借用英语或西医文化中现有的词汇和表达方式。例如，在开始研究中医药名词术语英译时，尽管存在着许多不同意见，其中也不乏主张直译或异化的，但经过反复讨论，还是把中医英译的标准统一为“与世界接轨”上，这无疑就是“中医西医化”。李照国[4]曾在《中医英语翻译技巧》中指出，“中医英译不能为了保持中医的民族特色而与全人类的文化发展对立起来，或者割裂开来。这样做的结果只能是将中医孤立起来，使之裹足不前。”他因此把中医英译的原则总结为“薄文重医、依实出华，比照西医、求同存异，尊重国情、保持特色”。虽然他也主张“尊重国情、保持（中医）特色”，但这是建立在“薄文重医、比照西医”的基础之上的，是针对那些在英语中找不到对应词的中医术语“不得已而为之”的办法。试以“气”和“五脏”等中医术语最初的英译为例。起初，译者借用英语词汇把“气”译成 air 或 energy，后来改为 vital energy。“心、肺、肝、脾、肾”等也均采用与西医解剖部位相关的词语 heart、lung、liver、spleen、kidney 来翻译[5]。魏迺杰[6]在《汉英英汉中医词典》总论中提出，译者偏好使用西医对应词，是由于他们认为西医学已然在整个世界建立了医学的标准，西医的概念具有较高的“可信度”。诚然，“借用西医固有的词汇翻译，能消除外国人对中医的陌生感和隔膜感，中医能够走出国门，这种归化的译法功不可没。”[7]但其缺点也是显而易见的，当时译文总体上倾向于西方读者原有的接受水平，不但中医所承载的文化内涵没有在译入语文化中体现出来，而且造成中医文化缺省的现象，出现了许多诸如“带下医”被译成 doctor underneath skirt、五脏六腑被译成“五个仓库六个宫殿”之类的笑话。

Even-Zohar[1]认为多元文化系统是一个动态的系统，其中各个子系统也会因时间的推移相互转化。随着我国的改革开放政策不断深入，我国的经济、政治力量逐渐壮大，中国在国际上的地位也得以提升，中国文化，尤其是中医文化也备受瞩目。中医的辨证论治及针灸、推拿等独特疗效以及其在养生、保健等方面的优势，使中医得以与西医分庭抗礼，虽不能说中医文化已在西方医学文化中处于强势，但足以说明国际社会对中医文化更加认同、更加热衷。许多译者也已经意识到现阶段中医译介的新局面，他们多采用“保持原作不动，让读者接近原作”的异化法，向译入语文化输入异质性的中医文化，将中医独特的文化价值真正地介绍给世界。正如麦考尔·雅蒲[8]所言，“现在中医西传的程度开始超过其初期的状态，如果坚持用西医化的译法则会抹杀中医本身的优点，应该用非西医化的翻译法保留中医自身的特点和优势，这样更容易让中医在西方落地生根。”魏迺杰[1]也建议“应该在翻译过程中保留中医概念系统的完整意象”。李照国等[9]更主张用“名从主人”的“语言国情学”来解决富有中医文化内涵的词语在英语里找不到对应语的问题，让中医英译真正做到名副其实。“气”和“五脏”等中医术语英译的变化就是最好的例证。众所周知，“气”作为中医所独有的概念，它不仅是生命活力，也是脏腑等组织的活动，air、energy 或 vital energy 这些英语对应词已经不能传达出中医“气”的这种本质。英国翻译家李约瑟借用汉语拼音，把“气”直译为“Qi”，使“气”的文化内涵得以完整地传达，这种译法已为译界普遍接受。中医五脏不仅代表人体五个系统的生理功能、病理变化，还包括其相互关系，只是大体上与西医实体解剖器官近似，因此，许多专家建议采用直译并在其后加注汉语拼音，如 Heart（Xin）、Lung（Fei）、Liver（Gan）、Spleen（Pi）、Kidney（Shen），这样，就能完整地传达出它们的中医文化内涵了。类似这类富有中医文化内涵的词如“阴阳”“三焦”“脏腑”“刮痧”等均采用了这种音译的异化法，目前这些词的音译已被普遍接受并已成为鲜活的英语，这在一定程度上丰富了英语文化，为英语输入了新的异质性成分。

3. 结语

在当今跨文化交流日益频繁的全球化语境下，中医文化以其独特的疗效和优势在国际上受到更多人的欢迎和青睐。从多元文化系统的视角来研究中医英译，对于我们了解和把握中医文化在西方医学文化中的地位有重大的指导意义，从而帮助我们更好地传承和弘扬中医文化。相信在不久的将来，中医文化会以其独特的魅力和价值，在国际文化这个大系统中绽放出更加绚烂的光彩。

参考文献

[1] Even-Zohar I. Polysystem studies. Tel-Aviv：Porter Institute for Poetics and Semiotics，1990：11.

[2] 王东风．翻译文学的文化地位与译者的文化态度．中国翻译，2000，21（4）：2-8.

[3] Munday J. Introducing translation studies. London and New York：Routledge，2001：27-29.

[4] 李照国．中医英语翻译技巧．北京：人民卫生出版社，1997：16-20.

[5] 兰凤利．论中西医学语言文化差异与中医英译．中国中西医结合杂志，2007，27（4）：368-370.

[6] Wiseman N. 汉英英汉中医词典．长沙：湖南科学技术出版社，1995：21-24.

[7] 罗枫．中医术语翻译的“归化”和“异化”．成都中医药大学学报，2007，30（2）：26-27.

[8] 麦考尔·雅蒲．中医英译“比照西医”原则的分析．福建中医学院学报，2003，13（2）：94-96.

[9] 李伟彬．从中英文化差异看中医英译的基本原则——兼评李照国、朱忠宝《中医英语翻译技巧训练》．上海科技翻译，2004（4）：57-59.

［原载《中国中西医结合杂志》，2010，30（7）：776-777.］

中医名词术语英译中的信息密度与翻译策略和方法

王洁华

信息密度是指在计算机记账中储存的单位信息所占用的空间越小，运载这一单位信息之间的信息密度就越高；单位信息从发送者到接收者所需要的时间越少，运载这一单位信息的信息密度就越高[1]。这一概念同样可用于指导中医名词术语英译。即在翻译过程中注重汉语中医术语与英译文信息密度的比较及其有效信息运载的能力，以降低语言翻译过程中主要信息传输的干扰因素。

从中医语言的特点来看，其文学色彩浓郁、字词精炼、寓意丰富，信息载量大，故其信息密度相当高。如形容患者恶寒、恶风之状：“啬啬恶寒，淅淅恶风”[2]；揭示阴阳转化、物极必反的规律：“重阴必阳，重阳必阴，寒极生热，热极生寒”。以往英译者为了最大限度地体现中医术语“原汁原味”，表达其内涵，采用了释意法（解释性译法），结果使英译文显得冗长，将运载信息的源语词，即中医语言分解成多个译语词，致使译语词的信息密度大为降低。以中医术语“辨证施治”为例，按译文先后时间为序，可见以下几种译文：

例 1：determination of treatment based on the differentiation of symptoms and signs[3]（信息密度为 0.364）

例 2：planning treatment according to diagnosis[4]（信息密度为 0.8）

例 3：treatment based on syndrome differentiation[5]（信息密度为 0.8）

例 4：syndrome differentiation and treatment[6]（信息密度为 1）

（注：信息密度＝源语词的意义单位数÷译文词的意义单位数）

由上述例子可见信息密度越高，译文越精密（0.364→0.8→1 ）。这正符合了科技英语语言特点，即：科技作品叙述要简洁明确、逻辑严密。换言之，要遵循 A（accuracy，准确）、B（brevity，简练）、C（clarity，清晰）的原则。在中医术语汉英互译时，采取哪些翻译策略与方法才能有效地达到较高的信息密度，或尽可能与原文相对应的信息密度？笔者通过对 2007 年世界卫生组织推出的“传统医学国际标准名词术语（WHO International Standard Terminologies，WHOIST）”的分析、比较先前中医术语的英语译文，认为以下几种策略与方法是行之有效的。

1. 模糊策略与表意化的方法

在日常生活中，模糊现象普遍存在。适当的模糊能使问题简化。如表述“长与短”“美与丑”“清洁与污染”等这样一些对立概念时，前者对于后者都是相对而言，并没有绝对分明的界限。中医某些术语也具有这一特点。类似“虚”与“实”，“燥”与“湿”，这样一些对立概念之间，什么程度才算是虚？何种程度才称为实？“燥”与“湿”的精确度是多少？毋庸置疑具有模糊性。模糊性是语言的一个基本属性。既然英汉两种自然语言背景都具有模糊性，在中医术语英译时就可采用表意化方法，即英译时仅对原文做文字层面上的处理，完成表层信息语言转换。

例 5：温病学 warm disease (study)[6]，英译没有将“温病学”译为 doctrine of epidemic febrile disease（流行性发热疾病学）。“warm”一词的英文释意为：having fair1y high temperature，between cool and hot，使人联想到温度、发热，同时又模糊了精确的“温度”。

例 6：泌别清浊 separation of the clear and turbid[7]，而不是译为 separating the food essence and water from the waste matter。WHOIST 译文不去体现究竟“清”和“浊”各为何物，但 clear、turbid 两个词基本足以表明其相对的差异。

例 7：天人相应 correspondence between nature and human[6]，将“天”淡化为“自然”，用通俗易懂的语言翻译抽象的概念。采用忽略源语言中的确切含意，仅翻译字面意。运用模糊策略，可使读者见词则明白其表层意思。

2. 避“虚”就“实”策略与多用实词少用虚词的方法

避“虚”就“实”的策略是指多用实词，包括名词、动词、形容词、副词；少用虚词，包括限定词、介词、连词和感叹词。在实词中，翻译中医术语时应首选名词。根据 Johansson 等[7]的研究，名词＋名词，每 100 万词中，这种结构在科普读物和一般读物的比是 11 507：5427。

例 8：太阳中风 attack of Taiyang channel by wind[6]

太阴中风证 greater Yin wind stroke pattern（完全采用实词）

例 9：气分湿热证 Qi aspect dampness heat pattern[6]（完全采用实词）

可见上述两个 WHOIST 译文均采用实词作定语，且大多是名词。“太阴中风证”英译文连用了 3 个名词作定语，例 9 的英译文中连用了 4 个名词作定语。

此外，还可利用实词的派生语素，即有效地使用实词的前、后缀派生形式创造出新词的多种形式，用尽可能简洁的语言传达最大的信息量。

例 10：肝火犯肺证 pattern of liver fire invading the lung [6]

例 11：清热解毒药

译文 1：heat-clearing and detoxicating medicinal[6]

译文 2：medicinal for clearing heat and removing toxic substances

通过比较上述例句的结构变化，说明解释性译文中如果虚词功能词用得多则会使译文冗长。WHOIST 译文就“实”避“虚”，恰当应用词性和结构变换，大大提高了信息密度。

3. 坚持民族性策略与音译法

“语言国情学认为一种语言中总有一些反映民族特有的事物、思想和观念而在别国的语言中找不到对应词的词语”[8]，如中医基础理论中的“阴、阳、气”，在翻译中如何处理这类词语呢？采用音译法。其实音译早已是各种语言借用外来语丰富自身词汇的一种有效的方法。现在我们的词汇中就有许多外来语，如logic（逻辑）、lymph（淋巴）、radar（雷达）等。

中医术语中哪些词较适合采用此种译法呢？按照“中医术语阴阳分类原则”，中医术语可分为阴性词汇（相对“惰性”的词汇），特点是活跃度较低，无论将其放在何种语境中，均相对稳定。如针灸穴位名、方剂名、中医典籍名，以及一些极具有民族特色的词，如阴阳、太阳等；阳性词汇（相对“活性”的词汇），特点是活跃程度高，词的内涵意深，如“虚”“实”“神”等。对于“阴性”词汇可采用音译法。目前国际标准化针灸穴位名称均采用汉语拼音加编号方法表示，方剂名和中医典籍名的英译也离不开汉语拼音[9]。有时我们在中医术语英译时采用半音半译法，中国著名语言学家张培基称它是一种“凑合”的办法。例如，汉语的“爱克斯光”是从英语 X-ray 用此法吸收过来的，其中“爱克斯”是 X 的音译，“光”是“ray”的意译[10]。中医术语译文也有此类现象，如手太阴肺经（lung meridian of hand Taiyin ）、心阴（heart Yin）、肝气（liver Qi）等。

中医是中华民族特有的医学体系，具有鲜明的民族性，在英译时应予以体现这一原则。

4. 西为中用策略与借用西医英语词汇法

西为中用策略是指借用西医现有的术语翻译中医学概念，此法既可减少母语非中文读者对中医的隔膜感，又可使中医获得一条走向世界的途径。

中医术语中的阴性词汇，如人体解剖部位、器官，一些病症和治法等有相应的西医术语参照物，如大肠（the large intestine）、膀胱（bladder）。另外还有中医的五脏——心、肝、脾、肺、肾，借用西医术语可分别译为英译为 heart、liver、spleen、lung、kidney，尽管对中医和西医来说采用了同样的名词，它们各自的内涵却是不同的。又如一些病名和治法：麻木（numbness）、便秘（constipation）、泄泻（diarrhea）、泄法（purgation），还有许多在此无法一一赘述。这些均可借用西医英语词汇法翻译，且目前已约定俗成。

5. 转换语言“移植”策略与直译法

转换语言“移植”策略是指在译文语言条件许可时，既保持原文的内容，又保持原文的形式——尤其指保持原文比喻、形象和民族的地方色彩等。在中医术语英译时，我们可采用直译法，即基本对应地将源语的词汇转换为另一种语言。如中医术语五行（five phases）、里寒（interior cold）、气病及血（Qi disease affecting the blood）、风火眼（wind-fire eye）、辨证施治（syndrome differentiation and treatment）等。

此种表象对应英译文是否会造成理解歧义？否。根据语言心理学"语义网络"的原理，"语义网络是由相互连接的要素组成的，这些要素就是概念和节点，它们通过各种关系，彼此连接"[11]。据此，syndrome differentiation and treatment 可简化为下位层网：

syndrome
/ \
treatment differentiation

此层网形成"证"为可辨、可治的语义网络模型。人们通过语义自然连接网络，顺势延伸、扩展，理解词意。可见最贴近的自然对等的译法是符合语言心理学原理的。

本文讨论了如何调动多种英译策略与方法，实现中医名词术语英译的信息密度的目标，达到最贴近自然对等的境界，使母语为非中文的读者正确认识、理解中医名词术语英译的表述。

参考文献

[1] 李照国．中医英语翻译技巧．北京：人民卫生出版社，1997，76.
[2] 杨鹏举，杨延巍，曹丽静注释．伤寒论．北京：学苑出版社，2007：27.
[3] 广州中医学院编写组．汉英常用中医词汇．广州：广东科技出版社，1982：247.
[4] 原一祥，任继学．汉英双解中医大辞典．北京：人民卫生出版社，1997：134，1086.
[5] 李照国，朱忠宝．中医英语翻译技巧训练．上海：上海中医药大学出版社，2002：94.
[6] World Health Organization. WHO international standard terminologies on traditional medicine in the western pacific region. Geneva：The Office of Publication，WHO，2007：10，13，26，134，155，159，259.
[7] Kennedy G. An introduction to corpus linguistics. Beijing：Foreign Language Teaching and Research Press，2000：270.
[8] 李照国，李萧红．医古文英语翻译技巧．上海：上海中医药大学出版社，1998：8.
[9] 王洁华．中医药术语英译标准之探讨．河南中医学院学报，2007，22（4）：73-74.
[10] 张培基．英语翻译教程．上海：上海外语教育出版社，1980：186.
[11] DW 卡罗尔著．语言心理学．缪小春译．上海：华东师范大学出版社，2007：108.

[原载《中国中西医结合杂志》，2010，30（1）：91-93.]

音译法在中医英译中的应用原则与策略

任荣政　丁年青

音译（transliteration）亦可称作译音，作为一种以语言的读音为依据的翻译方式，其一般是按照源语言语词的发音在目标语言中寻找与之发音相同或相近的语音进行替代翻译[1]。由于中医学自身的学科特点所决定，音译法在中医汉英翻译实践中的使用频率要远高于其他学科[2]。本文就结合音译法的相关理论以及翻译实例，对音译法在中医英译领域中的应用进行梳理和总结，为中医英语翻译和教学实践提供理论参考。

1. 音译法的基本理论

1.1　音译法的历史源流

有关音译法的应用与研究在中国翻译史上由来已久，可以追溯到汉唐时期的佛经翻译，而其中最系统、最具代表性的论述当属唐代玄奘法师的“五不翻”理论[3]。所谓的“不翻”并不是不翻译，而是指采用音译法进行翻译。有关玄奘法师“五不翻”理论的记述最早见于南宋法云所著的《翻译名义集》中[4]，其主要内容包括：①秘密故不翻，陀罗尼是。②多含义故不翻，如“薄伽梵”含六义故。③此无故不翻，如阎浮树。④顺古故不翻，如“阿耨菩提”，实可翻之，但摩腾已来存梵音故。⑤生善故不翻，如“般若”尊重，智慧轻浅，令人生敬，是故不翻。玄奘法师所提出的“五不翻”理论在实质上是关于音译法的五条应用原则。其中，除第一条“秘密故”原则比较局限于佛经等宗教翻译领域之外，其余四条原则对于今天我们进行中医汉英音译实践仍颇具指导意义。

1.2　应用音译法的必要性

翻译过程中最基本、最常规的手段就是在目标语言中寻找源语的对应词进行替代，也就是所谓的对应翻译法[5]，或称意译法[6]（此处的意译是广义上的概念，并非指与“直译”相对应的狭义“意译”概念）。然而，在语际转换中还存在着无对应语的情况，即在目标语言中找不到与源语意义一致的词语。在这样的情况下，主要的解决手段有迁移法（transference）和音译法两种。其中，迁移法是将源语原封不动地移植到目标语言中[7]，如将法语词“traceur”（跑酷）、意大利语词“pizza”（比萨饼）照搬到英语译文中。应用形译法的基本条件是源语与目标语言必须属于相同的文字体系，如法语、意大利语和英语。由于汉语与英语属于迥然不同的文字体系，两者之间无法使用形译法进行转换，因此，应采用音译法。

1.3 音译法的应用形式

在英汉语际交换中，英汉翻译和汉英翻译中均可采用音译法。英汉音译主要是选择与英语发音相近的汉字进行替换，而由于汉字是形、音、意结合的文字，如果能在表音的同时兼顾达意，则更是理想之选，如在西医学、生物学领域中，基因（gene）、克隆（clone）等词语的音译。由于受学科特点的制约，中医翻译领域中的音译法应用基本为汉英音译。汉英音译主要有两种应用形式，除了我们目前所熟悉和使用的汉语拼音方案外，另一种则是由英国人 T. Wade 在 1859 年首次提出，并由 HA. Giles 进行改良之后所形成的“威妥玛-翟理斯式”（Wade-Giles）拼音法，也简称“威氏拼音法”[8]。在我国的《汉语拼音方案》公布前，汉英音译一直都采用的是威氏拼音法。从 1982 年起，我国提出的《汉语拼音方案》被联合国标准化组织接受，确定为拼写中国人名、地名和一切中文文献的国际标准，原有的威氏拼音法被废止[9]。应该承认，威氏拼音法的发音比较符合英语的发音习惯，因此，更加容易为西方人所接受。但是它也存在一符多用等弊端，如“chu”同时对应“居”和“朱”等，容易造成混乱和不便。况且根据名从主人的原则，其为《汉语拼音方案》所取代也是理所当然。近年来，WHO 所颁布的针灸穴位[10]以及传统医学名词术语的国际标准方案[11]中所使用的音译也都是采用《汉语拼音方案》。但是，由于威氏拼音法毕竟在汉英音译中应用了一百余年，受语言约定俗成规律的影响，至今仍有一些汉语专有名词和普通名词的音译保留了威氏拼音法的形式，如清华大学（Tsinghua University）、青岛啤酒（Tsingtao Beer）、功夫（Kung Fu）、荔枝（litchi）等。中医术语的“气”和“太极拳”，除了音译为“Qi”和“Taiji”外，也可以见到“Chi”和“Tai Chi”的形式。其中“Chi”多见于较早出版的中医英文书籍，正逐渐被“Qi”所取代，而“Tai Chi”则呈现和“Taiji”并存的局面。

2. 音译法在中医英译中的应用范围

中医学作为我国的传统医学，在数千年的发展历程中融汇了中国古典哲学和传统文化的精髓，并形成了自己独特的理论体系和实践方法，因此，相比西医学等其他自然科学领域，中医学包含了更多具有鲜明民族特色的事物和概念，在其对外翻译中，音译法自然就有了更为广阔的应用范围，以下按照学科内容分类对音译法在中医英译中的主要应用进行梳理。

2.1 基础理论的翻译音译法

在中医汉英翻译中最为典型的应用是用来翻译中医基础理论中所独有的一些基本概念和专业术语。如前所述，相对于英汉音译，汉英音译就其应用形式本身而言相对固定，可供选择的余地并不大，关键在于对其适用原则的理解和把握。

在前面有关应用音译法的必要性的论述中提到的无对应语的情况，究其原因就是源语中的词汇所反映的事物为该民族所特有，其在目标语言的民族文化背景中并不存在，所以没有相应的指代用语。这也就是“五不翻”理论中的“此无故”原则，可以说是对音译法应用原则的最本质的概括。具体到中医基础理论的汉英翻译实践，要正确地判断哪些中医术语适合采用音译法翻译。中医基础理论作为中医学体系的基础部分，阐述了中医学的哲学基础、中医学关于正常生命现象以及疾病的认识等，因此，必然会蕴含一些为中医理论体系所独有的基本概念和术语，其在英语等其他民族语言中找不到恰当的对应语，因此，宜采用音译法。

以“阴阳”一词为例，其来源于中国古代哲学的范畴，是对自然界相互关联的某些事物或现象对立双方属性的概括[12]。阴阳概念的内涵丰富而外延宽广，虽然阴阳的对立属性可以用“negative and positive”“female and male”以及“dark and bright”等英语词语来进行解释，但是这些词却都无法全面反映阴阳概念的内涵与外延，因此，将其音译为“Yin Yang”是唯一的选择。需要指出的是，在翻译实践中，并不是所有的“阴阳”都应采用音译，只有当其作为古典哲学中表示相互对立的概念而使用时，阴阳才同时具有“动静、寒热、天地、日月、男女”等丰富而宽广的含义，才符合“此无故”原则，因此，适合采用音译翻译法；而当阴阳在一定的语境中分别指代“日月”“男女”“昼夜”等具体的事物，则应意译出其确切含义，而不应以拼音代之。比如中医古典医籍《诸病源候论》中论述“阴阳过度，则伤包络”，此处的阴阳实际为性生活的委婉语，因此，应意译为“sexual activities”才恰当[13]。

“气”也是中医基础理论中所特有的一个概念。一些学者依据中医学中的气具有不同种类以及气的一词多义性来论证气采用音译的必要性，其实并未抓住问题的本质[14-16]。实际上，中医学中的气的基本内涵是来自中国古代哲学，其被认为是构成宇宙万物的基本物质，同时气的运动变化也是推动万物发生、发展的基本动力。当“气”最初被介绍到西方时，人们主要是基于气对宇宙万物以及人体生命活动的维持和推动作用，而将其意译为“vital energy”。在《新世纪汉英大词典》中，所给出的中医气的英语对应词仍为“vital energy”[17]。但是，随着交流的不断深入，人们发现这个意译无法表达其丰富的内涵，故最终放弃了意译而改用音译“Qi”来代替[18]。

总之，基于以上分析，不论是“阴阳”还是“气”，都是中医学所独有的概念，符合“此无故”原则，在英语等其他语言中无法找到与之内涵和外延相同的对应语，所以需要采用音译，这也是在中医汉英翻译中应用音译法需要首先把握的基本原则。

2.2　中药、方剂的翻译

中药名称的标准翻译是采用拉丁语进行标识，并应包含药用部位、药材来源的属名（来自同属的可加种名）以及炮制手段等基本信息[19]，具体标识应以《国家药典》的规定为准，对于药典中未收录的中药也应仿照药典的格式进行翻译标识。除了使用拉丁语外，为了方便信息的快速传递与有效交流，近年来中药名称翻译越来越呈现出辅以英文名称和汉语音译的标注趋势，如大青叶为：[da qing ye] Folium Isatidis（拉）；Dyers Woad Leaf（英）[20]。使用汉语音译的好处是能够反映出中药在中医中的原始应用状态，方便外国使用者根据其发音与中医师进行口语交流以及确定相应的中药。需要注意的是，由于有些中药名称发音完全相同或相近，如斑蝥与斑茅均为 [Ban mao]、地筋与地锦均为 [Di jin] 等，则其音译形式也就完全一样。但是，由于同时配有拉丁语和英语标识，造成混淆的可能性并不大。

与中药的翻译不同，方剂名称的翻译要更为复杂。中医方剂的命名方式多样，有以组成方剂的全部或部分药物命名的，如桂枝汤、麻杏石甘汤；有以方剂的功效、主治命名的，如温脾汤、止嗽散；有以药物剂量比例命名的，如六一散、九一丹；有以服药时间命名的，如鸡苏散、鸡鸣散；有以功效比喻命名的，如玉屏风散、泰山磐石散；还有以象征、隐喻方式命名的，如白虎汤、大小青龙汤等。除此以外，还有综合运用几种方式命名的，以及将药物炮制、煎服方法等信息融入方名中。这些都使得中医方名异彩纷呈，富含中医学理论以及传统文化内涵，从而给其英译带来了极大的挑战。以相对简单明了的按组成药物命名的方剂为例，有译者按照方名中的药物拉丁语译名进行翻译[21]。但是，考虑到拉丁语的繁复性，用其来译“桂枝汤”这样的方剂尚可接受（但是也存在理解和使用不便的问题），而如果是翻译“麻杏石甘汤”或者方名组成更为复杂的方剂，那么其译名的冗长难免令人望而生畏。至于文化内涵丰富的方剂名翻译则更是争论激烈，难以达成共识。以白虎汤为例，其方名中的“白虎”来自中国传统文化中的四象，以其应秋而炎暑自解来表征方药具有清热的功效，与实际的动物白虎并没有直接关系，因此，一些学者认为本方名如果直译为“White Tiger”，不但无法传递其深刻内涵，甚至有导致误解的可能，而主张从功效主治的角度意译为“Decoction for Removing Pathogenic Heat”[22] 或“Decoction for Eliminating Heat”[23]。然而亦有学者反对这种译法，并从保持文化内涵以及翻译的异化角度坚持采用“White Tiger”的翻译方法[24-26]。由此可见，在目前的中医方剂翻译中，无论是直译还是意译，都很难在短时间内实现对方剂简洁、统一的英译，因此，也就无法起到有效标识方剂的作用。在现阶段，音译法是对方剂英译的基本和主要途径，只有在统一进行音译的基础上才能进一步探索方剂名称贴切、合理的意译翻译。在具体的音译过程中，方名的翻译通常采用方名音译加剂型直译相结合的方式，如桂枝汤的音译为“Guizhi Decoction”。虽然也有学者主张方剂的音译应采取彻底音译法，如将桂枝汤音译为“Guizhi Tang”[27]，但是按照音译的一般规则，剂型作为指类词并没有进行音译的必要。此外，在音译的过程中还要注意汉语拼音发音的准确性，尤其是对多音字的发音进行鉴别，例如中成药知柏地黄丸的音译在已发表的文献中出现“Zhibai Dihuang Pill”和“Zhibo Dihuang Pill”并存的现象。分析该方剂是由六味地黄丸加知母、黄柏（黄檗）两味中药配伍而成的，而黄柏中的柏字应读作 bò，因此，知柏地黄丸的正确音译应为“Zhibo Dihuang Pill”[28]，但是在 2004 年全国科学技术名词审定委员会颁布的《中医药学名词》[29]以及 2010 年版的《中华人民共和国药典》[30]中，知柏地黄丸的音译却均为“Zhibai Dihuang Pill”，值得商榷。

2.3 经穴名称的翻译

中医学的对外传播在针灸领域开展得最为成功，这极大促进了针灸学相关理论的英译；反过来，针灸理论的英译和国际标准化对海外“针灸热”的形成可以说是功不可没，这反映出中医国际化进程与中医英译事业间密不可分、相互促进的关系。目前，经穴名称的英译翻译是整个中医英译中开展的最为成功、争议最少的领域，通行的英译方式为汉语拼音音译加所属经脉的英文缩写及编码。例如“足三里”是足阳明胃经的第三十六个穴位，而“足阳明胃经”的英文缩写为“ST”，因此，“足三里”的国际标准译名为 Zusanli (ST 36)[10]。在实现国际标准化的全部 361 个经穴中，有几组穴位因为汉语发音相同而有相同的音译，包括“伏兔”与“扶突”，“腕骨”与“完骨”，以及“中渚”与“中注”，但是由于配合使用了经脉定位编码，并不存在混淆的问题。除了经穴采用音译外，对于那些有特别含义的特定穴位的翻译则采用音译与意译相结合的方式，如五输穴的英文翻译为井穴（Jing-Well）、荥穴（Ying-Spring）、输穴（Shu-Stream）、经穴（Jing-River）、合穴（He-Sea）。可以看出，其中“井穴”和“经穴”的音译完全一样，但是因为配合了意译，同样也不至于混淆。对于穴位名称采用音译的翻译方法，也有一些学者提出了不同的看法。古人在为穴位命名时，运用古代天文、地理、建筑学等知识进行比喻和类比，将穴位的解剖定位、生理功能、主治功效等信息融入其中，如孙思邈在《千金翼方》中就曾指出：“凡诸孔穴，名不徒设，皆有深意”，因此，采用音译翻译法难以体现出原中文名称所蕴含的深刻含义与美学价值。对此，有学者提出如果听任目前针灸穴位翻译的现状继续下去，针灸穴位含义所富含的中国特有文化的内容会随时间的推移而在境外慢慢淡忘甚或消失，并认为这有悖于对外传播中医药学的初衷[31]。此外，著名的外籍中医翻译专家 Nigel Wiseman 也是穴位名称意译的积极倡导者，在其编写的《实用英文中医辞典》[32]中，他对所有的针灸穴位名称都作了意译，如将“睛明”穴意译为“Bright Eyes”。应该说，这些专家学者希望通过意译体现穴位名称的文化内涵的主张是值得肯定的，但是，这必须是在保证穴位译名的标准化和规范化的前提之下，必需首先要满足在不同国家开展统一、规范的针灸医疗的需要，因此，音译在目前以及今后相当长的一段时间内都是穴位名称翻译的主要方式。

2.4 医家、医著的翻译

在中医学漫长的发展历史上涌现出众多杰出的代表性人物，这些医家所开创的理论以及所撰写的中医著作都是构成中医理论体系的重要组成部分，要对外介绍中医学就不能不提及这些医家。从这个角度来讲，著名医家的名字也是中医英译的重要内容之一，这也是为什么在《中医药学名词》[29]和WHO公布的《WHO西太平洋地区传统医学名词术语国际标准》[11]两个规范性文件中都纳入了历代著名医家姓名英译的原因。作为专有名词，对医家姓名的翻译采用音译法无可厚非，但是由于英美人名的顺序与中国不同，为名在前而姓在后，为此，对于中国人名英译究竟如何处理姓和名的先后顺序问题，在认识上有一定的分歧，在实践中也存在不统一的现象。实际上，姓名的先后顺序是一个民族历史文化传统的具体体现，根据名从主人的原则，在译入其他语言时，无论是书写形式还是在口头交际中，都应尊重源语民族的历史文化传统而保持原有的姓名顺序[33]。在我国正式对外发行的英文报刊（如*China Daily*）以及我国领导人出席的国际会议上，中国人姓名的英译顺序是非常明确的，即都是姓在前而名在后，因此，中医医家的翻译也应该按照这个顺序进行音译，如“张仲景”的标准音译为“Zhang Zhongjing”。另外一个在人名音译过程中应该注意的问题是有些医家的名字是“复姓＋单字名”的形式，如西汉医家淳于意，复姓“淳于”单名“意”，魏晋医家皇甫谧，复姓“皇甫”单名“谧”，在翻译中应注意区分姓和名，分别翻译为“Chunyu Yi”和“Huangfu Mi”。有关中医学著作名称的英文翻译属于书名翻译的范畴，本不应采取音译法，但是由于中医学领域中的情况特殊，应当区别对待。对于近现代尤其是新中国成立后出版的中医类书籍，其书名翻译应采取意译法，并确保同一本书英语译名的统一性，如果书籍在出版时本身已经带有英语译名的，则应该尊重原作的英译名。而对于那些在漫长的历史长河中积淀下来的中医古籍，其中文书名常常用词古奥、含义隽永，如《审视瑶函》《格致余论》《重楼玉钥》等，要对其进行恰如其分的翻译实属不易，更加难以对其英译名实现统一。以中医学奠基之作《黄帝内经》为例，其英译名就有“The Yellow Emperor's Classic of Internal Medicine”“The Yellow Emperor's Inner Canon”“Huangdi's Canon of Medicine”等近10种之多。这里暂不评论这些译名的孰优孰劣，单单是译名如此庞杂本身就会造成指代不清，给传播与交流造成一定的混乱，带来诸多的不便。《黄帝内经》书名本身文字质朴，其英译研究也开展得相对较多，书名英译尚且如此混乱，那么对于数量巨大的中医古籍来说，要想在短时间内寻找到恰当的英译并达成统一显然难以实现。鉴于中医古籍作为中医学的经典性著作，经受了漫长的历史考验而留存至今，远非普通的医学书籍可比，其书名具有显著的专有名词性质，因此，在翻译中，不妨在意译的同时，保留书名的音译，从而明确指代对象，方便交流与传播，如此也有助于推动书名意译的学术争鸣。

3. 中医汉英音译应遵循的基本原则

音译翻译应遵循两条基本原则，即名从主人原则和约定俗成原则，在中医翻译领域应用音译法也同样要遵守这两条原则。

3.1 名从主人

名从主人原则的主要含义是指人名、地名等专有名词以及富有民族特色的词语在音译时都应按照其来源民族语言的发音来译，例如“金日成”不能译为 Jin Richeng，而应根据朝语译为 KimIl-sung[34]。名从主人原则本身比较好理解，而且因为我国是中医的发源地，绝大多数词汇的音译只需按照汉语拼音进行音译即可。需要注意的是，在中医中有少数用语来源于佛教，而佛教传入我国的历史较为久远，这些用语已经融入了汉文化之中，因此，很容易被误认为是汉语词汇而按汉语拼音进行音译，如“菩萨”一词的正确音译不是“Pusa”而应是“Bodhisattva”，因此，中医方剂“菩萨散”的音译应为“Bodhisattva Powder”，这才是真正做到了名从主人。

3.2 约定俗成

“约定俗成”一词语出自荀子的《正名》篇，“名无固宜，约之以命，约定俗成谓之宜，异于约则谓之不宜。名无固实，约之以命实，约定俗成谓之实名。”约定俗成作为语言的一个基本特征，它反映了当某一事物的名称为社会所普遍接受并长期使用后，就带有了某种约束力和一定的强制性，而不能随意进行更改。约定俗成原则对音译的影响既体现在如“五不翻”理论中“顺古故”原则所说的对某些已经约定采用音译的词汇不再进行意译，也体现在对一些约定进行意译的词汇不再采用音译。如中医学术语“三焦”一词，其英译翻译采取音译更为合理[35]，但是，WHO 在 20 世纪 90 年代初制定的翻译标准就将“三焦”的标准译法规定为“triple energizer”。经过多年的使用，“triple energizer”已经成为了“三焦”一词在英语中的实际对应词。除此以外，约定俗成原则还体现在当人们认识到一些词语的音译由于历史的原因存在一定的偏差时，仍然难以进行纠正而继续沿用原有的音译。如有学者考证，“艾灸”一词的英译为“moxibustion”，其中表示“艾”的词根“moxi”来自日语中“艾”的音译“moxa”，故而根据“名从主人”的原则提出应按照“艾”的汉语发音“ai”而将“艾灸”的英译改为“aibustion”，以彰显中国是艾灸治疗的发源地[36]。然而，“moxibustion”一词已经使用了数百年，早已经为国内外人士所熟悉，要重新调整必然会带来诸多不便，也很难达成共识。由此也可以看出，在一定条件下，约定俗成原则对音译的支配和影响力要高于“名从主人”原则。在认识到约定俗成原则对音译实践存在影响的同时，还应该认识到这种影响是相对的，而不是绝对的、一成不变的。随着不同民族间的交流日益深化，人们对异国文化背景中的事物会获得更加深刻和具体的认识，因此，其在总体遵循“约定俗成”的同时，会对局部的不合理的翻译进行调整和修正，也就是“再约定”的过程[37]。这种再约定体现在音译翻译实践中，既可以是某些词语原来采用的意译逐渐被音译所代替，如前面所举的“气”的翻译从“vital energy”到音译为“Qi”的例子；也可以是某些原来采用音译的词语逐渐找到了或创造出合适的对应语，如中医“证”的翻译，从最初音译为“Zheng”演变到目前的意译“pattern”或“syndrome”。这种在翻译实践中的“约定与再约定”过程也表明翻译是一项需要不断反思与创新的事业。

4. 中医汉英音译应避免的误区

在中医汉英音译过程中除了要遵循上述的基本原则外，还要注意避免两大误区，或者说走向两个极端，一是惧用或拒用意译法，二是对音译法的滥用。

4.1 拒用或惧用音译

由于音译一直以来被当做翻译过程中的“变通之法”和“权宜之计”，而缺乏足够的重视，一些译者担心如果使用音译法会被人质疑自己的翻译水平而尽量避免使用音译法。此外，也有一些译者过度担心国外读者对音译词的接受能力，不敢使用音译法，而在目标语中勉强寻找与之类似或接近的对应语或是自行造词进行替换，如将“太极拳”翻译成“shadow boxing”。这样做的弊端是以偏概全，导致源语信息的缺失，甚至背离了源语的真实含义。

4.2 滥用音译

与拒用或惧用音译法相对的另外一个极端，就是译者人为地扩大音译的使用范围，导致对音译法的滥用。出现这种局面的原因有两类。一类是译者过分强调中医内涵的独特性，如有学者认为中医五脏的概念偏重功能性而与西医的五脏不同，反对采用“heart”等意译法；还有的学者提出 acupuncture point 或 acupoint 失去了“穴位”一词原有的空间概念，应将“穴位”音译为“Xuewei”[38]。另外一类滥用的情况则是由于音译法本身比较容易操作而会使译者养成避难就易的习惯[5]。如前文所述，对于阴阳的具体语境不加鉴别，凡是遇到“阴阳”就统统音译。无论是出于上述哪一种原因，过多、过滥地使用音译，都会影响信息的有效传递，不应当提倡。上述两个误区在中医汉英音译中都应该极力避免，而其关键还是在于对音译适用原则的正确理解与严格把握，并在翻译实践中对具体语境进行深入细致的分析，从而作出准确的判断。

5. 中医汉英音译的优势

最后，音译法作为中医汉英翻译中的一种必要的翻译手段，不但可以有效解决无对应语的意译困境，如果使用得当，还能发挥出意译法所不具备的优势。一方面，采用音译翻译法能够实现译语的统一和规范，而这是名词术语翻译需要满足的最基本要求，如前文所提到的方剂、穴位以及医著等的音译都体现了这一点。另外一方面，随着中外交流的不断深化，西方人士对汉语音译词的接受能力也在不断提高，适当使用音译词可以激发他们的兴趣和探求精神，从而有利于进一步推动中医药乃至中华传统文化的对外传播与输出。

参考文献

[1] 维基百科．音译（2013-10-16）/［2013-11-12］．http：//zh.wikipedia.org/wiki/%E9%9F%B3%E8%AF%91.

[2] 任荣政，朱玉琴，许琪，等．从玄奘"五不翻"理论解读中医汉英音译．上海中医药大学学报，2012，26（5）：16-18.

[3] 徐丽萍．玄奘"五不翻"理论解析．牡丹江师范学院学报：哲学社会科学版，2008，（5）：61-63.

[4] 方广锠．玄奘"五种不翻"三题．法音，2006，（10）：11-15.

[5] 刘宓庆主编．新编当代翻译理论．北京：中国对外翻译出版公司，2005：178.

[6] 维基百科．意译（2013-03-9）［2013-11-12］．http：//zh.wikipedia.org/wiki/%E6%84%8F%E8%AF%91［EB/OL］.

[7] 黄粉保．论音译的语用功能．中国科技翻译，2005，18（3）：53-55，43.

[8] 张庆荣．中医术语英译中的音译．中国中西医结合杂志，1997，17（6）：369-371.

[9] 范铮．如何转换成妥玛式音译中文刊名．大学图书馆学报，1991，（5）：47-51.

[10] 世界卫生组织（西太平洋地区）主编．世界卫生组织针灸经穴定位．北京：人民卫生出版社，2010.

[11] 世界卫生组织（西太平洋地区）主编．WHO西太平洋地区传统医学名词术语国际标准．北京：北京大学医学出版社，2009.

[12] 孙广仁．中医基础理论．北京：中国中医药出版社，2005：34.

[13] 兰凤利．中医古典文献中"阴阳"的源流与翻译．中国翻译，2007，（4）：69-72.

[14] 梁忠宝．中医名词术语英译方法浅议．锦州医学院学报，2001，22（6）：78，87.

[15] 蒋建勇．中医英译中的音译现象与翻译的等值理论．中国中西医结合杂志，2004，24（8）：750-751.

[16] 李照国，李相敏．言不过其辞，动不过其则——谈谈中医英语翻译中的音译问题．中西医结合学报，2007，5（6）：712-714.

[17] 惠宇．新世纪汉英大词典．北京：外语教学与研究出版社，2003：262.

[18] 李俊梅．词汇空缺与中医术语的翻译．中国中西医结合杂志，2007，27（3）：272-273.

[19] 薛俊梅．中药名称的译法探讨．亚太传统医药，2011，7（8）：174-175.

[20] 谢竹藩．新编汉英中医药分类词典．北京：外文出版社，2002：233.

[21] 隋慧娟．中医方剂翻译略议．中医药学报，2001，29（3）：6-7.

[22] 申光．中医方剂名英译问题探讨——格式及其内涵．中国中西医结合杂志，2004，24

(8)：751－752.
[23] 康广盛，周洪伟. 浅谈中医英译中方剂名称的翻译. 中国中西医结合杂志，2008，28 (6)：555－556.
[24] 罗磊. 中药商品名称的美学特征与英语名称的翻译. 中国中西医结合杂志，2003，23 (3)：225－226.
[25] 蒋基昌，邓家刚，杨书兰. 中医常用方剂名称英译错误探讨. 中西医结合学报，2009，7 (8)：794－796.
[26] 朱函亭. 中医方剂英译中的异化翻译法. 浙江中医杂志，2009，44 (10)：773.
[27] 魏迺杰，冯晔. 对《中医药常用名词术语英译》的一些意见. 中国中西医结合杂志，2006，26 (10)：953－955.
[28] 刘九茹. "Zhi Bai Dihuang"还是"Zhi Bo Dihuang"? ——也谈中医方剂名英译. 中国中西医结合杂志，2010，30 (11)：1221，1226.
[29] 全国科学技术名词审定委员会主编. 中医药学名词. 北京：科学出版社，2004：205.
[30] 国家药典委员会主编. 中华人民共和国药典. 北京：中国医药科技出版社，2010：820－821.
[31] 朱函亭，李亚平，郑芳子. 针灸穴位翻译与中医文化传承. 中国中西医结合杂志，2008，28 (6)：556－557.
[32] 魏迺杰，冯晔. 实用英文中医辞典. 北京：人民卫生出版社，2002：747.
[33] 王丽. 音译法使用中的"对等"原则. 山东外语教学，2010，(4)：110－112.
[34] 蔡寒松. 汉、英词语音译的语言学与社会语言学因素. 中国翻译，1991 (6)：20－22.
[35] 赵英. "三焦"英译应以音译为好. 国医论坛，2005，20 (4)：45－46.
[36] 牛喘月. 早期中医西译者的翻译思路与方法. 中西医结合学报，2003，1 (4)：309－311.
[37] 张顺生. 对翻译中"约定俗成"的再思考. 上海翻译，2009，(2)：57－60.
[38] 胥荣东，张永旺. 关于"穴位"一词英文翻译的看法. 中国针灸，2005，25 (8)：598.

[原载《中国中西医结合杂志》，2014，34 (7)：873－878.]

浅议连字符在中医术语英译中的使用

范奎玲　丁年青

通过对现行的多本中医术语英译词典以及 WHO 西太平洋地区 2007 年颁布的《传统医学名词术语国际标准》（以下简称 WHO 标准）的调查与研究，笔者发现有关连字符在中医术语英译中的使用较为混乱。对于同一词条译法中的连字符加与不加的问题，不同译者之间存在很大分歧，甚至同一译者，对于一些中文语法结构相同的不同术语，也存在连字符使用上的差别。并且，从近年来中医术语翻译学的建设和发展来看，连字符的重要性并没有得到充分的重视。杨静[1]指出中医术语英译需符合简洁性原则（conciseness principle）。连字符复合词的运用符合现代英语日趋简化的趋势，运用到中医术语翻译中，可以表现出术语语义的整体性、单一性、简洁性的特点。本文欲先探讨普通英语中连字符使用的一般原则，再根据中医术语选用的英译用词的词性构成，试图归纳总结出在中医术语英译中连字符的一些使用规律。

1. 英文连字符使用的一般原则

英语构词法主要有复合法、缀合法、派生法、拼缀法、缩略法、逆成法、转化法、拟声法等，而在复合法、缀合法、缩略法、逆成法等构词中有许多词汇都是通过连字符来实现的[2]。结合连字符在中医术语英译中的使用，本文主要针对复合型连字符构词中的复合形容词结构现象进行分析。

1.1　复合型连字符构词（表 1）

由表 1 可以看出形容词性连字符复合词的使用情况比较复杂，但要注意的原则是其作为前置修饰语使用，为了更好地体现复合词的语义单一性和感官的整体性，并避免歧义，一般需加连字符。如 small-businessman 意为“做小买卖的商人”，而 small businessman 则表示“身材矮小的商人”。

1.2　缀合型连字符构词

英语派生词是在词根上加上前缀或后缀构成的词，它的使用情况也较为复杂，但其中尚有一些规律可循。结合中医术语英译，在此仅对以下两种情况进行分析。①前缀与词根的第一个字母是大写，前缀与词根之间应加连字符，如：Pan-African。②通常在 self-、half-、quarter-、all-、well-为词缀的缀合词各部分之间应加连字符。如：self-control、self-respect、half-asleep、quarter-share、all-round[2]。

表 1　普通英语中复合型连字符构词的使用

构词情况	使用举例
肝名词＋过去分词	custom-built（定制的）
形容词＋现在分词	easy-going（随和的）
形容词＋过去分词	new-born（新生的）
副词＋现在分词	forth-coming（即将到来的）
副词＋过去分词	well-dressed（穿着讲究的）
形容词＋形容词	deaf-mute（聋哑的）
名词＋形容词	war-weary（厌战的）
数词＋名词	15-minute（15 分钟的）
数词＋名词＋ed	four-legged（四条腿的）
名词＋名词＋ed	lion-hearted（狂妄自大的）
形容词＋名词＋ed	short-sighted（目光短浅的）
过去分词＋副词	worn-out（磨损的）
名词性连字符复合词	pain-killer（止痛剂）
名词＋副词	looker-on（旁观者）
动词＋副词	take-away（外卖）

2. 中医术语英译连字符的使用现状

由表 2 可见国内外中医翻译者对连字符的使用总体情况存在显著差异。另外，对于同一术语的英译，连字符的使用也存在明显区别。如“半表半里”的英译，就存在以下诸多翻译：half-superficies and half-interior、midstage penetration、semi-exterior and semi-interior、half-external and half-internal part、between exterior and interior、half-exterior and half-interior，可见即使在统一将“表里”译为 exterior and interior 的前提下，诸位译家仍然存在连字符的使用与否、使用几个连字符以及复合词的词性问题等方面的差异。由此可见，连字符使用的统一问题值得中医翻译工作者的重视，规范地使用连字符将给我们的工作带来诸多方便，同时更加有利于中医的对外交流。

表 2 现行主要中医词典中连字符的使用现状

中医词典（著者）	总词条（条）	连字符词条（条）	比例（%）
WHO 标准[3]	3044	370	12.16
魏迺杰[4]	21 666	3053	14.09
李照国[5]	23 001	1386	6.02
方廷玉[6]	6017	574	9.54
谢竹藩[7]	3270	462	14.13
欧明[8]	4367	932	21.34

3. 中医术语英译连字符使用优劣举例分析

笔者认真比较了 6 本中医英语词典中连字符的使用，其中有很多可借鉴学习的例子。比如“提插补泻”一条，WHO 译为 lifting-thrusting supplementation and draining，将两个动名词用连字符连接，极具整体感，用以修饰其后的 supplementation and draining，准确地传达出源语的内在含义。再如“半身汗”一词，很多译者选用了 hemilateral sweating 或 hemihidrosis 来翻译。但笔者考究古文献，清・徐大椿所著《医略六书》卷二十“半身汗者，汗不遍身，或上或下或左或右”，可见“半身汗”并不只含“偏侧”之义，因此，hemilateral 或 hemihidrosis 不能全面传达源语的意义，而 WHO 译为 half-body sweating，是为优例。但笔者也发现了一些尚显不足的术语翻译，特举例分析如下。“八纲辨证”，在 6 本词典中收录了不下 8 种翻译：eight principle pattern identification/syndrome differentiation、eight-principle pattern identification、differentiation of syndromes with eight principles、differentiating syndromes with eight principles、eight principle syndromes differentiation、eight-principles syndrome differentiation；differential diagnosis in accordance with the eight principle，读者见此着实难辨孰正孰误、孰优孰劣。该条术语选用的英译词为 eight、principle 和 differentiation，符合复合型连字符构词中“数词＋名词”的使用条件，因此，用连字符连接，eight-principle 作为前置修饰语修饰 syndrome differentiation，符合科技术语的整体性的特点。并且为体现术语的简洁性原则，应尽量少用 of、with、in accordance with 等介词（词组），因此，笔者建议“八纲辨证”应译为 eight-principle syndrome differentiation。对于“肝火上炎”，在 6 本词典中同样存在诸多不同的翻译：liver fire flaming upward、upflaming liver fire、upflaming of liver fire、hyperactivity of liver fire、flaming of liver-fire、up-flaming of liver fire、flaming-up of liver-fire。“肝火”译为 liver fire，当属无异，但是否加连字符，众译家则存在分歧。笔者认为 liver fire 首先符合名词性连字符复合词中“名词＋名词”的使用情况，所以“肝火”不论单独使用或用于构成其他四字术语，加连字符均应属规范使用。“上炎”，选用的英译词为 up 和 flaming，符合连字符复合词中“adv＋v-ing”，因此，可译为

up-flaming。另外，将 up 置于 flaming 之前，起到强调“肝火向上之势”。综上，笔者建议“肝火上炎”译为 up-flaming of liver-fire。“天人相应”是中医基础理论中的重要术语，但在各个词典中的译法亦不统一，共有以下几种：correspondence between nature and human、heaven and humankind are mutually responsive、correspondency between man and nature、correspondence between man and universe、relevant adaptation of human body to natural environment、correspondence between human and the universe、the relationship between human body and enviornment。该条术语同样符合连字符构词中“名词＋名词”的使用情况，故译为 human-nature correspondence 更能体现术语的整体性与简洁性。对于“大肠寒结”，该条术语在有些词典中均译为 large intestinal cold bind，此译法易造成“large”修饰“bind”的歧义。故建议将“大肠”作为整体翻译，用连字符连接，译为 large-intestinal cold bind。

4. 中医术语英译中连字符的使用情况归纳

通过以上分析，笔者特将中医术语英译中通常需要使用连字符的情况归纳如下：

（1）名词＋名词：①阴阳理论相关术语，如：阴阳理论 Yin-Yang theory；阴阳平衡 Yin-Yang balance。②两种病邪合称，如：风寒证 wind-cold pattern/syndrome；风寒咳嗽 cough due to wind-cold。当然，还可见于多邪合而致病，如风寒湿病 wind-cold-damp disease；风火热毒证 wind-fire-heat toxin syndrome。③两个脏腑合称，如：心肺气虚 heart-lung Qi deficiency；肝胆气郁 liver-gallbladder Qi depression。④气血津液辨证相关术语，如：气血失调证 Qi-blood disharmony/syndrome；气阴两（亏）虚证 pattern/syndrome of Qi-Yin deficiency。

（2）名词＋分词：中医术语英译中，相对于过去分词，现在分词在构成连字符复合词时更常见。①采用此译法的中医术语最多见于治法、中药、方剂中，如：活血化瘀药/剂 blood-activating and stasis-resolving drugs/ formula；清热凉血药/剂 heat-clearing and blood-cooling drugs/ formula。②用于“十怪脉”“七绝脉”的翻译，如：雀啄脉 sparrow-pecking pulse；鱼翔脉 fish-waving pulse。③名词＋过去分词，采用此译法的中医术语不多见，如：齿痕舌 teeth-printed tongue。应注意：关于现在分词与过去分词的取舍问题，一般来说，表主动关系，或名词与动词构成动宾关系，采用现在分词；反之，如果表被动，则采用过去分词。

（3）形容词＋名词：例如，红丝疔 red-thread clove sore；下痢清谷 clear-food diarrhea；同名经配穴 combining same-name meridian acupoints。“下痢清谷”，如译作 clear food diarrhea，恐会贻笑大方。由此可见，如不加连字符，则对于形容词所修饰的名词成分会产生歧义，从而令整条术语的英译不能“达”意。

（4）形容词＋形容词：采用此译法的中医术语最多见于复合脉象、舌苔、面色等的描述以及复合针刺手法，例如，浮数脉 floating-rapid pulse；舌淡红 light-red tongue；面色嫩红 tender-red complexion；疾徐补泻 quick-slow supplementation and draining。

（5）前缀＋名词：中医术语英译中常用的前缀主要有 half-、non-、counter-、para-等，如，半表半里 half-exterior half-interior；心肾不交证 heart-kidney non-interaction pattern；脐旁 para-umbilical region；相侮 counter-restriction。

（6）数词＋名词：如，八纲辨证 eight-principle syndrome differentiation；六经辨证 six-meridian syndrome differentiation；五更泻 five-watch diarrhea；七星针 seven-star needle。

（7）音译＋名词：目前，此种译法仅用于脏腑相关术语中，如，脏 Zang-organ；腑 Fu-organ；奇恒之腑 extraordinary Fu-organ。另外，尚有一些在中医术语英译中不太常见的连字符用法，如"数词＋名词-ed"形式，例如：三棱针 three-edged needle，与普通英语中的 four-legged table 结构一致。

5. 结语

通过对英语中连字符的构词功能以及中医术语英译中连字符的使用情况可以得出以下结论：第一，中医术语英译中连字符的应用应根据英语连字符的基本构词功能即英译采用的单词的词性来判定；第二，和普通英语连字符的使用一样，中医术语英译中连字符的应用应本着"若修饰词对后面成分的修饰作用易产生歧义，此时应尽量使用连字符来连接"的原则；第三，中医术语的英译应规范使用连字符，以促进中医术语英译国际标准化进程。

参考文献

[1] 杨静. 中医术语英译的优选论分析. 海外英语，2011（10）：23.
[2] 李砚霞. 连字符构词探索及其翻译. 湛江师范学院学报，2009，(4)：66－68.
[3] WHO 西太平洋地区传统医学名词术语中英对照国际标准. 北京：北京大学医学出版社，2009.
[4] 魏迺杰. 英汉汉英中医词典. 长沙：湖南科学技术出版社，2005.
[5] 李照国. 汉英中医药大词典. 世界图书出版公司，1997.
[6] 方廷玉，陈锋，王梦琼. 新英汉中医学辞典. 中国医药科技出版，2003.
[7] 谢竹藩. 新编汉英中医药分类辞典. 北京：外文出版社，2002.
[8] 欧明. 汉英中医辞典. 广州：广东科学技术出版社，1986.

[原载《中国中西医结合杂志》，2014，34（4）：496－498.]

中医名词术语英译标准化应用之因“地”制宜

叶　晓

中医名词术语由于古老、精炼和多义性，其英译标准在制定开始，学界就一直存在争鸣，至今仍未达成一致标准。世界各地不同的出版社也采用了不同的标准，从而造成了读者对术语理解的片面性和不统一性，增加了外籍学员学习中医的难度，有碍于中医学在国外的传播。

1. 现状分析

2000—2007年，随着期刊文章、中医名词术语英译标准化会议、专业国际会议上的学术争鸣，多个中医名词术语及其英译标准化项目取得一定进展[1]。笔者认为比较权威的中医名词术语英译标准主要有：北京大学谢竹藩教授主持完成的国家中医药管理局“中医药名词术语英译标准化”课题，其成果之一《中医药常用名词术语英译》在2004年由中国中医药出版社出版[2]；中国中医科学院王永炎院士、梁菊生教授、朱建平教授牵头实施的国家科技部2000年度科技基础性工作基金立项项目“中医药基本名词术语规范化研究”之研究成果，经全国科学技术名词审定委员会审定公布，由北京科学出版社2005年出版[3]；2004年，WHO启动了“传统医学术语国际标准化”工作，于2007年10月16日，WHO西太平洋地区首次正式公布了《WHO西太平洋地区传统医学名词术语国际标准》(WHO International Standard Terminologies on Traditional Medicine in the Western Pacific Region)[4]；2007年12月，世界中医药学会联合会（World Federation of Chinese Medicine Societies，WFCMS）颁布《中医基本名词术语中英对照国际标准》(International Standard Chinese-English Basic Nomenclature of Chinese Medicine)，并向国内外推行[5]。

上述4套中医名词术语英译标准的设立无疑在很大程度上解决了现阶段中医国际交流中中医名词术语译文不统一、翻译不准确甚至误译等问题。

2. 存在问题及对策

通过比较上述几套术语英译标准，不难发现它们之间也存在许多不同之处，如参与标准制定者不同、采用英译原则不同、收词范围不同及部分相同术语的英译名不同等。到目前为止，上述几个“标准化”的方案均已经推行4年以上，但是差别仍较大，远未达成一致。

术语英译标准的不同必然会对各国中医的医疗、科研、学术交流、信息传播、经贸、教育等多方面带来困难。虽然 WFCMS 与 WHO 西太平洋地区办事处开始在翻译标准上开展合作，以提高世界卫生组织传统医学术语国际标准（WHO International Standard Terminologies，WHO IST）和中医基本名词术语中英对照国际标准的共同中医词条英译的一致性，但就其现状而言，中医药国际交流参与者应如何采用或者采用哪一套标准化的中医名词术语英译，以最大程度上减少中医药国际交流障碍，目前仍是一个重要问题。笔者认为需因“地”制宜，即通过情况具体分析，然后采用相应的具体策略。

2.1　单一标准的情况

采用单一标准的情况主要存在于英文版的中医学著作出版物和学术论文方面。现在，国内人民卫生出版社和上海科技出版社都主要采用 WFCMS 标准，而东方医学出版委员会（Commission for Oriental Medicine Publications，COMP）有两家出版社（Paradigm Publications 和 Blue Poppy Press）则规定使用魏迺杰博士制定的英文中医名词术语体系为其出版物的英文词汇标准[6]。在同一出版物中使用同一种术语英译标准无疑非常重要，这不仅能确保中医名词术语英译在全文中的一致性，又能减少译者的主观性，从而使译文更易理解。随着中医药国际交流的进一步开展，国内外英文版中医学著作的出版量和中医研究学术论文呈日益增多的趋势，因此，国内外出版社、中医学术杂志编辑部应相互协调，为其出版的中医英文出版物或论文指定权威性较高的一套中医名词术语英译标准。

2.2　混杂标准的情况

中医英语翻译的研究和教学本身就会对中医名词术语英译各套标准进行分析和比较，因此，必然会存在混杂使用各套标准的情况。对于中医双语教学和对外教学，由于各个教材出版社并未统一采取某一套术语英译标准，并且教学中为了从不同层面阐述某些术语，也会存在混杂使用各套标准的情况。另外，在中医临床口译中，由于涉及学科门类多，接触国外人员广，临场灵活性高，译者也不可能单一使用某一套术语英译标准，而往往要结合多个英译标准，甚至还可能完全抛弃标准化的英译术语，采取解释性翻译等翻译方法。不过，中医临床口译具有一定的学术性，实践中应尽可能采用某套中医名词术语英译标准，同时辅以结合其他各个标准。

2.3　无标准的情况

在中医药国际交流中，常常还涉及对中国文化或中医知识没有了解或了解很少的国外人士。对于用中医术语说明的中成药说明书、科普性的中医教育书籍等，即使采用某一术语标准并且英译得十分准确，国外人士也未必会理解什么是“clearing heat and relieving the exterior”或“resolving turbidity with aroma”等术语英译。对此类情况，笔者认为应抛开术语英译标准，以接受者为中心，以理解为度，采用意译或者让人容易理解的语言去阐述。

综上所述，笔者认为在多套中医名词术语英译标准共存的情况下，我们在实际运用中应该因“地”制宜，根据具体情况具体分析，从而灵活采用术语英译标准。

参考文献

[1] 洪梅，朱建平. 近30年中医名词术语英译标准化的历程. 北京：中国中医科学院，2008.

[2] 谢竹藩. 中医药常用名词术语英译. 北京：中国中医药出版社，2004.

[3] 中医药学名词审定委员会. 中医药基本名词. http：//www.cttcm.com.cn/zyyjbmc.htm.

[4] 世界卫生组织（西太平洋地区）. WHO西太平洋地区传统医学名词术语国际标准. 北京：北京大学医学出版社，2009.

[5] 世界中医药学联合会. 中医基本名词术语中英对照国际标准. 北京：人民卫生出版社，2008.

[6] 兰凤利. 中医名词术语英译：唯一还是多重标准？中国中西医结合杂志，2010，30（2）：188－192.

[原载《中国中西医结合杂志》，2013，33（9）：1290－1291.]

不同翻译手段在中医文献翻译中的辨证施用

左连君

翻译的主要手段是直译和意译。直译是基础，意译为辅助和补充。从翻译上的层次论来看，直译与意译的比重依文体的不同而不同。在通常情况下，翻译学术性科技文献基本采用直译法，注重较强的信息对应的准确性，而对文学作品则以意译为主，力求获得最佳可读性与艺术性。中医文献虽属学术范畴，却渗透着浓厚的民族文化和较强的古代哲理，任何翻译法的绝对化都是行不通的。鉴于中医学独具一格的医学理论体系及充满古代文学气质的表述形式，“辨证施用”不同的翻译手段，将直译、意译、音译等融合运用，是中医英译恰当的翻译策略。

1. 直译兼意译

在英汉双语的表层句式及深层内容都能相对契合的情况下，直译是最便利的语言转换模式。在《中医临床各科》《中国针灸》《中医药膳》《方剂学》等书的英译中，双语内容契合的情况十分普遍，尤其见于辨证论治章节中的主证与主治部分，从中略举一二：

（1）原发性高血压病中肝肾阴虚的主证为“头晕目眩，耳鸣目涩，心悸心烦，失眠健忘，手足心热，腰腿酸软，口干，舌质红，少苔或无苔，脉弦细”，直接转换为：Headache，vertigo，tinnitus，dryness of eyes，vexation，palpitation，insomnia，poor memory，feverish sensation in the palms and soles，aching and lassitude of the loins and legs，dry mouth，red tongue with little fur，fine and string-like pulse。

（2）各个穴位的主治部分，如曲池穴的主治为“咽喉肿痛，腹痛吐泻，痢疾，水肿，眩晕，湿疹，伤寒余热不退，半身不遂，手臂肿痛”，直接转换为：Sore throat，abdominal pain，vomiting，diarrhea，dysentery，edema，dizziness，eczema，residual fever after febrile disease，hemiparalysis，swelling and pain of the hand and arm。当然，这种对应式转换只是相对而论的，大多章节中的直译部分包含着必不可少的意译成分。如在病因病机、证候分析章节的翻译中，同样是词组式的行文，但词语之间隐含的逻辑关系却需要融入意译手段方可完成。例如：“［证候分析］：肝气郁结，日久化火，则口苦口干，坐卧不宁，烦躁不安。火盛伤肝，则右肋灼痛，火盛伤津，则大肠失润，大便干燥。”对这一段需要调整转换才能表达出行文中的主次因果关系：“(Analysis of Syndromes)：Prolonged accumulation of liver-Qi tends to be transformed to fire with manifestations of bitter

dry mouth, restlessness and irritability. And excessive fire will impair liver collaterals marked by burning pain in the right hypochondrian and also impair body fluids, which can result in the loss of moisture in the large intestine marked by dry stools。"
这种直译与意译相融的翻译方法在中医推拿针灸的介绍中大量运用。例如：头面部穴位（天门）的位置为两眉中间直上，至前发际呈一条直线。操作：用两拇指桡侧面或两拇指面自下而上交替直推，称为"开天门"，亦称"推攒竹"。主治：发热，头痛，感冒无汗，或汗出不畅、精神委靡、警惕不安等。(Tianmen) Location: The part above the line between the eyebrows up to the anterior hair line. Manipulation: Pushing straightly with radial surface or face of thumbs alternatively from below to above is called "opening Tianmen", also known as "pushing Zanzhu". Indications: fever, headache, cold without sweating or with obstructed sweating, listlessness, vigilance and restlessness。

2. 意译兼音译

中医理论术语作为祖国医学文化源远流长的结晶，与西医文化概念大相径庭。理论术语的表层结构十分简练，但溢于字面之外的含义却极为丰富。要做到准确翻译，应摆脱字面句式的束缚，透过表层，探究深层的实质含意。阐析性转换模式是翻译中医理论术语的有效手段。如"辨证施治"这一术语蕴含着深刻的语义信息，意思是：将四诊所搜集的临床资料，运用脏腑、经络、病因等基础理论，加以分析、归纳，从而作出诊断和定出治疗措施。只有运用意译方法才能较全面地传达出术语的实质内容，译成：Diagnosis and treatment based on an overall analysis of symptoms and signs, the cause, nature and location of the illness and patient's physical condition according to the basic theories of traditional Chinese medicine。"急下存阴"这一术语指的是治疗实热证的一种疗法，其实质内容是：使用具有清热作用的峻猛泻药，迅速通便泻热、清除燥结，以保存津液，适用阐析性译法：Using drastic purgatives to eliminate heat for the preservation of body fluids。"发表不远热"指对于风寒表证须用辛温药以解表散寒，称为发表不回避热药，阐析性译成：Medicines of hot nature are not contraindicated in dispelling the superficial factors。但有一些中医基础理论术语，如"阴阳""五行""气""标本""虚实""三焦""五脏""六腑"等是中医独特思维方式的体现。这些术语含义丰富、概念独特，在英语中找不到等值词，意译又过于冗长繁杂，影响行文的可读性。对于此类"译作语言"词组空缺的情况，运用音译加附注阐析的手段是比较妥当的做法。如在行文中只出现"Yin""Yang""Qi""Sanjiao""Wuxing"等音译词，应另在合适位置加附注进行详解。

3. 音译兼英译

音译兼英译是指在中医英译的某些内容上音译占了相当大的比例，在中医推拿针灸的介绍中运用广泛。例如《中国针灸学》中的穴位名称全部采用音译：shaoyang（少阳），zhongfu（中府），hegu（合谷），lieque（列缺），shousanli（手三里），xiaguan（下关），neiting（内庭）等。在《中国药膳》译本中，介绍食疗药膳的辨证施食方面运用了不少音译兼英译手法。例如对食疗中药的介绍：wuji（black chicken），shengjiang（fresh ginger），gaoliang（Chinese sorghum），baimal（white wheat），shanyao（Chinese yam），congbai（green Chinese onion）。从翻译的效果上来看，笔者认为中医英译文中夹杂着一些音译词在一定程度上促进了“中国英语”步入英语外来词的行列，与此同时也维护了中医文体语言的原始气质与色调。例如，在“病毒性肝炎”一病的英译文中，可见直译、意译、音译的融合运用：Viral hepatitis，caused by hepatitis viruses，can be divided into three types：Type A，Type B and Non-A，Non-B hepatitis... In TCM this disease belongs to the categories of “huangdan（黄疸）”（jaundice）“ganyu（肝郁）”（stagnation of liver-Qi），“xietong（胁痛）”（hypochondriac pain）and “zhengji（癥积）”（mass in the abdomen）。

4. 英译兼拉丁语译

不同翻译手段的有机结合充分表现在中医临床处方、中成药、中药方剂的译文中。根据药理专家的意见，同一种中草药，英文可能会有不同的名字。鉴于草药的汉名与英文名不能达成完全一致，国际上通用拉丁语统一标准比较准确，因此，在中药英译中融入拉丁语，构成一词二式（或一词三式）的译法在《中国名优中成药》《中国药膳》《中国临床各科》《方剂学》等系列译本中广泛使用。如：人参（renshen）ginseng—Radix Ginseng，陈皮（chenpi）immature bitter orange—Fructus Aurantii Immaturus。另举一食疗处方为例：（桂姜人参粥）：桂枝 6g，干姜 6g，人参 3g，大枣 8 枚，煎煮，沸后改文火煎成浓汁（略）。译文形成（Gruel of Cinnamon Twig，Dried Ginger and Ginseng）：cinnamon twig（Ramulus Cinnamoni）6g，dried ginger（Rhizoma Zingiberis）6g，ginseng（Radix Ginseng）3g，Chinese-date（Fructus Ziziphi Fujubae）8 pieces，decocted together. When the water comes to the boil，decocted with slow fire until the juice becomes thick.

实践证明，不同的翻译手段并不是相斥的，而是相互关联、相互渗透、相互补充的。“翻译方法论的辩证法就在于扬弃绝对化，树立整体观”。在中医的英译中，不同翻译方法的“辨证施用”是推动中医英译工作健康发展，将传统中医文化推向世界的重要策略。

（原载《中国中西医结合杂志》，2004，24（4）：364－365.）

中医名词术语翻译层面观及其译语特点

林　岩　何丽艳　郑寒松　王朝辉

众所周知，现代语言学把语言单位划分为音位、词素、词、词组、句子和语篇 6 个层面。我们可以根据语境的不同使用不同的翻译层面，可以根据需要选择在这 6 个层面中的一个或几个层面上进行翻译。无论是在哪个层面上进行翻译，要求译语必须准确、科学、简洁和规范，科技翻译尤其如此。

关于中医名词术语的翻译层面目前国内外研究得很少。中医名词术语从语言学角度可划分为音位、词素、词和词组 4 个层面，因此，中医名词术语是在这 4 个层面上进行翻译的。

1. 中医名词术语的翻译层面及其译语特点

1.1　中医名词术语的音位翻译层面及其译语特点

中医名词术语的音位是指字位，其本身没有独立意义。在翻译中当名词术语的音位需要在译语中获得对应时，就应成为翻译单位。中医药学中中医基础理论方面的名词术语是中医学理论体系的重要组成部分，其内涵独特。正确地翻译这部分术语对于中医名词术语翻译的规范化有着重要的意义。但由于中西文化及中西医之间存在着巨大的差异，所以这部分术语在英语中很难找到对应语，因此，这类中医名词术语只能将音位作为翻译单位，只能在音位层面上进行翻译。例如：气，Qi；气功，qigong；阴阳，yinyang；太阳，taiyang；少阳，shaoyang；阳明，yangming；太极拳，taijiquan；合谷，hegu；人迎 renying。

适用于在音位层面上翻译的这类中医名词术语为数不多，而且译语也已固定，基本上为国内外公认。

1.2　中医名词术语的词素层面翻译及其译语特点

英语词素是构成词汇的最小语义单位，绝大多数不能独立存在。一个词可以含多个词素。大多数科技专业术语，尤其是西医术语多半是由词素构成的。在词素层面翻译中，构成原文词的每一个词素在译入语的对应词中都有一定的相应词素，因此，科技英汉翻译尤其是西医英汉翻译中大量的是在词素层面上操作的。例如：psycho/biology（“/”表示隔开词素），心理生物学；gastro/entero/pathy，胃肠病；erythro/penia 红细胞减少。

同样，我们可以根据这一原则，尝试将词素层面翻译应用到中医名词术语的翻译中。例如：风秘，anemo/genous constipation；湿泻，hygro/genous diarrhea；

心气虚，hypo/cardic/Qi；肾虚不孕，nephro/asthenic sterility；外感胃脘痛，exo/genous stomach/ache；得气，acu/esthesia。

由此可见，在词素层面的英汉翻译中，词素层面既是分析词汇的基础和依据，是学习和掌握英语词汇的钥匙，又是中医名词术语词素层面汉英翻译中的有效翻译成分。而且，采用词素层面翻译的中医名词术语译语具有简洁规范、科学性专业性强、信息密度高、交际功能强等特点。

1.3　中医名词术语的词层面翻译及其译语特点

所谓中医名词术语词层面的翻译指的是将词作为翻译单位，即用英语语言中相应的相近对应词代换等值的或无等值的中医名词术语的组成部分。举例如下：

第 1 组：里热，interior heat；舌强，stiff tongue；风秘，wind constipation；湿泻，wet diarrhea；心气虚，insufficiency of cardiac Qi。

第 2 组：真牙，true teeth；小舌，small tongue；血厥，blood syncope；肺热，lung heat；失神，spirit depletion。

上述两组中的中医名词术语均是采用词层面翻译法翻译的，其特点是术语中的每个词在英语语言中都能找到相应或相近对应词。如术语中有“里”“风”“泻”“血”“舌”“真”等，而英语中相对应有“interior”“wind”“diarrhea”“blood”“tongue”“true”等。那么，采用词层面翻译法翻译中医名词术语的效果如何？其译语具有什么特点？大量翻译实践证明，词层面翻译包含两种情况：①在词层面翻译中，如果英语中相应或相近的对应词能代换等值的中医名词术语的组成成分，那么这种翻译法具有汉英词对应性强、取词方便、译语直观、通俗简洁等优点。第 1 组的词都具有这些特点。②在词层面翻译中，如果英语中的相应或相近的对应词代换无等值的中医名词术语的组成成分，也就是说不能代换等值的中医名词术语的组成成分。换句话说，术语中的每个词虽然在英语中都有对应语，但这些对应语组成的译语意义并不能表达术语整体词汇组成的意义，那么这种词层面翻译法往往会歪曲术语原意或不符合译入语的规范，容易造成歧义，不能提倡和采纳。第 2 组就是这种情况，其中的术语采用词层面翻译法进行词对词直译，其译法无法从整体上揭示术语的正确语义。比如，英语中有“真”(ture) 和“牙” (teeth)，却没有“true teeth”，有“小” (small) 和“舌”(tongue)，却没有“small tongue”。 “真牙”和“小舌”的正确译语分别为“wisdom teeth”和“uvula”。

在中医对外交流初期，这种词层面翻译法应用广泛，虽然在一定程度上解了当时的燃眉之急，但由于这种词对词的直译法只适合少部分中医名词术语，因此，也造成了很多混乱。随着中医翻译科学性及其译语规范性的提高，无论是从微观上纠正原来采用词层面翻译的中医术语译语的错误还是从宏观上指导准确选择词层面翻译法都十分重要。

1.4 中医名词术语的词组层面翻译及其译语特点

所谓词组层面翻译指的是在中医名词术语翻译中以词组为单位也就是翻译是在词组层面上操作。这种翻译法至今在中医名词翻译中仍相当普遍。该翻译法也包含两种情况。

1.4.1 中医名词术语词组层面上的描述性、解释性翻译 例如：风秘，constipation due to wind evil；湿泻，diarrhea due to wetness evil；肾虚不孕，sterility due to the deficiency of the kidney；外感胃脘痛，stomachache caused by external pathogen factors；得气，getting the feeling of needling。

中医名词术语的这种在词层面上的描述性、解释性翻译不能简捷其译语。与原术语相比，译语冗长，信息密度低，交际功能差，规范程度低，缺乏专业性，除非不得已，否则不应采纳。

1.4.2 中医名词术语词组层面上的意义综合性翻译 一些中医名词术语，其意义并不等于组成术语的各个词意义加起来的总和，因此，不能按其组成成分来翻译。只能把各个词的意义综合起来作为一个语义单位翻译出来，才能较好地再现原术语的信息，揭示术语的准确意义。例如：辨证论治，treatment with syndrome differentiation；泾溲不利，dysuria；肌肉不仁，numbness；筋骨痿软，flaccidity of extremities。

由此可见，词层面上的意义综合性翻译不仅能较好地表达术语的实际内涵，而且能有效地简捷译语，因此，值得推广。

2. 中医名词术语不同层面翻译法译语的比较

以下各术语是分别从词素、词、词组 3 个层面或其中的两个层面进行翻译的，试比较以下各例：风秘，anemogenous constipation wind constipation/constipation due to wind evil；湿泻，hygrogenous wet diarrhea/diarrhea due to wetness evil；外感胃脘痛，exogenous stomachache/stomachache caused by external pathogen factor；得气，acuesthesia/getting the feeling of needling；辨证论治，treatment with syndrome/differentiation；心气虚，hypocardio Qi/insufficiency of cardiac Qi。

可见，中医名词术语可以有 4 个翻译层面，固定采用某种翻译层面的术语为数极少（多限于中医基础理论部分）。多数情况是中医名词术语不同，其翻译层面也不尽相同。值得注意的是同一术语可以采用不同翻译层面，因而获得的译语也不同。比如，“湿泻”“辨证论治”“肾虚不孕”等，其翻译层面不尽相同。而同是一个术语“风秘”，可以在 3 个翻译层面上进行翻译，但获得的译语特点不同。很明显，采用词素翻译层面翻译的译语“anemogenous constipation”既简明、规范，又能反映原术语内涵，为专业用语；采用词层面翻译所得的译语

“wind constipation”虽然也可以，但俗了些，只是普通用语；采用词组层面描述性，解释性翻译的译语“constipation due to wind evil”，虽然能表达原术语的内涵，但译语过长，规范程度低，缺乏专业性，因此，信息密度低，交际功能差。由此可见，术语“风秘”虽然可以在3个层面上进行翻译，但采用词素层面翻译法所获得的译语最理想、最规范。术语“心气虚”可以在词素或词层面上进行翻译，所得译语分别为“hypocardio Qi”和“insufficiency of cardiac Qi”，显然前者优于后者。又如，既可采用词素层面又可以采用词组层面进行翻译的“肾虚不孕”“外感胃脘痛”和“得气”，所得译语显然采用词素层面翻译法较词组层面更为理想、规范，因此，词素翻译法可能是中医名词术语翻译标准化的最佳方法之一。

我们认为，只有了解了中医名词术语的翻译层面及各层面译语的特点，才能在中医名词术语的翻译中选择最佳翻译层面，从而获得最理想的译语。这对于中医名词术语的翻译标准化、译语规范化可以起到实质性的推动作用。

［原载《中国中西医结合杂志》，2001，21（12）：937－938.］

论名词化在中医文本英译中的运用

李　虹　董敏华　徐亚萍

关于名词化（nominalization），不同的语言流派从不同的视角进行了研究，包括结构主义、转换生成语言学派、功能语言学派和认知语言学派等。在《现代语言学词典》中，“名词化”被定义为“从其他某个词类形成名词的过程或指从一个底层小句得出一个名词短语的派生过程”[1]。韩礼德（M. A. K. Halliday）则认为名词化是“用名词来体现本来用动词体现的‘过程’或形容词体现的‘特征’”[2]，认为它属于语法隐喻的范畴。简单地说，所谓名词化就是用名词短语的形式来表达句子、动词短语、形容词短语所要表达的内容。由于名词短语通常表示静止的状态，比较正式、客观，不如动词短语和形容词短语生动形象，所以在不同文体中的应用频率是有差异的。科技英语要求语言简洁、结构严谨、文体正式，强调客观性，而名词化结构正好能满足这样的需求。“名词化的使用和发展最初很可能源于科技文体之中”[2]。王晋军[3]通过对语料的定量分析，发现名词化比例在科技英语中高达 72.6%，而在英语小说中则仅占 27.2%，得出的结论是：名词化的比例越高，语篇的正式程度也就越高，由此可见，名词化是科技英语的重要特点之一。关于名词化结构的作用，各派也各有侧重。其中功能语言学派比较全面地研究了它在语言各个层面上的体现，如小句内部的功能、语篇功能、语类功能、语义功能等[4]。中医英语和医学英语一样，属于科技英语的范畴。但两者又有所不同，医学英语的源文本为英语，多数情况下需要从英文翻译成中文；而中医英语则不同，不存在地道的中医英语，所有现存的中医英语文本都是从中文翻译成英文的，因而汉译英成为主要任务。对科技英语中名词化结构的汉译已经有大量的探讨和研究，而对如何运用名词化结构进行中医文本的英译鲜有报道。本文主要通过举例来说明中医文本英译时名词化的方法、作用和适用条件等。

1. 名词化结构与中医文本英译

认知语言学家兰盖克（R. W. Langacker）提出了名词化的三种形式：①词汇名词化：通过词汇名词化，产生新的词汇，用于表示某种行为或事件的总称；②动词名词：将带有其他成分（除主语外）的动词名词化；③句子名词化：将动词以及与之相关的所有成分（包括主语）名词化，形成事件的表达[5]。其中第①和第②类形式在中医术语的翻译中非常常用，而第③类多见于中医语篇的翻译。由于科技英语的重点在于描述现象、状态，而名词化结构主要呈现静态特征，故大量使用名词化结构符合其文体特征，使整个语篇显得客观而正式，个人主观意识较少。与之不同的是，汉语是一种缺乏屈折形态的语言，其语法结构表现较强的相似性，并具有“板块”特点。意义决定于语序，有“以动词为中心”的语法特征[6]。连淑能认为“英语倾向于多用名词，因而叙述呈静态；汉语倾向于多用动词，因而叙述呈动态”[7]。中医语言也不例外，在中医文本中也经常出现主谓结构、动宾结构来表示症状、病机、治法等术语或者在句子中充当主语、宾语，因而在将中医术语或语篇翻译成英语时经常需要把汉语中的动词结构翻译为英语中的名词化结构，以符合英语语言和英语科技文体的要求。但这种转换并非单纯的词性改变，而是在整个术语或整个句子结构、语义表达等方面都发生相应的变化。以下就从中医术语和语篇的英译两方面来探讨如何应用名词化结构及其所起的作用。

1.1 词组层面的名词化

在翻译中医术语时常常需要将中文的主谓结构、动宾结构转换为英语的名词结构，因为症状本身强调的是某种病理状态，而不是强调动作过程。以下以中医表示症状的短语为例说明名词化的过程和方法。如：吞酸 swallowing acid，流涕 runny nose，畏寒喜暖 aversion to cold and desire for warmth，拒按 tenderness。以上症状中，中文都是用动宾结构来描述的，而在翻译成英语时，都采用了名词性结构。其中 swallowing acid 是用动名词＋名词的形式，把动词“吞”翻译成动名词 swallowing，后接宾语 acid。runny nose 属于形容词＋名词的形式，不仅有词性和结构的改变，而且是对整个词组进行了视角的切换和意象的替代。“涕”这个词的英文对应语 nasal mucus 没有出现在译文中，而是用 nose 这个意象来表现，采用了韩礼德所谓的隐喻式而不是一致式，符合英语的惯用表达法。aversion to cold and desire for warmth 以名词＋介词短语的形式，把动词“畏”和“喜”翻译成名词 aversion 和 desire，然后根据两个词的惯用搭配，分别选用介词 to 和 for，后面接介词宾语 cold 和 warmth。tenderness 对原术语进行了重新整合，把原来的动宾词组直接用一个名词表示出来，在结构和语义表达方式上与中文有明显的区别。

上述例子均属于名词化隐喻的体现，但名词化的方法有别，表现为结构和形式上的差异。可见在翻译中医术语时需根据具体语义和表达的需要，选择合适的名词化结构。再看下面的例子：①寒热往来 alternation of chills and fever；②身热不扬 unsurfaced fever；③语声低微 faint，low voice；④腹痛 abdominal pain；⑤营卫不和 disharmony between Ying Qi and Wei Qi。以上术语中文均属于主谓结构，在译成英语时则采用了名词化方法。其中①～③均以中文的主语（名词）作为中心词，而把谓语（动词）译成了修饰语（定语），分别由现在分词、过去分词和形容词来承担。④则将中文的主语“腹”（名词）译成了修饰语 abdominal（形容词），而把谓语“痛”（动词）译成名词 pain 充当中心词。⑤也是把谓语“不和”（动词）译成名词 disharmony 充当中心词．而将中文的主语“营卫”（名词）译成了介词短语 between Ying Qi and Wei Qi 作后置定语。在这些例子的翻译中，都存在表达视角和结构的转换，而不仅是词性的改变。

1.2　语篇层面的名词化

范文芳认为“名词化隐喻体现参加者和过程两种语义，这种结构有事物的特征又体现参加者意义；有动词特征又体现过程意义”[8]。这一点在以下例子中可以得到体现。如：

例 1：风寒袭表，郁遏卫阳，肌表失于温煦则恶寒。

（1）When wind cold attacks the exterior and stagnates the defensive Qi，the fleshy exterior will fail to be warmed，causing aversion to cold.

（2）Stagnation of defensive Qi from exterior attacking of wind cold will create failure of the fleshy exterior to be warmed，causing aversion to cold.

（1）由两个小句构成，使用了主从复合句的结构，词汇密度较小。另一方面突出了动作，结构和用词与源语非常接近，表示当前一个动作发生后就会产生后一个动作。

（2）则将复合句变成了一个简单句，但词汇密度增大。而且把中文三个小句中的前两个小句“风寒袭表，郁遏卫阳”翻译成名词性短语，充当主语成分，替代了从句。（1）中的第 1 小句的作用用于说明谓语动词发生的条件。相应动词“袭”和“郁遏”（stagnate）转换成了动名词 attacking 和 stagnation，发生了词性的改变，语义功能也发生相应变化。同时由于这两个名词之间又存在因果关系，其中 attacking 是因，而 stagnation 为果，两者用介词 from 来连接，并作为主语部分。而第 3 小句“肌表失于温煦则恶寒”又是前面 2 个小句的结果，故也将其翻译成一个名词性结构。在这个名词性结构和前面的主语之间增加了动词 create 来做谓语。也就是说通过词组结构、小句层次的变化及重新组合使得小句及语篇中的信息结构发生相应的变化，使得语篇结构更紧凑，关联更密切，语言更严谨、更正式，充分体现了名词化隐喻的效果。因而（2）的译法不仅是词性的改变，而且从不同的视角对原文本进行了解读和诠释，因此，名词化使非已知非共有的信息在形式上变成已知的共有信息，从而隐蔽地向读者或听者传达信息[9]。正如胡壮麟所说的那样，名词化隐喻是意义表达的变异，不仅仅是词汇的选择[10]。名词化结构正是通过切换认知视角使短语或句子的意义重心发生相应的变化，而逻辑关系则体现得更为明确，这就顺应了科技英语的文体特点。

例 2：阴阳离决，精气乃绝。

（1）If Yin and Yang dissociate from each other，essential Qi will be exhausted.

（2）Dissociation of Yin and Yang will lead to Qi exhaustion.

原文出自《黄帝内经·素问·生气通天论》。（1）在句式上采用了复合句，语义明确易懂，但结构比较松散，词汇密度小，信息量不高；而在选择体现这些小句功能的词类时，采用了韩礼德所谓的一致式，即用动词词组表达过程，用名词词组表达参与者。（2）则使用了1个小句，即简单句的形式，把中文的两个主谓结构分别译成两个名词性结构，然后鉴于两者之间存在因果逻辑关系，增加了“lead to”来充当谓语，体现这种关系。此结构比较紧凑，语言简洁，词汇密度大，信息量高，表达准确、精练，逻辑关联更密切。在词类选择上，采用了名词化隐喻式，即将含有动词的主谓词组转化为名词词组来体现过程，更能体现科技英语的特色，符合其表达习惯。（2）的译文对原句进行了重新组合，在结构上明显不同于原文本，语义也就从不同的角度得到了表达。

例3：阴平阳秘，精神乃治。

（1）Only when Yin is calm and Yang is sound can essence spirit be normal.

（2）Calmness of Yin and soundness of Yang ensures normal essence spirit.

本句原文也出自《黄帝内经》。古汉语语言非常简洁，但比较深奥费解。首先在结构上，通过分析考证，可以知道前一句是后一句的条件；在词义上，要特别注意“平”“秘”“治”这些词的理解和翻译。在译文中，例3（1）采用主从复合句来翻译，把前句译成条件，后句译成结果，结构相对松散，但语义清晰明了。例3（2）则把原文的两个小句分别译成名词性短语，增加了谓语动词，用一个简单句来体现这种条件和结果的关系。对应于原文的言简意赅，译文结构也非常紧凑，语言精炼，符合目标语的语言习惯和思维方式。从以上例子可以看出，在翻译中医文本时，常常需要用名词性短语来表达某些小句，对源语的结构和表达方式进行转换，并找出名词化背后的逻辑关系，以体现中医文本的高度概括和凝练。可以说，科技语篇为了表达更复杂的经验和更高度的认知，已完成了从简单的小句被“打包”（pack）成词组的过程，或从两三个小句“打包”成一个小句的过程[11]。

2. 名词化在中医翻译中的作用

不同学派在论述名词化的作用时有不同的视角和侧重点，以下主要就名词化在中医翻译中的语义表达和语篇衔接功能进行讨论。

2.1　改变语义表达的视角和方式

乔姆斯基（IV. Chomsky）[12]曾指出，名词化使“语言文字的表层结构通过转换规则，在结构深层产生出新的语义来”。

例4：如果脾不统血，就会导致各种出血。

Failure of the spleen to control blood leads to a variety of bleeding.

在这个句子中，我们可以看到，Failure of the spleen to control blood 中，of 后接的 the spleen 是这个短语动作状态的发出者，而原文中的整个条件状语从句转换成了一个名词性短语，充当主语。表达的视角从假设至结果变成一个陈述判断，语言结构非常简洁，语义也很明了，逻辑关系清晰。或者说名词化是“一种对语法结构和语义常规的偏离”，以期实现“突显目的”的作用[13]。

例 5：精气夺则虚。

Deprival of essential Qi leads to deficiency.

（注：例 1～例 5 选自李照国主编的《中医英语》[14]）。

R. W. Langacker[15] 曾对名词化的迂回表达问题（periphrasis）进行了研究，指出在名词化过程中，涉及语言的迂回表达问题时，“of”是一个常用的语法标记语，但它不仅标记语法结构，也意味着语义变化。如例 5 中的“deprival of essential Qi”和“the cause of disease”从表面结构上看是相同的，但“of”所体现的关系却大相径庭，后者只表明参与者之间的静态关系，而前者则提示过程，包括动作的状态和动作的对象，没有参与者。句子中“of”后面接的 essential Qi 是 deprival 这个动作状态的接受者，以静态的名词形式表示出动作的过程。

2.2 衔接语篇

名词化隐喻在语篇中的功能主要体现在语篇衔接。这种衔接功能主要是通过建立“主位一述位”衔接而实现，即充当前一句的述位部分的动词名词化后可以充当下一小句的主位部分，“主位一述位”的衔接是实现语篇衔接和连贯的重要手段之一[8]。

例：随着生理活动的变化，血液在各组织器官之间重新分配，这种重新分配也与肝的功能密切相关。

The blood needed by different organs and tissues constantly varies with the change of physiological activities. Such a variation constant variation is also closely related to the function of the liver to store blood[16].

在这个语篇中，前一小句的谓语动词（述位）varies 在后一小句中变成了名词 variation，充当主语（主位）。通常情况下，要想使前句中动词包含的内容变成后句中的主位，在语法结构上就需要将该动词结构转换成名词结构，即把表示动作的动词转换成表示状态的名词，这样就把两个小句在语义上衔接起来，因为词汇结构上的变化也会产生语义表达上的相应变化，这也是名词化语法隐喻的效果之一。

综上所述，名词化结构是进行中医文本英译的常用手段，它主要通过翻译视角的切换、句子结构及词性的变化、语义表达方式的改变来体现语篇的客观、严谨和高度逻辑性。但在使用这一手段时，不能仅仅停留在表层结构或词汇含义的对应上，也不仅仅是单纯的词性转化，必须从深层次剖析原文的意义，理清句与句之间以及词组与词组之间的关系，确定哪些结构需要名词化以及如何进行名词化。同时要对整个句子进行重新整合，并根据需要删减或添加某些成分。尤其是医古文，由于语言非常简洁，句法上也有别于现代汉语，有时甚至给人晦涩之感，所以首先必须花足够的时间和精力透彻理解原文的中文意义，其次再考虑如何选择恰当的句式和词汇将其翻译成英文，使原文的精髓得到充分的体现。由于英语名词化隐喻是一种比较抽象且正式的书面语言，而中医语言一般都高度抽象，概括性强，所以在翻译成英文时适合大量使用名词化短语，使译文和原文在语言风格上也能保持一致。但另一方面，也要把握好名词化的度，而且要考虑潜在的读者群，不能无限制无条件地使用，避免造成语篇信息密度过大，晦涩难懂，甚至造成误解，这就违反了翻译的根本原则，也达不到翻译的基本目的和应有效果。

参考文献

[1] 戴维・克里斯特尔编. 现代语言学词典. 沈家煊译. 北京：商务印书馆，2000：240.
[2] Halliday MAK. Introduction to functional grammar. London：Arnold，1994：352－353.
[3] 王晋军. 名词化在语篇类型中的体现. 外语学刊，2003，113（2）：74－78.
[4] 范文芳，汪明杰. 论三大流派对英语名词化现象的研究. 外语研究，2003，79（3）：15－18.
[5] 杨小虎，王君，吴雅凤. 名词化的主流学派研究. 重庆大学学报（社会科学版），2004，10（5）：101－106.
[6] 谢遐均. 医学英语语篇中名词化隐喻的功能及翻译. 西北医学教育，2009，17（5）：1019－1012.
[7] 连淑能. 英汉语对比研究. 北京：高等教育出版社，2006：104.
[8] 范文芳. 名词化隐喻的语篇衔接功能. 外语研究，1999，（1）：9－12.
[9] 靖安典. 名词化语法隐喻及其理解. 宜春学院学报，2011，33（1）：177－179，139.
[10] 胡壮麟. 语法隐喻. 外语教学与研究，1996，108（4）：1－7.
[11] 胡壮麟. 评语法隐喻的韩礼德模式. 外语教学与研究，2002，32（2）：88－94.
[12] Chomsky N. Language and mind. New York：Harcourt Brace Jovanovich，1968：107.
[13] 胡壮麟. 语篇的衔接与连贯. 上海：上海外语教育出版社，1994：262.
[14] 李照国. 中医英语. 上海：上海科技出版社，2009：108，26，51，116.
[15] Langacker RW. Foundation of cognitive grammar（VOl. Ⅴ）：descriptive application. California：Stanford University Press，1991：22－50.
[16] 吴昌国. 中医基础理论. 上海：上海浦江教育出版社，2002：59.

［原载《中国中西医结合杂志》，2013，33（5）：701－704.］

“东方情调化翻译”在两套中医名词术语英译标准化方案中的体现

李永安

中医翻译在走过漫长的道路之后，终于在2007年和2008年迎来了两套译名标准化方案：WHO亚太西区的传统医学名词术语国际标准[1]（主要为中医译名）和世界中医药联合会的中医基本名词术语中英文对照国际标准[2]。这两套译名标准化方案的问世是中医翻译和中医对外交流史上的一个重要里程碑。纵观两套译名标准化方案，有许多译名显现出“东方情调化翻译”方法。

1. 什么是东方情调化翻译

“东方情调化翻译”是从西方翻译家L. Venuti的“异国情调化翻译”（exoticization）演变而来的。所谓“异国情调化翻译”就是“翻译的效果产生一种表面的差异，一般涉及外国文化的一些特征，如地理、风俗、烹饪、历史人物和历史事件；保留外国地名和人名，或者一些怪异的外国词汇。”[3]顺应这种思路，我们不妨将汉籍英译中的“异国情调化翻译”更具体地称为“东方情调化翻译（orientalization)”。我们以C. Birch翻译中国经典《牡丹亭》里的例子加以说明：①“一名廪生陈最良，年可六旬，从来饱学。”（第5出）“…a scholar by the name of Chen Zuiliang. He filled his belly with books. ”[4] ②“虽然是饱学名儒，腹中饥，峥嵘胀气。”（第13出）“Scholar of note，though stuffed with learning. ”[4]③“经史腹便便，昼梦人还倦。”（第6出）“…mine too/bulging with weight of classics and histories. ”[4]以上3个例子中，C. Birch运用“东方情调化翻译”方法，直接仿照汉语，将两处“饱学”译成“filled his belly with books”和“stuffed with learning”，将“经史腹便便”直译成“bulging with weight of classics and histories”。这种东方情调化翻译方法不但充分揭示出其语义，而且完全保留了其汉语表达方式，使得译文隐喻的意象充满了东方情调，生动而表现力强，同时也丰富了英语的表达习惯和方法。再看以下两个例子：④“正如此想间，只见那生向前说了几句伤心话儿，将奴搂抱去牡丹亭畔，芍药东边，共成云雨之欢。”（第10出）“But just as this was in my mind he came close and began to speak fond words to me，then taking me into his arms he carried me to a spot beside the peony pavilion beyond the railings lined with tree peonies，and there together we were fond of the joys of cloud and rain. ”[4]⑤“则为这断鼓零钟金字经，叩动俺黄粱境。”（第27出）“But all these random drumbeats，/striking of bells，/intonings of precious scriptures / break in upon my yellow-millet dreams.[4]在这2个例子中，C. Birch将“云雨之欢”和

“黄粱境”译成“joys of cloud and rain”和“my yellow-millet dreams”。众所周知，“云雨之欢”是男欢女爱的隐讳说法；而“黄粱境”也就是“黄粱梦”，意为想要实现的愿望落空。这种按照汉语字面意思的翻译，不加说明和注释的方法，通过大胆、奇异、出人意料的译文，让读者可以强烈感受到原文的神秘、怪异、情趣和美感，给人留下了无限遐想的空间，使人充分感受这来自东方语言情调的魅力。有时，为了追求这种东方情调化翻译效果，西方一些翻译家尽量模仿汉语的表达形式，甚至不惜出现一些语法错误。请看以下例子：⑥“两情和合，真是个千般爱惜，万种温存。”（第10出）“Passion was matched by passion, and indeed a thousand fond caresses, a million tendernesses passed between us.”[4]在此句中，众所周知，tenderness是一个抽象名词，不可数，但C. Birch用a million修饰tenderness，出现a million tendernesses。这种不顾译文语法错误，一味保留原文形式的东方情调化翻译，做到了向英语读者传达原文的语言和文化，感觉到原文的语言和文化的异质性，以及异国情调。

2. 东方情调化翻译方法在两套标准化方案中的体现

根据笔者统计，两套标准化方案中大约1/3的译名体现了这种东方情调化翻译方法。限于文章篇幅，只能分门别类，说明东方情调化翻译方法在中医名词术语翻译中的几种应用（文章译例选自WHO亚太西区的传统医学名词术语国际标准[1]者标记为WHO；选自中医基本名词术语中英文对照国际标准[2]者标记为WFCMS）。

2.1 一些中医疾病的译名

例如，在WHO方案中，“青风”“雷头风”“慢脾风”等被分别翻译成“bluish wind”“thunder head wind”“chronic spleen wind”等。事实上，“青风”相当于西医中的“开角型青光眼”（angle-opening glaucoma）。WHO方案并没有将这个病名按照交际翻译法译成西方人容易明白的“angle-opening glaucoma”，而是采用东方情调化翻译法，对应汉语译成“bluish wind”，可以让读者了解中医独特的病因病机理论。同样，“雷头风”和“慢脾风”也没有按照两个病名的实际含义，释义性译成“swollen head with thundering sound and ache”和“chronic infantile convulsion due to dysfunction of spleen”，而是对应汉字，采用东方情调化翻译方式译成“thunder head wind”和“chronic spleen wind”，也是出于同样的原因。

2.2 一些独特的疗法以及与五行学说有关的译名

中医基础理论建立在中国古代哲学，特别是阴阳学说和五行学说的基础上，因此，中医名词术语中充满了哲学术语。例如，在两个标准化方案里，“釜底抽薪”“培土生金”“土不制水”等分别被对照汉语直接译成“taking away firewood from under the cauldron”（WFCMS，WHO），“banking up earth to generate metal”（WFCMS），“earth failing to control water”（WFCMS）等。两套标准化方案没有将上述 3 个名词释义性翻译出其医学含义，而是按字面对译，这种东方情调化翻译保留了中医语言中独特的哲学色彩和特有的文化信息。

2.3　一些与儒学有关的译名

儒学丰富和发展了中医学，因此，中医语言里也有不少儒学词汇。例如，“君药”“臣药”“君火”等充分体现了中医里的儒学理论。两个标准化方案将这几个名词分别直接译成“sovereign medicinal”（WFCMS）、“minister medicinal”（WFCMS，WHO）、“sovereign fire”（WHO），而没有按归化翻译法分别译成西方读者更容易懂的“principal medicinal”“adjuvant medicinal”“heart fire”，这样的译名保持了中医文化的特异性，体现了东方情调化特色。

2.4　一些解剖部位译名

由于中医学理论的独特性，加上在早期中医学理论形成时人体解剖知识的欠缺，这样就形成了中医中一些独特的表示解剖部位的名词，例如，“寸关尺”“膜原”“宗筋”“玄府”等。“寸关尺”指中医诊脉时布指的具体部位，桡骨茎突处为关，关前腕端为寸，关后肘端为尺。不论是两个方案中的音译“cun，guan，chi ”（WFCMS，WHO），还是字面对译的“inch，bar and cubit”（WFCMS，WHO），都体现了东方情调化翻译方法，使译名保留了中医学理论特色。这种翻译在对外交流中，可以充分体现中医与其他医学体系的不同。同样，将“膜原”（胸膜与膈肌之间的部位）、“宗筋”（阴部或阴茎）、“玄府”（汗孔）对照汉语分别译成“membrane source”（WFCMS，WHO），“ancestral sinew”（WHO），“mysterious mansion”（WHO），也体现了东方情调化翻译方法。

2.5　一些中医方剂的译名

我们看看下面一组中药方剂学名词的翻译：十八反——eighteen antagonisms（WFCMS，WHO），十九畏——nineteen incompatibilities，四气——four Qi（WHO），辛甘发散为阳——pungent and sweet with dispersing effect pertaining to Yang（WFCMS），辛甘化阳——pungent and sweet transforming into Yang（WFCMS）等。这一组名词的翻译和前面的例⑥一样，为了保持与汉语用词和结构的一致，甚至不惜出现译名中的语法错误。众所周知，“antagonism”“incompatibility”“Qi”等在英语中一般为抽象名词，无复数，而“antagonism”和“incompatibility”都用了复数；“Qi ”前面有数词“four”，却没有用复数；“pungent”只是形容词，其名词为 pungency。在“辛甘发散为阳”的译名“pungent and sweet with dispersing effect pertaining to Yang”中，按照语法“pungent”应为名词“pungency”；“辛甘化阳”译名“pungent and sweet transforming into Yang”中，“pungent”同样应为“pungency”。这种为了与汉语对应，不惜牺牲英语语法规

范的译名，在两个标准化方案中还有不少。这些译名都充分体现了东方情调化翻译方法。

3. 如何看待东方情调化翻译

作为东方情调化翻译的代表人，C. Birch 采用这种方法翻译的《牡丹亭》在西方的反应如何？当 1980 年 C. Birch 翻译的《牡丹亭》问世后，许多人怀疑这种近乎死译式的翻译是否能够适合舞台表演的需要。然而，出乎人们意料，这个译本很受欢迎，以此为基础的舞台表演也大获成功，而且经久不衰[5]。这说明 C. Birch 抓住了西方人的心理需要，其充满东方情调化翻译的语言符合他们对东方作品的文化心理的预期。那么，两套中医名词术语译名标准化方案中的这部分体现了东方情调化翻译方法的译名，其效果到底怎么样？自从两套方案问世两年多来，至今尚未有明显的反对声和批评文章。相反，我们看到的是大家都在努力维护和推广这一来之不易的成果，这本身就是对两个标准化方案的认可。正像语言没有优劣性一样，世界上的文化也无优劣之分。中医语言作为中国语言的一部分，同时也是中国文化的一部分。两套标准化方案中的东方情调化翻译方法的体现是保持中医特色的有效方法，也是向世界传播中医文化和中国文化的重要途径。21 世纪是一个多民族文化共存、齐放异彩的世纪。随着中国的经济地位和综合国力的提升，中国文化必将越来越备受关注，影响也会越来越大。积极大胆地向世界传播中国文化是广大翻译工作者义不容辞的任务。东方情调化翻译方法同样是传播中国文化的重要途径之一。

参考文献

[1] World Health Organization. (WHO) international standard terminologies on traditional medicine in the western Pacific region. Geneva: The Office of Publication, WHO, 2007.

[2] 李振吉，贺兴东，王奎主编. 中医基本名词术语中英文对照国际标准. 北京：人民卫生出版社，2008.

[3] 蒋骁华. 典籍英译中的“东方情调化翻译倾向”研究. 中国翻译，2010，30 (4)：40-45.

[4] Birch C. The peony pavilion. New Pelhi: Indiana University Press, 2002: 12, 20, 51, 63, 152.

[5] Wang RP. The peony pavilion. Beijing: Foreign Languages Press, 2000: 119.

[原载《中国中西医结合杂志》，2011，31 (11)：1570-1572.]

中医英译的语言学思考

江　楠

罗曼·雅各布森（R. Jakobson，1896—1982）是布拉格语言学派的代表人物，他对翻译理论的主要贡献体现在《论翻译的语言学问题》（*On Linguistic Aspects of Translation*，1959）一文中[1]。雅各布森将翻译分为语内翻译（intralingual translation）、语际翻译（interlingual translation）和符际翻译（intersemiotic translation）。语内翻译是指用同一种语言中的一些语言符号解释另一些语言符号，即释义。语际翻译是我们平常所理解的翻译，是指用一种语言符号解释另一种语言符号，即不同语言之间的翻译。符际翻译是指用非语言符号，如图标、手势、美术、音乐等解释语言符号。中医英译目前存在很多争论，如术语问题，使用拉丁语还是现代英语来命名，如何统一这些术语；文体问题，要不要保留“四字格”；文化问题，中医英译是不是文化翻译，等等。本文借鉴 R. Jakobson 对翻译的分类，从语内翻译及语际翻译出发，对比佛经翻译的语素化现象来说明中医学的语内翻译和语际翻译，以最佳关联作为翻译新标准，建议采用希腊语、拉丁语词素和合成法创立术语。

1. 语内翻译

我们在讨论普通的翻译活动时，语内翻译通常被忽略。但是，就中医翻译而言，语内翻译显得尤为重要。在中医药典籍的翻译所面临的诸多问题中，无善本居其首。“清季萧延平曾为此发过一番议论：‘自来校书，苦无善本，医书尤甚。盖中国自科举制兴，凡聪明才智之士，多趋重词章声律之文，即间有卓荦异材，又或肆力于经史汉宋诸学，於医学一门，辄鄙为方技而不屑为。故自林亿等校正医书后，从事此道者实不多觏，晦盲否塞，几近千年，纰缪纠纷，问津无路’（《黄帝内经太素·例言》），因此，古代医书中的文字讹误现象便尤胜他书，校勘整理任务极其艰巨，工作亟待深入，意义至关重大。”[2]目前，中医古籍白话文版本非常少，这对中医药典籍的英译工作带来不小的压力。白话文的重要性体现在它是古代汉语与外语之间的一个重要中介。白话文的句法结构有许多西方语言的句法特征，而这一转向又直接来源于“五·四”时期翻译文体对古代汉语的影响。把医古文翻译为白话文，有利于我们对于医古文词组之间逻辑关系的把握。我们应该抓住并利用白话文的这个特点，这样才能使译文读起来更流畅，更像英文。中医药典籍之“善本”对于热衷于中国传统医学以及致力于中医药翻译事业的后辈们来说将大有裨益。

2. 语际翻译

2.1　对等与翻译的标准

“道”与“逻各斯（logos）”这对中西哲学的最高范畴引出东西文化系统各自的特点。从符号取向上看，“道”与“尚象”的思维方式相关，采用“言象互动”的符号系统；“逻各斯”则同理性思辨相关，采用语言逻辑符号系统。中西方文化在此分道扬镳。既然它们之间不能对等，那还能够翻译吗？赵彦春把翻译定义为“一个对源语进行（语内或语际）阐释的明示——推理活动，an act of ostensive-inferential (intralingual or interlingual) interpretation of a source text”[3]。赵彦春是在关联理论的框架下对翻译进行定义的。在关联理论看来，交际基于两个基本条件：①交际双方的“互明”（mutual manifestness）；②最佳的认知模式，即关联性。这两个基本条件构成了关联理论的明示——推理模式。翻译是一个交际过程，翻译过程是动态的，因为交际双方的认知结构和认知环境是不定的；源语交际者和译者构成交际的双方，译者和译语接受者构成的第二轮的交际双方，其认知结构和认知语境又有了进一步差异。此外，不同语言构成的语篇或文本因语义和文化等因素的限制，不可能完全对等。我们认为中医英译的任务不仅仅是完成语码转换这个过程，而应该在源语作者和译语接受者不同的认知语境之间，尽一切可能创造最佳关联。最佳关联最基本的要求是中医英译创造的符号系统是自我完备的，对中医理论的叙述是准确有效的，英译文本具有较高的可读性并有利于译语接受者进行推理。直译、意译、音译等都只是为建立最佳关联所应用的手段罢了。通过翻译，建立最佳关联才有利于译语接受者加深对中医学的认识。

2.2　词、概念和事物

语言是具有表征性的。语言不能穷尽事物的所有特征，所以只能以符号代表某一事物。词、概念和事物之间的关系如图 1 所示：词与事物通过概念相连。语言的形式与意义之间是“一”与“多”的关系，这是人类语言的特点。比如：土豆、洋芋、山药蛋都是指同一事物；而“北京”这一个词既指一个城市，又指我们的首都，在新闻媒体中又特指中国政府。正是这样的一与多关系，使我们的语言变得经济，体现出有限的手段无限的运用。中医语言更是如此，阴、阳无所不指。阴、阳是对所有相关事物的相对属性或同一事物本身存在的对立双方属性的概括。从阴、阳衍生出阴气与阳气、心阴与心阳、肝阴与肝阳、少阴与少阳等词汇来表达中医的概念。

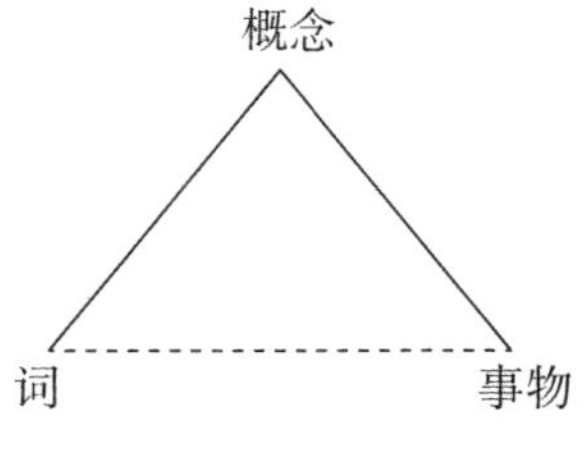

图 1　词、概念事物之间的关系

袁洪仁在《谈经络学说术语的英译》一文中认为“文献中将‘经络’译作‘channels and collaterals’或‘meridian’，这种意译令人费解。根据《黄帝内经》对经络的论述及现代经络研究的结果，表明经络结构包括血管网络（血行脉中）、神经网络（气行脉外）和感传网络（经气游行），故‘经络’应译作‘neurovaso-Qiduct’，意为‘神经血管性气导管’。这种译法既表达了经络原有神经血管解剖学基础的事实，又表达了经络‘内属于脏腑，外络于肢节’之类神经血管必然的网络形态。加上后缀‘-Qiduct’又区别于解剖学上的神经血管，表达了中医经络‘行气血’的功能特征”[4]。我们对于同一事物的理解可能千差万别。对“经络”一词下定义，一百个人就有一百种说法。但是，理解上的千差万别只体现于内涵，而不是外延。语言不能穷尽事物的所有特征，即便是把“经络”翻译成neurovaso-Qiduct，这个符号真的就完全体现出经络“血行脉中、气行脉外、经气游行”的意思吗？经络是人体运行气血的通道，“通道”二字是不会变的。外延决定了其词义相对稳定的成分。把“经络”翻译成 channels and collaterals 或 meridian，不是不准确，而是给大家留下进一步阐释的空间。如果不这样做，势必出现一个形式对应一个概念的情况。但是，经络的内涵每丰富一次，我们的术语就要修改一次，术语就永远都固定不下来。阴阳五行、气血津液、脏象、经络等中医学基本概念的内涵相当丰富，这些词的英译，无论采用拉丁语，还是现代英语，都只能翻译其词义稳定的部分，即外延，只有这样，术语才能够相对固定下来。

2.3 拉丁语与现代英语之争

李永安认为“不应提倡使用已经死亡的拉丁语来翻译中医，而应该使用国际上广泛使用的现代英语”，“也许这些术语的译文是准确的，但是却难记、难读、难写。拉丁语是一种死亡的语言”[5]。长期以来，M. Porket 教授致力于用拉丁语翻译中医术语，如：风 ventus、实 replete、寒 algor、肾 orbisrendlis、涌泉 fons-scateus、心 orbis、虚 inanis 等。

我们认为，中医术语的英译可以用希腊语、拉丁语词素（affixation）和合成法（compounding）来创立，用汉语拼音甚至是中文汉字作为辅助，而用现代英语为其作出解释，以此建立最佳关联。首先，西医术语大多都是由希腊语或拉丁语词素合成、派生而成的。在为新发现的疾病和症状命名时，医学家总是寻找希腊和拉丁语词素构成新词，这一点是西医术语的特征。其次，我们以佛经翻译来做对比。外来词的单音节语素化[6]在佛经翻译中起到非常大的作用。梵语是拼音文字，汉语是象形文字。梵语往往是多音节的，而汉语音节简单。语素化的结果是被缩略的多音节词，比如以“佛”代替了“佛陀、浮屠”，可以作为语素参与汉语构词，构词能力大大加强。仅以“佛”为例子，就有“借花献佛、立地成佛、佛眼相看、泥多佛大、择佛烧香”等。汉语中约有 35 000 个词汇出自佛经翻译。这些词汇被进入汉语系统，沿用至今，可见其影响力之大。

刁骧谈到了用希腊语、拉丁语词素构建的中医术语具有简洁、专业、规范、交际性强、便于掌握、便于检索的特点[7]，例如“里热”endopyrexia（heat-syndrome in the interior of human body）与“风眩”anemogenous dizziness（dizziness due to the wind-evil）。如果编写一本英汉中医词典，我们总是需要一个西文符号来代替“里热”作为head word收入词典。如果用heat-syndrome in the interior of human body，那么这是一个很长的词组，而不是一个词。endopyrexia却更像一个词，更具有术语味。在词典中，我们用拉丁语词素构成的语言符号endopyrexia或者合成词interior heat作为首字，heat-syndrome in the interior of human body作为其解释，并且附上“里热”二字以及其汉语拼音，甚至可以列出“里热”的来源，这样做就可以建立最佳关联。

笔者认为使用拉丁语来翻译是不切实际的，而用希腊语、拉丁语词素和合成法来创立中医英译术语是可行的，并且体现了有限的手段且无限的运用。这与中医学的从阴阳、五行衍生出一切的思想相契合。可以设想，如同佛经翻译所经历的单音节语素化一样，用希腊语、拉丁语词素和合成法创立的中医学术语是可以进入西方语言体系的。目前越来越多的西方人士对中医充满兴趣。随着人们的使用，这些词汇中的一部分将逐步稳定下来，正式进入英文词库，这难道不是文化交流吗？德国哲学家海德格尔曾经说过“语言是人类存在的家园”。还有什么东西比语言更具有影响力？这些词汇虽然“形”是西方的，可“神”却是中医的。

3. 结语

中医的语内翻译是对中国传统医药文化进行丰富，使民族文化得以传承的过程。外国人用“死”的希腊语、拉丁语来创立中医术语，其实质也是为了使希腊语和拉丁语在一定范围内得以复兴，是从语言上丰富本族文化的一种途径。一个民族的文化如果得不到丰富、发展与交流，必将消逝。中医的语际翻译中所出现的种种问题是东西方文明碰撞、冲突的体现。这些问题有待在进一步的文化交流中，即在中医英译的过程中慢慢理解，逐渐交融，并得以解决。

最后，以荀子的话来结束本文的讨论，“名无固宜，约之以命。约定俗成谓之宜，异于约则谓之不宜。名无固实，约之以命实。约定俗成谓之实名。名有固善，径易而不拂，谓之善名。”

参考文献

[1] Jakobson R. On linguistic aspects of translation// L. Venuti. The translation studies reader. London and New York：Routledge，1967：113－118.

[2] 段逸山．比较异同寻求确据——古医籍校勘方法举要．医古文知识，2004，(1)：42.

[3] 赵彦春．翻译学归结论．上海：上海外语教育出版社，2005：121-128.
[4] 袁洪仁．谈经络学说术语的英译．中国中西医结合杂志，2001，21（3）：198.
[5] 李永安，李经蕴．奈达的翻译理论在中医翻译中的应用．中国中西医结合杂志，2006，26（9）：858.
[6] 苏新春．当代汉语外来单音语素的形成与提取．中国语文，2003，（6）：549-558.
[7] 刁骧，胡幼平．浅谈词素翻译法在中医翻译中的应用．中国中西医结合杂志，2006，26（3）：266-268.

[原载《中国中西医结合杂志》，2009，29（6）：551-552.]

中医术语英译标准化讨论

杨伊凡

从 20 世纪 70 年代针灸热开始，中医术语英译标准化的问题就一直受到各国同行的关注，不少专家为此做过很多努力。国内外学者也出版了不少有关这方面的辞书，各种中医、针灸书籍和教科书的英译本更是大量发行。对于中医术语英译的讨论也长期进行，《中国中西医结合杂志》的相关栏目也进行了大量讨论。通过大家的努力，中医术语英译标准化得到不断的完善，从而产生了《针灸教育中医术语英译标准词汇》（以下简称《标准词汇》）。应该说，这是目前最好的版本。其主要特色表现在：保持中医术语的特色，词能达意，简明、简洁，容易理解，用词标准化，易被国外同行接受等。

1. 拼音

《标准词汇》强调应该尽量少使用拼音，我认为这个原则是对的。但对于用英文词汇确实不能清楚、明了或不能传神地表达的一些中医词汇，使用拼音表达仍不失为是一个较好的方式。如本书中的“阴阳”（Yin，Yang），“气”（Qi）等保留拼音是很好的。但有一些词汇如完全取消拼音则觉得不能完全表达原来中医术语的意思，如把“营”这个常用中医术语完全改成用“nutrition”或相关的词则有时不能表达原意。如“nutritive Qi”表示“营气”则没问题，但用“nutrient-system syndrome”来表达“卫气管血”的“营分证”则未能很好地说明疾病传变和程度的原意。如保留拼音，用“Ying syndrome”或“Ying level”或许更原汁原味。同理，“卫分证”译为“defense-system syndrome”也没有“Wei syndrome”表达得那么全面。又如“神”，《标准词汇》使用“vitality”和“mind”，“精神”则使用“spirit”。但中医“神”这个词的含义非常广，在生理、病理、治疗、健康上又侧重不同的意思。我发现澳大利亚当地的中医针灸师非常喜欢和常用“Shen”来表达中医术语中有关“神”的意思。如临床上要表达“神不守舍”“热伤心神”“养心安神”等，以上英语单词好像不能完全概括所要表达的意思。还有“寸、关、尺”，如果使用“inch、bar、cubit”似乎还没有原来的“Cun、Guan、Chi”那么好。

2. 字母

《标准词汇》中全部中医术语的英译词汇都用小写，我不太理解其中的用意或规则。教科书和文献亦有不少使用小写的。中医术语是和一般语言或者是西医专业用语是有区别的。即使用同一词汇，但它们往往表达了不同的意思和内涵。这些不同是通过什么形式表达出来呢？我认为采用词头大写的方式比使用括号或粗体、斜体好些。如中医五脏的“心、肝、脾、肺、肾”与西医的脏腑器官“heart，liver，spleen，lung，kidney”采用完全相同的词汇，但中医同行都知道，中西医五脏的内涵是有很大不同的，而我们却用一模一样的方式来表达！如果使用“Heart，Liver，Spleen，Lung，Kidney”，即词头大写的方式来表达中医的五脏又如何？对内行者来说即使是用字母小写的词汇也能明白含义，但中医的英文出版物有可能面对的是广大群众和西医专业人员，如果没有不同的表达，他们很容易感到困惑。同理，书中还有大量这类词汇均可考虑用词头大写以示区别。如“风、寒、暑、湿、燥、火”——“wind，cold，heat，damp，dryness，fire”。如果“wind”“cold”用小写词头，你认为它指天气吗？如果换成大写词头“Wind”“Cold”，则比较容易理解为中医的风寒感冒。对中医而言，“热毒”证（Heat and Toxin）患者在西医检查时可能全部指标正常。但如果说“toxin，poison”在某人体内，他会感到怎么样？又如中医的“郁证”可译成“depression”，但是西医的“抑郁症”并不贴切中医的原意，不过如果没有特别贴切词汇的话，就使用词头大写“Depression”，那意境就好得多。许多中西医的同一词汇其含义同中有异，这一点是肯定的，如何表达这种异，应该是中医术语英译标准化所要尽量体现到的。

3. 词意

中医术语英译实质是东西方文化交流的一部分。东西方文化之间存在不同是肯定的。如何用英语的词来达到中医术语的意是一项很艰巨的工作。《标准词汇》在这方做得很出色，当然也还存在一些值得进一步推敲的地方。中医词汇有“嘈杂吞酸”。本书将“吞酸”译为“acid swallowing”，把“反酸”译为“acid regurgitation”。按照临床实际，以上两词应均指胃酸反流的意思。实际上使用“acid regurgitation”即可，而“swallowing”则不免觉得有点儿牵强。“纳呆”也是临床常用的术语，译成“anorexia”（“厌食症”也是这个词）似显得过重，如果使用“poor appetite”或“loss of appetite”似比较贴切一些。将“虫积证”译成“worm accumulation syndrome”又显得太过直译一点，如果采用“parasitic worm syndrome”可能会显得更医学专业化。“气滞血瘀”在中医术语中使用率特别高，被译为“blood stasis due to Qi stagnation”（血瘀是由于气滞所引起），而临床上所要表达的意思则多是气滞和血瘀同在，因此，不如建议使用“Qi stagnation and blood stasis”或者“Qi and blood stagnation”。还有一个常用术语是“五心烦热”，《标准词汇》的译文是“vexing heat in the chest，palms and soles”，意思是中医所说的“烦热在胸口、手掌和脚心”，这个词的另一个常用译文为“five heart hots”，极为形象化。我问学生以上两个词要选哪个，他们选择后者。又如“止泻”，用“checking diarrhea”似乎又觉得生硬了一点儿，可考虑译为“relieving diarrhea”或“stopping diarrhea”。

总之，标准化的意义在于为一个中医术语选择一个最恰当的英译，在多个英译词汇都可以表达这个词的情况下，就需要讨论推敲需要考虑的因素，包括保持中医特色、词能达意、简洁明了、习惯用语、专业化、形象化、约定俗成等。

［原载《中国中西医结合杂志》，2004，24（6）：569.］

中医文献英译的文化对等

梁俊雄

翻译是两种语言沟通的桥梁，译者在翻译时必然会介绍与传播源语所体现的文化。但是由于不同民族之间文化差异的存在，文化意蕴的传达必然会成为翻译中的难点和障碍。美国著名的翻译理论家 E. Nida 就说过："对于真正成功的翻译而言，熟悉两种文化甚至比掌握两种语言更重要，因为词语只有在其作用的文化背景中才有意义"[1]，所以他又指出："Language and culture cannot exist without each other"[2]。语言是文化的组成部分，是文化的载体，各民族的语言必然反映出该民族所处社会的特定文化，使用不同语言的民族之间必然存在文化差异，而这种文化差异就构成了翻译的障碍。从这个意义来说，翻译的目的之一就是要在源语（source language）和目的语（target language）之间建立文化对等（cultural equivalence）。在构成翻译对等的诸多方面，文化对等是一个不可或缺的重要对等。文化对等的原则要求译者积极介绍源语的文化意蕴，努力传达原作的文化特色，忠实地再现原作的整体文化氛围。

文化因素在中国典籍（当然也包括中医文献）的翻译中都可能遇到，与此相关的一些词语也是翻译中最难处理的，其一，涉及对此类词的理解问题，其二，涉及如何使其译文既能为外国读者所理解，又能与原文的意思"对等"。严格地说，医学属于文化范畴，医学的发展实系于其文化母体，与文化母体有着千丝万缕的联系。中医学与中国的人文地理条件及主导的传统文化有着相互依存的关系。在中医文献中，许多术语言简意丰，经历了历史文化的积淀，反映了汉族的社会状况、宗教信仰、价值观念等，蕴含着丰富的文化含义，往往难以在英语中找到同等的表达方法。作为"文化使者"的译者，应遵循文化对等的原则，使用各种翻译方法最大限度地传递源语中的文化意蕴，因此，进行翻译方法的研究就有着很大意义。下面我们试图从最基本的翻译方法——音译、直译和意译来探讨如何在中医文献英译过程中保持文化对等。

就文化对等而言，能够最忠实地传递原文的文化意蕴的翻译方法就是音译。现代英语词汇的一个特点就是来源广，外来词多。它已向世界各国语言借用了50多万个外来词，差不多是英语总词汇量的一半。在各民族之间的文化交流中，对外来文化中独特的现象、概念，如在本民族语言中难以找到对应的词汇翻译，采用音译的方法不失为一种明智的选择，因此，笔者提出，对一些最基本的中医术语，应采用音译的方法[3]。但这种方法有一个缺点，英语和汉语是不同体系，没有专门知识的人看了这种音译术语，根本不知所云。但随着中医影响的扩大，这些术语是能够逐渐为英语学术界所接受的，当然这需要一个过程。目前，运用这种方法应该有所限制，数量由少而多，随着中医影响的扩大，可以逐渐地增加音译的数量。

在译文语言条件许可下，可以用直译法。例如中医的“提壶揭盖”，这是一种治疗方法，意即通过宣通上焦的气机而使下焦腑气畅通，进而达到排出大小便的目的。这个术语非常形象生动，有着很浓厚的中国文化特色。显然，在西医中没有类似的疗法，如果直译为“lifting the lid to pour off water in the pot”，未尝不是一种好方法。这样翻译的好处很多，既保留了源语文化的情调，使读者感到新鲜生动，还传播了源语文化，更加有效地促进文化交流，扩大了读者的知识视野。当然，如果在该术语首次出现时用括号加上解释（opening the lung Qi to treat constipation or dysuria），这样读者就容易明白了。在中医术语英译时，能采用直译法处理的例子很多，例如，“热结旁流”可译为“fecal impaction due to heat with watery discharge”，“风寒束肺”译为“wind-cold tightening the lung”，“风热犯肺”译为“invasion of the lung by wind-heat”，“热胜则肿”译为“excessive heat bringing about swelling”，“炅则气泄”译为“heat may consume vital energy”等就是很好的例子。但是，我们必须认识到，文化对等是相对的，而不是绝对的。在很多情况下，译文与原文能达到的只是一种动态或功能上的对等。例如，中医有脉应四时（seasonal variations of the pulse）的现象，如春应中规（normal taut pulse in spring）、夏应中矩（normal full pulse in summer）、秋应中衡（normal floating pulse in autumn）和冬应中权（normal deep pulse in winter）。何为“规”“矩”“衡”“权”，英语中完全没有相应的概念，如果硬译，势必令人感到如堕五里雾中，所以，我们采用了直译加上某些词素解释性转换的方法是可取的。翻译的时候，同时应该注意到英语民族的文化背景和思维习惯，采用他们能够接受的方式，以减轻读者的阅读负担。译者可以在译文读者思维能力所能接受的情况下，适当地把原作中特有的由异域文化、环境、形象等因素铸成的思维方式再现出来[4]。

在音译法和直译法都不能解决问题的时候，就要求助意译法了。意译要求译文表达原文的意思，但可以不拘泥于原文的形式。例如，中医的“转筋”（俗称抽筋）译成 spasm；“转胞”（指胎儿压迫孕妇的膀胱所致的小便不通）处理为 dysuria due to the pressure of the fetus。语言反映文化，并受着文化的制约。采用意译法时，同样也应考虑到文化等同。在不同的文化里，相同的词语可有不同的文化含义。最典型的一个例子就是龙的概念。在东西方文化里，龙和 dragon 有着完全不同的文化内涵，不同的词语也可以有相同的含义。例如英语 kill two birds with one stone 和汉语的“一箭双雕”，还有 teach one's grandmother to such eggs 和“班门弄斧”等。这样就有了替代的翻译方法，这就是用目的语中带有文化色彩的词语取代源语中带有文化色彩的词语（replace the cultural expressions of the source text with those of the target language），这种翻译方法有利于使目的文读起来像原作一样。英语和汉语分属于不同的文化体系。语言是民族的，但思维是全人类的。对同样的事物，不同的民族可以有同样的认识，而采用各自带有鲜明民族文化色彩的表达形式，如在中医文献英译的时候，能够恰当地运用这种文化转换的替代译法，往往会有意想不到的效果。另外，谚语是语言的食盐，它是人们在自身的实践中锤炼出来的最生动、精练的语言。英语中的谚语更是不胜枚举，其中有一些与中医文化中的一些术语有异曲同工之妙。例如，英语的“a cracked bell can never sound well”与中医的“金破不鸣”，“a great ship asks deep waters”与“增水行舟”就是很好的例子。在翻译这些术语时，恰如其分地运用这些英语民族非常熟悉的谚语，可以加深读者的理解。

我们所说的文化等同，用于中医英语翻译，就是要着眼于译文读者的感受，强调译文对译文读者所起的作用，应与原文对原文接受者所起的作用大体对等。这不能要求译者限于某种固定的译法，而应从各种可能的译法中挑选最接近原文信息、效果和功能的译法。

总之，成功的译者应该有强烈的文化意识，认识到翻译是跨越语言文字、跨越文化的信息交流。而文化的差异和语言的差异一样，可以成为交流障碍。在实现语言转换的同时，还要克服文化差异的障碍，以保证信息交流的顺利实现，因此，我们不仅要精通语言，还要了解和研究语言背后的文化，在正确翻译的前提下，考虑处理文化差异和文化障碍的问题。

［原载《中国中西医结合杂志》，2004，24（3）：269－270.］

从接受理论浅谈中医翻译中的文化传达

张晶晶　戴　琪

美国翻译理论家 E. Nida 指出，“翻译是两种文化之间的交流。对于真正成功的翻译而言，熟悉两种文化甚至比掌握两种语言更重要。因为词语只有在其作用的文化背景中才有意义”[1]，他又指出“Language and culture cannot exist with each other”[2]。这说明翻译要将中西文化结合起来，而离开文化背景去翻译则不可能达到两种语言之间的真正交流。

医学属于文化范畴，医学的发展实系于其文化母体，与文化母体有着千丝万缕的联系。作为医学科学的群体，中医学和西医学研究的都是人体及其疾病的规律，目的都是为了保持和增进人类健康，防病治病。就其研究的主体来说，都是具有特定文化素质的人。英语民族习惯于将事物分解为各个部分，把具体问题从总体中分离出来，把复杂的问题划分为比较简单的形式和部分，然后进行各个部分的研究，从而形成个体或分析思维模式，因此，英语民族在思维形式上具有一种重分析、重形式、讲求精确的显著特征。与西方哲学的分析思维方式不同，汉语民族的思维方式深受儒家、道家与佛教影响，语言重意合、重悟性、重从事物之间总的联系上去认识和把握事物，在思维模式上有重整体、重含蓄、重综合的特点。古人一向有“文以意为主”“意在笔先”“以意役法”的文辞观。中国古代的语言研究也讲究“神而明之”，追求一种意会与顿悟，在语言表达中较注意语言背后的意向，重“意”而轻“言”，得“意”可忘“言”。

中医药是我国的国粹之一，具有鲜明的中华民族特色。中医英译对外交流的实质是一种传统文化的输出[3]。许多中医术语言简意丰，经历了历史文化的沉淀，反映了汉民族的社会状况、宗教信仰、价值观念等，蕴含着丰富的文化含义，往往难以在英语中找到同等的表达法。中医理论产生于古代，是受朴素唯物主义思想支配，以客观的观点综合逻辑思维的方法而建立和发展起来的基础医学理论。如何准确地将中医药学的理论、实践与科研成果介绍到国外，使国外学者能正确理解和接受，以促进中医药国际化，是中医界面临的问题之一。

我们都知道，具体的翻译实践走的是这样一条道路：文本（含有原文化内涵）—译者—译者构造的文本（含有被译者理解的文化内涵）—译者传达的文本（包括译者能够传达的文化内涵）—读者的接受（包括读者所能理解的内涵）。也就是说翻译的终点是读者，而文化翻译更是针对读者而进行的，因此，翻译的成败只能由读者来校验，也就是说，读者是所有以上因素的综合衡量者。安德列·

勒菲弗尔（A. Lefevere）认为翻译的首要任务是译文要让读者看得懂。理想的翻译还要表达原文的言外意义，其中就包括文化效应，所以，文化效应的终点也是读者。由此可见，读者在翻译中的地位是绝对不容忽视的，文化传达更应该是以读者为第一优先考虑。

对于具有文化内涵的中医理论，翻译中一般有两种出路，即归化策略（domesticating method）和以美国翻译理论家 L. Venuti 为代表的异化策略（foreignizing method）。归化是采用民族中心主义态度，是外语文本符合译语的文化价值观，把原作者带入译语文化，在强势文化中较多采用这种方法。在中医名词术语的翻译中也不乏这样的例子。比如借用英文词汇 cold 表示寒，heat 表示热。《韦氏词典》对这两词的解释为："Cold，naturally without heat—used in ancient and medieval sciences to describe one of the four qualities of the four elements. Heat，one of the fundamental qualities of body's elements，or humors recognized in medieval physiology"，这与中医寒、热的内涵相吻合。

与归化相比，在现代中医的翻译中，异化的手法更加常见。异化是指在文化价值观偏离主义的压力下，接受外语文本的语言及文化差异，把读者带入外国情境。20 世纪 80 年代，在 WHO 的组织下，国际上对针灸经穴英译名采用汉语拼音作了统一规范。又如目前等于文化输出的音译造词法[4]，阴、阳、五脏六腑、寸关尺三部、风气命三关、三焦、卫气营、六经病等，这些词表面看来似乎存在相应的英文词语，但从它们所表达的丰富中医内涵而言，却无法找到相应的译语。一般都主张将相关词汇音译为：Yin、Yang、Zang、Fu、Cun、Guan、Chi、Feng、Qi、Ming、Tri-jiao、Wei、Qi、Ying、Taiyang disease、Yangming disease、Shaoyang disease 等。又如用汉语拼音法表示中药方剂名已经完全可以满足交流的需要，并且可以避免不必要的误解[5]。这些异化的方法明显得到认可，在一定程度上促进"中国英语"步入外来词的行列，同时也维护了中医文体语言的原始气质与色调[6]。

E. Nida 将翻译过程分为 4 个阶段：分析、转换、重组与检验[7]。在检验的阶段无疑读者才具有最大的发言和评判的权力。校验的标准就是 E. Nida 的著名的"动态对等"或后来的"功能对等"。翻译是力争朝着"最高层次的对等"的靠近，而"最低层次的对等"则是基本要求。这些对等都受读者的文化背景知识限制。当代读者反映论和接受理论都强调读者对译文的参与作用。在功能对等翻译中，译文受者是一个重要因素，是交际活动的参与者（位于翻译道路的最后一环，也是决定性的一环）。当读者理解一篇译文时，他们因受姚斯的"期待视域"（horizon of expectation）的制约会不可避免地对应他们母语的用法或他们本民族文化习惯的知识。所以说中医译文的读者能否正确理解译者所要传达的意思关键不在于语言而在于文化，因此，对文化差异的处理，即是归化还是异化就成了理解译文文化内涵的决定性因素。

我们认为归化和异化各有道理，各有各的用武之地，不能绝对地摒弃任何一方。总体说来，归化大都表现在语言的层面上，为了跨越语言理解的障碍，为了让读者充分理解中医文化，大多数译者同意采用异化策略[8]。但是，说到底，在文化传达问题上的异化是为了最终使得读者做到真正的归化，也就是说使读者把源语经译者所传达的异域视野经自身的文化视野过滤、对比、沉淀而后引起视野的重新定位，在对比中做到对自身文化和源语文化的再认识，即在文化意义上完成真正的归化。著名的英国翻译家魏迺杰先生说，“在西传的过程中，中医并不能为了配合西方人的需求而有所改变。而西方意欲学习中医的人也绝对无法经由一种‘以其本身较为熟悉的知识系统将中医学重新过滤’的学习方式获得成功，他们必须真正地进入中医的世界。总之，只有当翻译者遵循中医原来被接受的传统方式去看待中医学并将中医忠实地翻译出来，才得以为西方真正想学习中医的人士开启一条迈入中医的大道”[9]。

参考文献

[1] Qiu MR. Culture and its translation. Beijing Foreign Languages，1998，(2)：19－22.
[2] Nida E. Language，culture and translation. Beijing Foreign Languages，1998，(3)：29－33.
[3] 周杰．关于中医英译作品内容的思考．中国中西医结合杂志，1996，16（1）：55.
[4] 张庆荣．中医术语英译中的音译．中国中西医结合杂志，1997，17（6）：369－370.
[5] 陆胜年．中医英译方法刍议．广西中医药，1994，17（4）：39－40.
[6] 左连君．不同翻译手段在中医文献翻译中辨证施用．中国中西医结合杂志，2004，24（4）：364-365.
[7] 谭载喜．新编奈达论翻译．北京：中国对外翻译出版公司，1999：66.
[8] 兰凤利．借鉴国外翻译经验和理念，促进国内中医英译事业发展．中国中西医结合杂志，2003，23（8）：627－628.
[9] Nigel Wiseman. 英汉·汉英中医词典．长沙：湖南科学技术出版社，1996，35.

[原载《中国中西医结合杂志》，2005，25（5）：463－464.]

中篇　分论　中医英译实践

第一节　中医基础理论英译实践

试论中医基础理论名词术语英译的标准

余文海

纵观近 20 年来的中医药学术论文和辞书等的英文翻译，所存在的最突出的问题是译词混乱。同一中医名词术语却有各种不同的译语。如《黄帝内经》，笔者所见到的就有三种译法。20 年前，有人译作“The Yellow Emperor's Manual of Internal Medicine”，《汉英医学大词典》（人民卫生出版社，1987）则译作“The Yellow Emperor's Internal Classic”和“The Yellow Emperor's Canon of Internal Medicine”，而 1983 年的《中医杂志》英文版却译作“The Canon of Medicine”。又如对“本草（学）”与“中药（学）”的英译分别为“Materia Medica”和“Chinese Materia Medica”。笔者以为此译法欠妥，虽然两者的含义同出一辙，但名称各不相同。不仅外国读者容易混淆，就是中国读者也不能分辨。为了使“本草（学）”和“中药学”的英译名有所区别，笔者认为“本草（学）”应译作“herbology”为妥。

中医英译的混乱，要求中医学界必须尽快将中医术语的英译统一起来，制定一个英译标准，逐步使之标准化，即规范化。本文就中医名词术语英译的标准及英译标准的具体方法制定进行阐述。

1. 标准

根据上海辞书出版社 1979 年出版的《辞海》的解释，“标准”的定义是：“①衡量事物的准则；②榜样；规范”。美国出版的权威性辞典——《韦氏第 3 版新国际英语足本词典》(*Webster's Third New International Dictionary of the English Language Unabridged*)（1961）对“标准”的定义解释得最为详尽，可扼要地归纳为：①法律性；②权威性；③普遍性（统一性）；④可行性（实用性）；⑤永久性；⑥价值性。以此为纲要，中医名词术语的英译标准同样也必须具有这 6 种特性，不然就不能成为“标准”。

确定一种事物的标准，国家政府的行政干预是一个首要条件，也就是说应具有法律保障。所以，要制定中医名词术语英译标准，必须要有政府的支持，由国家有关部门领衔，组织全国的中、西医专家和语言学家，并邀请国外具有较高英语水平的中医药研究者，共同研究编纂一部全国统一的中医药名词术语英译工具书。全国所有的中医药杂志社和出版部门在审稿时都应以这部工具书为蓝本。

2. 制定英译标准的具体方法

2.1 沿用法

沿用法是指把在含义上与西医完全相同的单词或词组直接套用过来，这是中医英译词汇的主要来源。如“血”译作 blood；“亡血”（即失血、出血、流血、溢血）译作 bleed、bleeding、hemorrhage 或 hemorrhagic；“汗”（即出汗、流汗、发汗）译作 sweat；“热”（即发热、发烧）译作 fever、fevered、feverish 或 febrile；“冷”（即恶寒、作冷、寒战、寒慄）译作 chill、chilliness、chilly 等。

2.2 合成法

合成法有两种方式：①按照英语构词法将英语、拉丁语、希腊语或意大利语的词缀（前缀和后缀）合成一个新词。如笔者合成的“卫、气、营”这三个新的英译词[1]采用的就是这种方法。这种译法用来翻译没有英文对应词的中医术语具有广阔的前景。②将词缀和汉语拼音合起来，构成一个新词，如“手太阴肺经”可译作“Chirotaiyinpulmonic Meridian”，“足太阴脾经”译作“Foottaiyinsplenic Meridian”。

2.3 拼音法

拼音法有两种方式：①汉语拼音：仅适用于含义极为广博精深并已成为一门独立科学学说的没有对应英文词的中医术语。如八纲中的“阴”“阳”分别译作“Yin”“Yang”，或“Yinyang”；六经的名称，如“太阳经”译作“Taiyang Meridian”。还有中药的成方——汤剂、丸、散、膏、丹等均可采用此法。如“桂枝汤”译作“Guizhi Decoction”等。②英汉谐音：挑选尽可能在音和义上与中医术语相一致的英语单词或词语，如脉象中的“浮”“沉”“迟”“数”分别译作“the floating”“the sinking”“the delaying”“the sharpness”等。

2.4 转化法

转化法有两种方式：①词名转化：就是将西医与中医病症完全相同而病名不同的英语单词转化为中医病名，并固定下来。如“结核病”这个西医病名的英文为“tuberculosis”，完全可以用作中医病名“痨瘵”的英译。同样，“肺结核”的英文“pulmonary tuberculosis”可用作“肺痨”的英译。又如“阑尾炎”与“肠痈”也可共用同一英文名“appendicitis”。②语种转化和词性转化：这是一个冲破语种禁锢格局的创举，也是中医术语特定性质所决定的。语种转化就是将含义广而精深并已成为一门独立科学学说的中医词语英语化。按照英语的词法规则将其转化成动词、名词、形容词或副词等为词性转化。如“阴阳学说”可将汉语拼音“Yinyang”按照构词法拼写为“Yinyangology”；[2]将“阴”和“阳”的汉语拼音分别动词化，但要结合词缀与汉语拼音合成法，如“滋阴潜阳”译作“reyin（ing）and deyand（ing）”，“养阴清热”译作“reyin（ing）and deheat（ing）”，“扶阳抑阴”译作“reyang（ing）and deyin（ing）；也可转化为及物动词并有自己的宾语，如“滋养肝肾”或“滋肝（肾）阴”译作“reyin（ing）the liver（kidney）”，“扶脾阳”和“助肾阳”分别译作“reyang（ing）the spleen”和“reyang（ing）the kidney”等，不一一列举。

2.5 派生法

派生法就是将英语原单词根据需要派生出符合中医名词术语的另一个新词。如《伤寒论》中的“汗家”可译作“sweater”，“亡血家”可译作“hemorrhager”。这样翻译比译成“sweating patient”和“bleeding（hemorrhagic）patient”要精练得多，并且保留了原来的风格。

2.6 缩略法

缩略法是指将已经定论的由多个单词组成的冗长句式如书名、病名、经络名或成方名等在文章中第一次全称出现后，取每个单词的第一个字母构成缩略语并注于括号内，下文再次出现时，均用缩略语，以取代全称。如“中医”的译名全称是“Traditional Chinese Medicine”，其缩略语为“TCM”。“TCM”已使用了多年，并为国内外中医学者所熟知，故已成定论，如同“世界卫生组织”的英文缩略语是“WHO”一样。

［原载《中国中西医结合杂志》，1995，15（1）：49－50.］

中医因果关系病名的特征及其翻译

王朝辉　林　岩

中医中有一类病名的特点是病名中的内涵是导致该病发作的致病因素，病名主要用来描述人体的各种病理变化，我们把这类病名统称为因果关系的中医病名。例如：肾虚月经过少（nephrasthenic hypomenorrhea）、肝厥头痛（hepitosgnocope headache）、风热腰痛（anemopyriclumbago）、血虚痹（hemopenic arthralgia）等均属于这类病名。

探讨并掌握其翻译特征有利于这类名词及其他类中医名词术语翻译的标准化。翻译这类中医病名涉及两个方面，一是这类病名本身的特征及其翻译，二是这类病名释文的特征及其翻译。

1. 因果关系病名本身的特征及其翻译

这类病名从词面上就可以领略到因果关系这一特征。目前我国各出版物（如《汉英中医词汇》《汉英中医辞典》《汉英双解常用中医名词术语》）对这类中医病名的翻译通常采用表示因果关系的后置短语来修饰中心词的表达方法。这类表达因果关系的后置短语通常为介词短语、分词短语和形容词短语等，因此，表达这种意义的常用结构为：

名词（中心词）due to 名词（介词短语）

名词（中心词）caused by 名词（过去分词短语）

名词（中心词）resulting from 名词（现在分词短语）

名词（中心词）attributable to 名词（形容词短语）

在翻译中以前两种表达方式为主，因此，"阴虚肺燥"译为"dry lungs due to deficient Yin"，"肾虚经闭"译为"amenorrhea due to the kidney deficiency"，"脏毒便血"译为"melena due to poison in the viscera"，"肾虚不孕"译为"sterility due to the kidney deficiency"，"肺热咳嗽"译为"cough caused by lung heat"。

从语义学上讲，这种译法基本上能将原病名术语所含意义表达出来，但是，作为术语，从词法及结构角度论来说这种翻译法也着实偏长，更欠规范。

西医中也有这类表示因果关系的病名，如细菌性痢疾、菌毒败血症、创伤性出血、尿毒症昏迷等。按上述翻译法，我们可以将这些西医病名分别译为 dysentery due to bacillus，septicemia due to toxemia，hemorrhage caused by trauma，coma due to uremia。

这种译法在语义学上也能表达原意，但是在已规范了的西医翻译中并没有采用上述这种表示因果关系的介词短语、分词短语或形容词短语等修饰语作后置定语修饰中心词，而通常只是将这些后置短语中的名词转变成形容词作前置定语修饰中心词来表达这类西医病名，即："细菌性痢疾"为 bacillary dysentery，"菌毒败血症"为 toxemic septicemia，"创伤性出血"为 traumatic hemorrhage，"尿毒症昏迷"为 uremic coma。

由此可见，西医病名的这种表达法既规范又能使翻译有章可循。与此相比，前述那类中医病名的译法不但在词法结构上偏长，也不符合英语科技术语的翻译，因此，我们可以仿照相应的西医病名的译法来表达这类中医病名。例如："肾虚月经过少"为 nephrasthenic hypomenorrhea，"肝厥头痛"为 hepitosgncope headache，"肾虚不孕"为 nephrasthenic sterility，"肺虚咳嗽"为 pulmopenic cough，"食积胁痛"为 dyspepsic hypochondrialgyia，"胆热多睡"为 cystopyric somnia。

采用这种表达方式后，不但从语义上能清楚地表达病名的意义，而且结构也十分简便。这种译法与同类西医病名的译法相符，无疑为这类中医病名的翻译规范化建立了可遵循的标准。

2. 因果关系病名释文的特征及其翻译

中医中因果关系病名的汉语语篇结构比较规范，通常由以下五部分组成：病名、类别、病因、症见和治则。

例如："闪跌血崩"，病证名。多因登高跌坠，或闪挫受伤，以致冲任失固，恶血下流。腹部按之疼痛。治宜行血祛瘀。

Trauma vaginorrhagia, a syndrome. It is often caused by falling from high, or injury from sprain and contusion which leads to debility of Chong and Ren Channels to release extravastated blood. The said syndrome is characterized by abdominal pain once pressed. It is advisable to follow such a therapeutic principle as promoting blood circulation to remove stasis.

由此可见，①表达"病因"的句型通常用 It is often (usually, mostly) caused by…。②表达"症见"的句型通常有：It is characterized by…；Its manifestations are…；It finds manifestations in…；The main symptoms are…；It is manifestated as…。③表达"治则"的句型往往有：It is advisable to follow such therapeutic principles as doing…；It is advisable to follow the therapeutic principles of doing…；It is applicable to do…

无论从语义学上还是从语篇结构上讲，这类释文汉语本身都比较规范，而且译文所用的句型也比较固定，因此，有利于中医翻译的标准化。这对于中止我国目前中医翻译在该领域的混乱现象，对于指导我国的中医翻译，对于中医翻译的标准化都是有益无害的。

[原载《中国中西医结合杂志》，1994，14（12）：749－750.]

试析中医“证”的几个常见英译名

汤思敏

中医英译目前还缺少一个标准原则，很多中医术语翻译不规范，而作为中医学特色之一，也是核心之一的“辨证论治”中的“证”字，也遭遇翻译不统一的难题。笔者就“证”的几个常见英译名作比较与分析。

1. “证”的内涵

“证”是中医学的特色，是中医学的特有概念。在辨证论治过程中，证的确定是立方、选方、遣药的重要依据。根据《中医基础理论》[1]，所谓证，是指“在疾病发展过程中某一阶段的病理概括。它包括疾病的原因、疾病的部位、疾病的性质和邪正关系，反映了疾病发展过程中，该阶段病理变化的全面情况”。每个具体的证，如痰热壅肺证、肝郁脾虚证、肾阴虚证、卫分证等，都是对疾病过程中所处一定阶段的病位、病因、病性及病势等所作的病理概括，是对致病因素与机体反应性两方面情况的综合[2]。

目前在中医学界，很多人把“证”与“证候”相等同，将“证”视作“证候”的缩写。候，《说文解字》释为“伺望也”。段玉裁在《说文解字注》[3]中提到，“凡觑伺皆曰候，因之以时为候”，此处“候”字应包含观察到的现象之义和对现象观察过程之义。在中医学里，最早把“证”与“候”连成一个词的是南北朝的陶弘景，他在《肘后方》序中提到了“证候”，其含义包括患者告诉的和医师观察的两方面病理状态及其变化过程[4]。1981 年版的《辞海 · 医药卫生分册》[5]把“证候”定义为“患病时出现的互有联系的一群症状，反映了疾病的原因和病理变化，可以了解疾病的部位，如表证、里证；正气和病邪的盛衰，如虚证、实证；疾病的性质，如寒证、热证；病机的变化，如闭证、脱证等”，因此，认为“证”完全等同于“证候”不是非常确切。

2. 几个“证”英译名的比较与分析

了解“证”的定义之后，再比较现在常见的几个“证”的英译名 symptom、sign、syndrome 和 pattern。

2.1 Symptom

symptom 是比较常见的“证”的英译名之一。《汉英分类字典》里的“证”基本都译成 symptom，如“辨证”被译为 differentiation and classification of symptom[6]。但是，用 symptom 翻译“证”是否准确呢？让我们再对比一下 symptom 的含义。symptom 在《剑桥国际英语词典》[7]中的释义之一为“any feeling of illness or physical or mental change which is caused by a particular disease”，并举一例“He's complaining of all the usual symptoms of flu——a high temperature，headache，and so on”。由例子和释义看来，symptom 应为疾病生理的或者精神上的变化症状，如感冒症状。《英汉大字典》[8]也将 symptom 解释为“症状”。那么 symptom（症状）是否就是中医“证”所对应的译名呢？

“症状”一词首见于西医文献，一般指患者“主观不舒适、不正常的感觉或某些病态改变，如头痛、发热、咳嗽、呼吸困难等，是认识疾病的向导，并能为诊断疾病提供重要的线索”[9]。比较“证”与“症状”的定义，可以发现两者在内容、范围等方面有明显不同。“症状”多是病发时主观不舒服的感觉或某些表现在外的状况改变；而“证”是阶段性病因、病位和病性的病理概括。同样，“证候”与“症状”的含义也不相同，证候的观察不仅着眼于现状，而且更关注疾病演变的过程、趋势和相互关系，是一系列症状的综合。比如头痛发热是症状，若与身痛及脉浮等结合起来，便为外感证候。形象地说，症状与证候的关系可以比作词语与其所在句子的关系。证候相当于一个有意义的句子，而症状则相当于句子中的一个词，弄清楚了每个词各自的意义及词与词之间的内在关系，才能完全清楚一个句子的意义，因此，把“证”或“证候”简单地翻译成 symptom 是不合适的，symptom 不能囊括“证”的所有含义。

2.2 Sign

“证”或“证候”被译成 sign 的场合也不少见。《英汉·汉英中医词典》[10]中就把“证候”译作 sign。笔者认为这种译法不可取。sign 对应的医学译名是“体征”[6]。“体征”与“症状”一样首见于西医文献，它是医师对患者体格检查到的客观病态表现，例如皮疹、心脏杂音、肝脾大等，而有的体征可被患者自行感知，例如皮肤黄染、水肿、包块等，因此，广义的症状也包括体征。从这个定义看，体征应该是包含在症状的范围内，比症状的范围要小。既然症状 symptom 不能囊括“证”的所有含义，何况体征 sign 呢？因此，把“证”或“证候”翻译成 sign 也是不合适的。

2.3 Syndrome

syndrome 应是最常见的“证”或“证候”的英译名。在《中医英语翻译技巧训练》[11]和《汉英分类词典》[6]等书中，都把“证”和“证候”翻成 syndrome。Syndrome 对应的英文解释为“a combination of medical problems that commonly go together，which may show the existence of a particular disease or mental condition”，即可以表明 syndrome 为一种疾病或精神状态的经常一起出现的一群症状。《英汉大字典》[8]里将其解释为“综合症状，症候群”。虽然此“症”非彼“证”，

但对比证候的定义“患病时出现的互有联系的一群症状”，还是基本对应的，因此，笔者认为可以把 syndrome 作为“证候”的译名。但前面提过，“证”不完全等同于“证候”，严格上说“证候”只是“证”的外候，如果“证候”对应的英文是 syndrome，那么“证”应该翻译成什么呢?

“证”的定义是“在疾病发展过程中某一阶段的病理概括”，按照字面翻译就是“pathogenesis generalization in a phase”。这样的翻译虽然比较确切，但很累赘。中医术语多数是 4 字结构，翻译的时候比较复杂，如果再加上如此复杂的“证”，就很拖沓了。然而，由于中西方文化背景和中西医两大医学体系各方面的差异，要在英语中找一个词可以囊括“证”的这个定义里所有的词和义，并不是一件容易的事。另外，目前中医学界很多人把“证”等同于“证候”，因而译者翻译时也大都把“证”与“证候”译成 syndrome，虽然不尽完善，但也不失为权宜之计。李照国先生在他的著作中提过，从目前的发展趋势看，“证”一般翻译成 syndrome。他认为，虽然中医名词术语的英语翻译目前还没有标准化，但却有明确的标准化趋势可循，翻译的时候应该遵循这些译法，尽量保持译名的统一[11]。针灸学中的穴位就是一个很好的例子。穴位一般译成 acupoint。acu-是前缀，为 acupuncture（针灸）的缩写，point 表示穴位。point 本义应为“点”，与中医经络上的“穴位”含义是不相同的，但译学界普遍采用这种译法，而国际上的针灸师也都习以为常而加以使用，那么再绞尽脑汁找出别的译法就显得多余了，因此，笔者认为把“证”翻译成 syndrome 是可取的，“辨证”可以翻译成 syndrome differentiation，而具体的证如“里证”“表证”则可分别翻译成“interior syndrome”和“exterior syndrome”。虽然这种译文是按汉语思维用词拼加而成，有中式英语之嫌，却很好地保留了中医概念的完整意象，反映了民族文化的特点。外国读者刚接触这种译文时可能觉得难以理解，但就像我们中国人也能理解“因特网”“艾滋病”“克隆”等外来词一样，他们在掌握了一定的中医学理论、经过一段时间的交流磨合后也应该能接受其深层含义，达成共识。正如魏迺杰所说，在西传的过程中，中医学并不能为了配合西方人的需求而改变，西方意欲学习中医的人必须真正地进入中医的世界，而翻译者也应该遵循传统方式去看待中医学并将中医学术语忠实地翻译出来。

2.4　Pattern

pattern 的释义之一为“a recognizable way in which something is done, organized or happens”，中文意思为“型”。魏迺杰的《英汉・汉英中医词典》[10]把“证”按照“证候”和“证型”分别译为 sign 和 pattern，并把热证、表证等证都归类到“证型”中。“证型”这个词在《中医诊断学》[2]的绪论中也有提到。临床较为常见、典型、证名规范的证，可称为证型。证型中的“型”确与 pattern 一词相对应，但翻阅《剑桥国际英语词典》《朗文当代高级英语词典》《英汉大字典》等权威大字典，都未发现 pattern 的释义中有医学上的“证型”这一条，因此，笔者认为 pattern 仅仅译出了“型”，但“证”的含义没有体现，“证型”这个术语还是翻译为 syndrome pattern 较为确切，正如“句型”不能只翻译成 pattern，而应翻译成 sentence pattern 一样。

3. 小结

以上笔者对中医术语“证”的几个常见英译名 symptom、sign、syndrome 和 pattern 做了一些比较和分析。通过比较分析，不难看出，symptom 和 sign 的对应名称应为“症状”和“体征”，与“证”的含义是不相同的，不能作为“证”的译名；而 pattern 意为“型”，也只能对应“证型”这一术语中的“型”，不宜作为“证”的译名；syndrome 对应的最贴切的术语应是“证候”，而因人们常把“证候”等同“证”，且目前尚无可以完全对应“证”的英语单词，译者通常把“证”同样翻译成 syndrome，笔者认为这也是可取的。

参考文献

[1] 吴敦序. 中医基础理论. 上海：上海科学技术出版社，1994：7.

[2] 朱文锋. 中医诊断学. 上海：上海科学技术出版社，1995：1－165.

[3] 段玉裁. 说文解字注. 上海：上海古籍出版社，2004：78.

[4] 韦黎. 證、证、症、候的沿革和证候定义的研究. 中国医药学报，1996，11（2）：5.

[5] 辞海编辑委员会. 辞海·医药卫生分册. 上海：上海辞书出版社，1981：57.

[6] 李开荣. 汉英分类词典. 南京：译林出版社，1996：1563－1564.

[7] Procter P. Cambridge international dictionary of English. London：Cambridge University Press，1995：1367－1481.

[8] 陆谷孙. 英汉大字典. 上海：上海译林出版社，2001：1735－1914.

[9] 张汉鹏. 诊断学基础. 北京：人民卫生出版社，1989：6－39.

[10] 魏迺杰. 英汉·汉英中医词典. 长沙：湖南科学技术出版社，1996：35.

[11] 李照国，朱忠宝. 中医英语翻译技巧训练. 上海：上海中医药大学出版社，2002：28.

[原载《中国中西医结合杂志》，2009，29（5）：464－465.]

中医学疾病的概念

——“病”“症”“证”的内涵与翻译

兰凤利

中国古人对疾病的认识源于一种直接的感觉。甲骨文中的病名多是根据某一部位生理功能失常命名的，如疾首、疾耳、疾口、疾齿、疾鼻等。《说文解字》对某些病症的认识已达到相当的水平，其中记录了许多种疾病，涉及内、外、妇、儿、五官、皮肤科及流行病等，仅《说文解字·疒部》就解释了102个与疾病相关的文字。《说文解字·疒部》中提到：“疒，倚也。人有疾痛也，象倚箸之形”，是病痛或患病的表征；“疾，病也”；“病，疾加也”[1]。英文用disease表达各种各样的“疾病”，如心脏病为heart disease。从字源来说，dis-有“相反”之义，ease则为“安乐”之义，所以disease义为“不安乐”。disease从前指“不愉快的事情”，后来特指“疾病”[2]。用disorder（dis＋order）表达身体、精神的“失调”，即轻微的疾病或身体不适。

关于疾病，现代人把它分为三个概念：①疾病（disease）：医学术语，指可以判明的人体生物学上的异常，可从体格检查、实验室检查或其他特殊检查确定；②病患或病痛（illness）：是一个人的自我感觉和自我判断，例如出现某种不舒服，认为自己有了毛病。在一些情况下，经检查可确定有疾病，但在很多情况下，则可能仅是一种心理学或社会学上的失调；③患病（sickness）：是对一种角色的社会地位的描述，即他人（社会）知道或承认此人现正处于不健康状态。大多数所谓的疾病实际上都是指病痛或患病[3]。

古人对疾病的认识一定程度上反映了当时的医疗水平。而中医学所涉及的疾病，实际上囊括了disease、disorder、illness（或ailment）的概念。此外，在现代西医学中视为“symptom”（即症状）的，有人解释为：Change in the way the body works or change in the body's appearance，which shows a disease or disorder is present and is noticed by the patient himself（Note：If a symptom is noticed only by the doctor，it is a sign.）[4]。即：患者本人感受到的预示疾病的身体功能状态或身体形态的改变（即“症”是医生发现的症状），如呕、咳、头痛等，在中医学中是“症”，也是一种疾病的概念。

“证”是中医学独有的认识疾病的概念，是机体在疾病发展过程中的某一阶段的病理概括。辨证论治是中医认识疾病和治疗疾病的基本原则，是中医学对疾病的一种特殊的研究和处理方法，也是中医学的基本特点之一。由于“证”包括了病变的部位、原因、性质，以及邪正关系，反映出疾病发展过程中某一阶段的病理变化的本质，因而它比症状更全面、更深刻、更正确地揭示了疾病的本质。国内普遍采用西方人容易理解的 syndrome 来表达这一中医学独特的概念，而西方则普遍使用 pattern 来表达。此外，还有译者将“证”译为 configuration、conformation等。

自中国中医科学院的吕维柏教授建议将中医学的“证”译为 syndrome、“辨证”译为 syndrome differentiation 之后，这一译法就得到了国内学界的普遍认同。然而，这一译法在国外出版的英文中医学著作中却很鲜见。国外学者或将“证”译为 pattern，或译为 configuration，或译为 conformation。其中以 pattern 最为常见，“辨证”则常译为 pattern identification。笔者认为，中医学中的“证”，用 pattern 来传达更妥。试想，我们如何对 climacteric syndrome（更年期综合征，中医病名为“绝经前后诸证”）再进行 syndrome differentiation（辨证），然后将患者再辨为肝肾阴虚 syndrome（证）或阴虚火旺 syndrome（证）?

正如 Kaptchuk 所说，“From a modern western perspective, it is tempting to translate the Chinese words as ‘differentiating syndromes’, but that rendering would distort the uniqueness and potential validity of the Chinese idea. ‘Syndrome’ is a purely descriptive term, suggesting an arbitrary grouping of signs and symptoms that is meaningless without an underlying cause. ‘Syndrome’ implies that something is missing.”[5]（译文：从现代西医学的观点来看，似乎应将“辨证”译为 differentiating syndromes，但是，这一翻译却歪曲了中医学思想的独特性和潜在的确定性。syndrome 仅仅是一个描写性的术语，提示没有根本原因的毫无意义的任意组合的一组症状和体征。如果用 syndrome 来传达“证”，不言而喻，丢失了一些意义。）

可见，中医学疾病的概念并不明确，来源也多种多样，包括了上文提到的各种各样的“（疾）病”“症”和“证”。其中，“疾”（病也）可译为 disorder，“病”（疾加也）可译为 disease。而今，往往以“疾病”并称，则可将轻微的疾病或失调译为 disorder 或 illness，将一般或较重的各种各样的疾病译为 disease。symptom 是“症”或“症状”的对应译语。对于“证”，则宜译为 pattern。

参考文献

[1] [汉] 许慎撰. [清] 段玉裁注. 说文解字注. 上海：上海古籍出版社，1988：348－353.
[2] 纪秋郎. 新知识英汉辞典. 北京：外文出版社；台北：远东图书公司，1997：311.
[3] H. P. 恰范特. 医学社会学. 上海：上海人民出版社，1987：14.
[4] Collin PH. Dictionary of medicine. Beijing：Foreign Language Teaching and Research Press，2001：574.

[5] Kaptchuk TJ. Chinese medicine: the web that has no weaver. Revised ed. London: Rider, 2000: 216.

[原载《中国中西医结合杂志》, 2010, 30 (4): 428－429.]

中医病症名称的英译方法

张登峰

中西医尽管分属于两种不同的医学体系，一些病症名称在含义上存在着很大的差异，但是，由于疾病及其症状属客观存在，不管人们如何命名，它总是实实在在地客观存在着[1]，所以，中西病症名称在一定的范围内有着共同或相似之处。正是这些共同或相似点，为我们借助于西医用语翻译中医病症名称提供了突破口。

这样做会不会引起理解上的混乱呢？我们认为绝对不会的，因为语言有它自己的使用范围，在什么范围应用，它就发挥着转达什么范围的内容。从语言学的角度来看，语言之间的相互借用是语言交际功能的正常发挥，是语言自身丰富与发展的一种标志。回顾西医传入中国的历史，当时的翻译工作者就是借用了中国传统医学固有的生理、病理知识和用语来翻译相应的西医概念。这不但没有妨碍西医在中国的传播，相反，促进了其在中国的发展，因此，在特定的中医语言环境中，当读者也是具备一定中医学知识的中外医药工作者时，借用西医用语来翻译一些中医病症名称是完全可行的[2]。当前的中医药对外交流与翻译实践也证实了这一点。

1. 中西医病症共同和相似之处

归纳起来，关于中西医的一些病症名称的共同或相似之处大体上有以下几类：

1.1 同名同义

同名同义指中西医一些病症名称的汉语命名和内涵基本相同或接近，见表1。

表1 中西医中同名同义病症名称对照表

中医	西医	中医	西医
疟疾	疟疾（malaria）	心悸	心悸（palpitation）
麻疹	麻疹（measles）	呃逆	呃逆（hiccup）
便秘	便秘（constipation）	遗尿	遗尿（enuresis）
痢疾	痢疾（dysentery）	白喉	白喉（diphtheria）
月经不调	月经不调（menoxenia）	纳呆	纳呆（indigestion）
失音	失音（aphonia）	肉瘿	肉瘿（exophthalmic goiter）

1.2　义同名异

义同名异即中西医病症的汉语名称各异，但意思大体相同或接近，这类名称主要包括骨伤和外科类的病症，见表 2。

表 2　中西医中义同名异病症名称对照表

中医	西医
颊车磋	下颌关节脱臼（dislocation of madibular articulation）
能远却近	远视（hyperopia ）
痨瘵	肺结核（pulmonary tuberculosis）
云雾移睛	玻璃体混浊（vitreous opacity）
木癞	瘤型麻风晚期（late lepromatous leprosy）
牛皮癣	神经性皮炎（neurodermatitis）
缠腰火丹	带状疱疹（herpes zoster）
脱肛	直肠脱垂（proctoptosis）

1.3　名同义异

名同义异即中西医病症的汉语名称相同，而含义不同。例如："伤寒"，中医是指各种外感热病的总称等，而西医则指的是由伤寒杆菌引起的肠道传染病；又如"结核"一名，中医是指形似果核的皮下包块，而西医则指的是由结核分枝杆菌所引发的疾病，如肺结核、骨结核等。

1.4　一名多病（症）

一名多病（症）即中医的一种病症相当于多个西医病症，反之，西医的一种疾病包含了数个中医病症。如：中医的"风疹块""瘖癗""鬼饭疙瘩"等病症相当于西医的"荨麻疹"（urticaria）。而中医的"目偏视"包含有西医的"斜视"（strabismus）、"共转性斜视"（concomitant strabismus）和"麻痹性斜视"（paralytic strabismus）三种疾病[3]。

2. 中医病症名称的英译方法

现代翻译理论表明，两种语言的词汇单位之间的语义对应情况可归纳为三大类型，即完全对应、部分对应和不对应。根据上述的归类比较，中西医病症名称在语义内涵上也大致如此，即基本对应、部分对应和不对应三种类型。"同名同义"和"义同名异"就属于语义基本对应，"一名多病（症）"属部分对应，"同名异义"等大多数用语则为不对应，因此，中医病症名称的具体英译方法如下。

2.1　借用翻译法

借用翻译法是指用含义上与中医病症基本相同的西医名称来翻译相应的中医用语，即"西为中用"。当前的中医对外交流与翻译实践也表明，借用某些西医用语翻译相应的中医名词术语是完全可行的。对于上文所列举的“同名同义”与“义同名异”这类中医病症名称，国内外基本上都是如此进行英译的。除此之外，在以下几种情况下，借用翻译法也可以用于英译中医学中的一些病症名称。

一病多名多译：就是说一种中医病症有数个名称，可以采用多个译语。例如：亡血，又称流血、出血、失血、溢血等，可英译成：bleed、bleeding、hemorrhage、hemorrhagic 等不同场合所需要的对应语。又如：白虎飞尺，又名附骨疽、多骨疽、朽骨疽等，其含义类似于西医的骨髓炎和骨结核，可译作 osteomyelitis and bone tuberculosis。一名多义合译，即一个中医病症名称包含了几个西医病症，可以借用多个西医病症名来英译。例如，内踝疽近似于西医的踝关节结核与骨髓炎，可英译为 tuberculosis and osteomyelitis of ankle joint。多名单义一译意思是多个中医病症名称指一个西医病症概念，可以借用一种西医名称进行英译，如：“湮尻疮”和“尿火丹”两种病症类似于西医的尿布皮炎，可借用 dermatitis 一词来翻译。

2.2　意译翻译法

意译翻译法就是根据原词的大意译出其深层的意思，而不是字面意义。例如，“木肾”指睾丸肿胀而无疼痛的一种症候，如果仅从字面理解译成 wood kidney，就让人难以理解，所以只能根据其含义译作 swollen testes；“木舌”译成 stiff tongue 就比较达意；“雀目”（又称雀目内障、鸡盲、鸡宿眼、鸡蒙眼等）含义与西医的夜盲症近似，可英译成 night blurred vision；“五色疡”——古人以五行配五色，将发于眼部的木疡、火疡、土疡、金疡、水疡统称为五色疡，因此，英译成 five ocular diseases 就比较达意[4]。

采用意译法来翻译中医的一些病症名称，不仅传神达意，而且具有回译性。下面一组中医病症名称就是典型的例子：白屑风 seborrheic dermatitis，缠腰火丹 herpes zoster around the waist，胬肉攀睛 pterygium，白陷鱼鳞 keratohelcosis，角弓反张 opisthotonos，白膜侵睛 phlyctenular keratitis。

2.3　直译翻译法

顾名思义，直译翻译法就是按照原文的字面意思进行逐字翻译的一种方法。这种方法的好处是使译语具有较显著的回译性，因而有利于交流。例如：“肾阳不足”“气虚不孕”“风热腰痛”等可分别英译成：insufficiency of kidney Yang、sterility due to Qi asthenia、lumbago due to wind-heat，这种直译也能够体现浓厚的中医特色[5]。

直译法的不足之处是，如果运用不当就会使译文显得生硬难懂或不符合译入语的表达习惯。例如，在现行的中医翻译活动中，有人将“白虎厉节”“鹤膝风”“天行赤眼”等分别英译为：white tiger joint running、crane’s knee wind、heaven-current red eye，在结构和表层意思上与原文都十分接近，应该说具有相当的回译性，但是读起来总觉得味同天书，因此，还是根据其实际含义意译为好，以免给读者的阅读和理解造成不必要的障碍。

2.4　音译翻译法

音译是翻译过程中不可缺少的技巧，其成功的例子不胜枚举。在翻译个别语义笼统模糊、内涵复杂的特殊中医病症名称时，音译是解决问题的最好途径。例如“阴阳”“气”等概念因其含义复杂，从一开始的意译已逐渐转变成目前的音译。又如病症名称“疝”和“痹”，无论是直译还是意译，其译文都会冗长烦琐，不便于行文，只有音译成 Shan symptoms 和 Bi symptoms，再加上必要的注解才比较理想。

2.5　综合翻译法

综合翻译法指同时采用几种翻译法来翻译中医用语的一种方法，也是中医药翻译中运用最普遍、最灵活的手法。例如：病名“消渴”，外国有人英译成 diabetes，also called Xiaoke in TCM；“奔豚”一词被英译成 Bentun syndrome (similar to gastroenteroneurosis)；“牛皮癣”被译成 oxhide lichen (psoriasis or neurodermatitis)。

除了上述几种译法外，还有其他译法，如释译法、描述翻译法等。然而，无论采用何种翻译方法，只要在忠实于原文的基础上，以科学求实的态度，我们就能够翻译出高质量译作。

参考文献

[1] 王振华，李凤英．中医“证、病”与西医的“症状、病”的比较．医学与哲学，1994，15 (7)：24－26.

[2] 李照国．中医英语翻译实践与技巧．北京：人民卫生出版社，1994：28－34，78－80.

[3]《中医大词典》编写组．中医大词典·外科分册．北京：人民卫生出版社，1982：9，15，28，30，42，51.

[4] 李照国．汉英中医药大词典．西安：世界图书出版公司，1997：21，54，76，217，301.

[5] 王朝辉，林岩，陈淑芬，等．中医基本名词术语英译探讨．中国中西医结合杂志，1994，14 (12)：749.

[原载《中国中西医结合杂志》，2006，26 (9)：855－857.]

中医病因学常用名词术语英译

张庆荣

目前中医药术语英译的研究和实践都有长足的进展，但并不统一。本文拟就病因学的英译进行初步探讨，以求对中医药术语英译的统一化和标准化略尽绵薄之力。

1. 病因及病因学

中医的病因（cause of disease 或 disease cause）又称病邪（pathogenic evil），病原（pathogen）、致病因素（pathogenic factor 或 etiological factor）又可称邪气（evil Qi 或 pathogenic Qi）、邪（evil）。evil 是一个非医学词汇，既可作形容词，又可作名词用，作为“邪”字英译词简洁而又恰当。pathogen 在英文字典多解释为“致病微生物”。例如，《道兰图解医学词典》（*Dorland Illustrated Medical Dictionary*，简称 DIMD）中将 pathogen 解释为 any disease-producing microorganism，但在早期的字典中亦有指其他致病物质的，如 1975 年出版的《现代科学词典》（*Modern Science Dictionary*）的解释为 disease-producing micro-organism or substance。所以，pathogen 作“病因（原）”译词较佳。“病因学”一般均用 etiology，但如用 etiology 作病因的译词则不恰当。

2. 外（感病）因和内（伤病）因

“内”与“外”的翻译主要有 endogenous 和 exogenous，internal 和 external，或 endopathic 和 exopathic。在意义上这 3 组词均没有问题，但第 1 组以医学应用为主，最为合适；第 2 组为普通词汇；第 3 组为医学专用词汇，但有时后接 pathogen 则显得 pathic 和 patho 重叠，故不如第 1 组适用。

这样，外（感病）因和内（伤病）因就可分别译为 exogenous pathogen 和 endogenous pathogen。

3. 六气与六淫

“六气”一般译为 six normal climatic factors、six climatic factors、six normal climates 和 six climates，以 six climates 为佳。normal 属超额用词，因“六气”本身内涵均有“正常”之意。“六淫”的译词有许多，有 six climatic pathogens、six climatic evils、six abnormal climatic factors、six climatic excesses、six excesses、 six pathogenic factors、six pathogens、six evils 等。六淫主要是影响人体的气候致病因素，一般用 climatic 修饰，故以 six climatic pathogens（evils）为佳。病因对人体就是异常的，故 abnormal 不需用。excess 的英文解释为“the state of exceeding that which is normal”（DIMD），是一种超常的状态，或超常量，而对六淫中医的解释中还含有正常的气候（非超常）对体质虚弱个体的影响；并且此词在病机学上多用作“实”的译词，故作为“六淫”的译词不合适。至于有时中医亦称“六淫”为“六邪”时，则又可简化为 six pathogens（evils）。

关于具体的六淫各邪，如“风邪”有两类译法，即 wind pathogen（evil）和 pathogenic（evil）wind 均可用，但以前者更符合原义。其他分别是寒 cold、暑 summer -heat、湿 damp、燥 dry、火（热）fire（heat）。注意，damp 和 dry 不能作名词用，用时需作 dampness 和 dryness。有人把“湿”译作 wet。wet 的英文解释在《钱伯斯 20 世纪词典》（*Chambers 20th Century Dictionary*，简称 CCD）中为“containing，soaked with，covered with water or other liquid；rainy”。故不合适。

4. 疠气

“疠气”的英译词主要有 pestilent pathogen（evil）、pestilential pathogen（evil）、epidemic pathogen（evil）、pestilent Qi、pestilential Qi、epidemic Qi。在 3 个修饰语中，pestilent 和 pestilential 两者同，以前者简单为佳。而 epidemic 还包括非感染性的，外延广，不符合中医原义。在三个主词中，Qi 不宜用，因易与作为组成人体和维持人体的气的译词 Qi 混淆。这样，“疠气”就应译为 pestilent pathogen（evil）。

5. 七情和五志

主要是“情”和“志”的译法不同，有 emotions、affects、passions、feelings、emotional factors 等。从语义和语用上讲，以 emotions 为佳。七情五志均为正常的情志变化。致病时的异常情志改变称作“七情内伤”或“内伤七情”，才是致病因素。中医的病因多是相对的，正如六气和六淫的关系一样。此时的七情是致病因素，当另有一译词，但实际上目前翻译界很少加以区别。本人建议致病的情或志当译为 affects，或 emotional pathogens 或 agents，以 affects 简单，既可作名词用，也可作动词用，其基本含义也有“影响人发病”的意思。例如 CCD 的解释为“to infect or attack as disease；to influence”。这样，“七情”和“五志”可分别译为 seven emotions 和 five emotions，而“七情内伤”则可译为 seven endogenous affects，或简作 seven affects。

具体的情志译词，如喜 joy、怒 anger 或 rage、恐 fear、惊 fright、悲 sorrow 或 sadness，一般多无异议。但其中的悲和忧，及忧和思的译词常相互交错不清，缺少界定。“忧”的译词有 melancholy、grief、worry、anxiety，或同“悲”之 sorrow 或 sadness。其中 melancholy 与 melancholia 相同，是一种精神疾病，不宜用。《朗文现代英汉双解词典》（以下简称 Longman）对“grief”的解释为“great sorrow”，《现代高级英汉双解辞典》（以下简称《双解辞典》）的解释为“deep or violent sorrow”，故不能用作译“忧”；sorrow 或 sadness 已作为“悲”的译词。剩下 worry 和 anxiety 哪一个合适呢？都可以，但以上 CCD、Longman 和《双解辞典》三本字典均用 anxiety 或 anxious 来解释 worry，且 CCD 对此词有 over-anxiety 的释义，故以用 anxiety 译“忧”为佳。关于“思”的译词有 anxiety、meditation、pensiveness、thought 和 thinking。其中 anxiety 已用作“忧”之译词。不宜用 meditation 的理由有二：其一，其动词的本意是“to think seriously or deeply”（Longman）；其二，Longman 和 DIMD 两字典给此词的释义中均有宗教色彩，如“the practice of deep religious thought”（Longman）。pensiveness 在上述字典释义中均用 thought 或 thoughtful 来释义。那么只有 thought 和 thinking 来译“思”适合。二者中用哪一个?《双解辞典》解释 thought 为“(power，process of) thinking”；CCD 为“a spell of thinking”；Longman 为“the act of thinking，product of thinking”。看来 thinking 最合适。所以上述七情可分别作：喜 joy、怒 anger、忧 anxiety、思 thinking、悲 sorrow、恐 fear、惊 fright。那么，当解释致病因素时则可在英文主词前分别加上 over、great、furious 或 excessive 修辞即可。但有四个英文词 rage [《双解辞典》解释为“furious anger”；Longman 解释为“(a sudden feeling of) wild uncontrollable anger”]、grief（《双解辞典》解释为“deep or violent sorrow”；Longman 解释为“great sorrow”）、terror（《双解辞典》解释为“great fear”；CCD 解释为“extreme fear”；Longman 解释为“very great fear”）、pensive（《双解辞典》解释为“seriously thoughtful”；Longman 解释为“deeply or dreamily thoughtful”）已经含有修饰意义了，故直接用之即可。那么七情（内伤）可分别译作：（过）喜 over-joy，（过）怒 rage，（过）忧 great anxiety 或 worry（CCD：over-anxiety），（过）思 pensiveness，（过）悲 grief，（过）恐 terror，（过）惊 excessive fright。

6. 痰饮和瘀血

“痰”的翻译比较一致，均译作 phlegm。“饮”的翻译有：fluid、fluid retention、rheum、retained fluid、stagnant fluid。其中 rheum 源于希腊语 rheuma fux，主要指排泄物（CCD 解释为“a mucus discharge”；DIMD 解释为“a watery discharge”），故不合适。fluid 多作为体内正常津液的译词；retention 是指某种状态、作用或过程（Longman 解释为“the state or action of retaining”），故 fluid 和 fluid retention 不宜。剩下的两个均可以，但以用形容词者 stagnant fluid 为佳。

“瘀血”的译词主要有 stagnant blood、stagnated blood、congealed blood；stasis（stagnation）of blood，blood stasis（stagnation）。首先要注意中医尚有“血瘀”一词，它是指一种病理状态。stasis（stagnation）of blood 和 blood stasis（stagnation）多作为“血瘀”的译词，因此，不宜作“瘀血”的译词。congealed blood 是指“blood in coagulation”或“blood clots”。诚然，这种凝固的血液或血块是瘀血，但中医的瘀血还包括运行迟滞缓慢的血液，显然用之不宜。同“饮”一样，stagnant blood 和 stagnated blood 两者中用前者 stagnant blood 为佳。

7. 外伤

“外伤”也有许多译词，主要有：trauma、wound、external damage、external injury 和 traumatic injury。其中 damage 为普通词汇。trauma、wound 和 injury 三词均为 DIMD 收载，看来为医学词汇，且三者意义有交叉。wound 在 DIMD、CCD、《双解辞典》、Longman 等字典中均有“正常组织结构断裂破坏”的含义（如 DIMD：“an injury or damage… with disruption of normal continuity of structure”）。而中医的外伤包括广泛，还有不出现组织结构断裂破坏的情况。另外，造成 wound 的常为 on purpose by a weapon（Longman）或 as the result of attack《双解辞典》，即为蓄意用武器或攻击的结果，而这些“伤”只是外伤的一部分。故用 wound 不合适。trauma 在 DIMD 中释义非常简洁：“①injury；②psychological or emotional damage”。在 Longman、《双解辞典》和 CCD 中的释义也多偏重于精神创伤，例如 Longman 的第一释义即为：“a damage to the mind caused by the body having been wounded”。看来，只有 injury 是最合适的了。但 injury 本身含义广泛（如 CCD：“wrong、damage、hurt、impairment、insult、offence”）。故用 external 限定一下很有必要，即“外伤”应译为 external injury。至于其他病因术语，如饮食失宜 improper diet、结石 calculus 以及寄生虫 parasite 等，一般翻译分歧不大，这里就不做探讨了。

［原载《中国中西医结合杂志》，2005，25（12）：1130－1131.］

中医“证”及其相关术语的英译

袁洪仁

证，又名证候，是机体在疾病发展过程中某一阶段的病理概括，包括了病变的部位、原因、性质及邪正关系，反映出疾病发展过程中某一阶段的病理变化之本质。证是在诊察（临床感知）病象的基础上，依据病因模式或辨证纲领等进行临床判断而获得的。现代关于证本质的研究表明，证是一种综合性的功能态，是全身多器官综合协调的结果，并随时间的推移而动态变化[1]。可见，证是疾病阶段性、状态性的病象概括。故将“证”译作“pathographihood”，意为“某一时期的病象”“某种状态的病象”。前缀“pathographi-”意为“病象”“用特殊方式对疾病记录的结果”[2]，不仅表达了“病藏于中，证形于外”的象数思维特征，而且表达了作为证候的病象并非停留于诊察——临床感知阶段，而是在感知的基础上作出的理性判断——“用特殊方式对疾病记录的结果”，即对疾病的病理变化之概括。后缀“- hood”表示时期、状态等意思，从而使“pathographihood”表达出证是疾病阶段性、状态性的病象概括之内涵。可将“pathographihood”缩写为 PGH，则“辨证论治”可译为“treatment decision according to PGH differentiation”，意即“治疗决策依据于证的辨别”，如“血虚证”“脏腑辨证”等可分别译作“blood-deficiency PGH”和“viscera PGH differentiation”。

参考文献

[1] 阎利，吴圣贤．证本质研究思考．中国中西医结合杂志，2000，20（5）：384.

[2] 袁洪仁．谈藏象与脏腑术语的英译．中国中西医结合杂志，2000，20（3）：164.

［原载《中国中西医结合杂志》，2005，25（7）：619.］

也谈中医术语“六淫”的英译

陈保蓉　李成文

六淫（the six pathogenic factors）是中医理论中阐发病因与发病的特有专用术语。印会河教授指出，“六淫，即是风、寒、暑、湿、燥、火六种外感病邪的统称。当气候变化异常，六气发生太过或不及，或非其时而有其气，以及气候变化过于急骤，在人体正气不足，抵抗力下降时，六气才能成为致病因素，侵犯人体而发生疾病，这种情况下的六气，便称为六淫”[1]。陆保磊认为，当六气变化失常或人体抗病能力下降，使人发病时叫六淫，又叫六邪。六淫必须通过人体的病理变化体现出来，否则不能称之为六淫。人体特定的病理状态是六淫的存在形式，如果没有这种病理状态，则六淫也就不存在了。所以，六淫既是病因又包含证候。病因由证候体现，证候代表病因。中医学认识外界病因的方法决定了这两方面的内容在六淫的定义中不能分割[2]。然而目前有关工具书对中医专业术语“风、寒、暑、湿、燥、火”的英译主要有：①wind，cold，dampness，heat，summer-heat，fire；②pathogenic wind，pathogenic cold，pathogenic summer-heat，pathogenic dampness，pathogenic dryness，pathogenic fire；也有人将其译作 unusual wind，unusual cold，unusual summer-heat，unusual damp，unusual dryness，unusual fire；或直接译为 Feng，Han，Shu，Shi，Zao，Huo[3]。

笔者认为 unusual wind、unusual cold、unusual summer heat、unusual damp、unusual dryness、unusual fire 中“unusual”的意思为“不寻常的”“杰出的”，如：He was an unusual film star even in Hollywood。由此可见，上述英译不能确切地表达中医病因学说中的六淫概念，影响了中医对外交流，这主要是对中医学中六气、六淫概念以及两者之间的关系把握上出现了偏差，曲解了中医学病因学说。

1. 六气概念

六气（the six climatic factors）是指自然界中风、寒、暑、湿、燥、火六种不同的气候变化，随季节变换交替出现。印会河认为，“它是万物生长的条件，对人体是无害的。故《素问·宝命全形论》谓‘人以天地之气生，四时之法成’。即是说人依靠天地之间的大气和水谷之气而生存，亦循四时生长收藏的规律而成长发育。同时，人们在生活实践中逐步认识了它们的特点，产生了一定的适应能力，所以正常的六气不易使人致病”[1]。

2. 六淫概念

六淫是中医学病因学说的重要内容，它不仅仅是病因，还应包含受邪后所表现出来的临床证候。病因由症候体现，症候代表着病因，证因一体，不能分割。所以由人体特定的病理变化体现出的风、寒、暑、湿、燥、火六种外感病邪的症候，才能称之为六淫。

3. 六气与六淫的关系

自然界的风、寒、暑、湿、燥、火六种气候随季节变换交替出现称作六气。外界气候不论是骤寒骤热，还是应寒反热、应热反寒，若人体功能能够适应这种变化而没有发病，这种反常的气候变化就不能叫六淫。只有当六气变化失常，太过或不及，或非其时而有其气，以及气候变化过于急骤，加之人体抗病能力下降时使人发病时才称为六淫，又叫六邪。即使没有明显的气候变化，若发生外感病，这种气候对于患者就叫邪气，因此，六淫概念的要点是能“使人发病时”的邪气，人体正气是发病关键，人体特定的病理变化是六淫的存在或外在表现形式，六淫体现了病因与邪正的关系。

4. 六气与六淫的英译

根据以上六气、六淫的概念以及六气与六淫的关系，因此，我们认为，将自然界中“风、寒、暑、湿、燥、火”正常的“六气”译为“wind，cold，summer-heat，dampness，dryness，fire”较译为“Feng，Han，Shu，Shi，Zao，Huo”合适，便于理解，虽然两者同义，但后者容易产生歧义，不利于中外交流。

我们认为六淫的“风、寒、暑、湿、燥、火”可以译为：① pathogenic wind，pathogenic cold，pathogenic summer-heat，pathogenic dampness，pathogenic dryness，pathogenic fire；② unhealthy wind，unhealthy cold，unhealthy summer-heat，unhealthy dampness，unhealthy dryness，unhealthy fire。

但是随着中医药对外交流的发展需求，是否可以把六淫直接译作“Pathogenic Feng，Pathogenic Han，Pathogenic Shu，Pathogenic Shi，Pathogenic Zao，Pathogenic Huo”，则更能反映出“风、寒、暑、湿、燥、火”这一中医学理论所特有的概念，便于理解中医学病因学说的深刻内涵，便于世人学习中医，接受中医，而且符合中医药专业术语英译的传统与特色。

参考文献

[1] 印会河．中医基础理论．上海：上海科学技术出版社，1984：93-94.
[2] 陆保磊．六淫新识．山东中医杂志，2003，22（10）：58.
[3] 刘伟．关于“风、寒、暑、湿、燥、火”中医术语英译的商榷．中国中西医结合杂志，2003，23（11）：872.

[原载《中国中西医结合杂志》，2005，25（3）：276-277.]

关于“风、寒、暑、湿、燥、火”中医术语英译的商榷

刘 伟

在从事中医英译工作所必备的工具书《汉英医学大辞典》中，“风、寒、暑、湿、燥、火”这六个中医术语的英译分别为“wind，cold，summer heat，damp，dryness，fire”。笔者在从事中医英译工作的过程中，对中医专业知识的了解逐渐增多，对中医专业术语的内涵也加深了理解。为此，感到《汉英医学大辞典》对这六个中医术语的英译有不妥之处，在此提出自己的看法，与同行们商榷。

在中医基础理论中，这六个中医术语指的是外感病因中的“六淫”。早在宋代，名医陈无择就明确指出：“六淫，天之常气，冒之则先自经络流入，内合于脏腑，为外所因。”《中医基础理论》把“风、寒、暑、湿、燥、火”区分为“六气”和“六淫”。“六气”指的是自然界中的风、寒、暑、湿、燥、火正常的气候现象，而“六淫”则是指正常的风、寒、暑、湿、燥、火自然现象超过了一定限度，或气候变化过于急骤，机体不能与之相适应而导致疾病发生的现象，并详细地阐明“六淫是超限度的六气”，“能否确定六淫与机体是否发病有关”，“气候的异常致人发病固然应该称其为六淫，但是气候变化基本正常，也会有人因其适应能力低下而得病，此时，对患病机体来说也只能将正常的六气变化称为六淫了”。

从上面的论述中我们可以确切地知道中医学的六淫中风、寒、暑、湿、燥、火六个专业术语指的不是自然界中正常的风、寒、暑、湿、燥、火六种自然现象。因为这六种正常气候现象是万物生长的条件，对人体是无害的。《素问·宝命全形论》说：“人以天地之气生，四时之法成。”人依靠自然界的大气、水谷之气而生存，并循着四时气候变化、生长收藏规律而生长发育。但是，如果气候变化反常，使机体不能与之相适应而导致疾病发生时，自然界中的风、寒、暑、湿、燥、火现象则由中医所指的“六气”转化为中医的“风、寒、暑、湿、燥、火”的“六淫”。

著名翻译家张树柏先生在《谈谈科技论文的翻译》一文中说：“科技论文上所用的普通字常有特殊的解释，如果没有科技方面的知识，只凭查字典或只知这些字的普通字意就会闹出笑话来。”《汉英医学大辞典》也只是把中医术语“风、寒、暑、湿、燥、火”英译成了其普通字意，用在中医英译中是不妥的。18世纪英国翻译理论家 AF. Tytle 曾讲过：“好的翻译是把原作的长处完全移注到另一种语言里，使得译文语言所属国家的人们能清晰地领悟、强烈地感受正像使用原作语言的人们所领悟、所感受的一样。”我们把中医进行英译，目的是让独特的

我国中医学走出国门，让世界人民了解中医，接受中医，让千百年来为炎黄子孙治病解疾的中医学为世界人民的健康事业做出应有的贡献；同时，也为中西医的结合进行学术交流做出贡献。正因为如此，中医术语的准确英译就显得至关重要。

笔者认为，《汉英医学大辞典》对“风、寒、暑、湿、燥、火”中医术语的英译，只是译成了自然界中的气候现象，仅符合中医里所指的“六气”，而未能译出“风、寒、暑、湿、燥、火”中医术语的真实内涵——“六淫”之意。《汉英医学大辞典》对“风、寒、暑、湿、燥、火”中医术语的英译显然是不合适的，也容易让母语为英语的人们对中医术语产生误解。因为他们无论如何也不能理解自然界中的“wind”与中医术语的“wind”的区别。即使是国内中医界的人士见到“风”这个中医术语被英译为“wind”时，也不禁哑然失笑。为此，笔者从下列3个方面提出“风、寒、暑、湿、燥、火”中医术语的英译：①从“风、寒、暑、湿、燥、火”中医术语在中医里指“六淫”的角度讲，应把这六个中医术语英译为“unusual wind，unusual cold，unusual summer heat，unusual damp，unusual dryness，unusual fire”。②从“风、寒、暑、湿、燥、火”六淫导致机体发病的角度来讲，还可把这六个中医术语英译为“pathogenic wind，pathogenic cold，pathogenic summer heat，pathogenic damp，pathogenic dryness，pathogenic fire”。③张树柏先生讲：“一个译名只要大家通用，就能成立。”中医源于中国，有着几千年的发展史，在长期的发展中，形成了世界上独一无二的中医理论，跻身于世界医学之林，为全人类的医学事业做出了贡献。在中医走向世界并逐渐被国外对中医感兴趣并对中医有所研究的学者所接受的今天，也可把“风、寒、暑、湿、燥、火”中医术语按音译而译为“Feng，Han，Shu，Shi，Zao，Huo”。

［原载《中国中西医结合杂志》，2003，23（11）：872.］

谈中医病因学说有关术语的英译

袁洪仁

中医病因学说有两个特点：一是整体观念，二是辨证求因。故中医的病因常是结合人体病理反应的综合名称，与证很难划分，临床上常按“治证即是治因”来行事。中医病因学说有关术语的英译必须忠实于此。

1. 六淫的英译

六淫是六气变化与体质差异所引起的外感病之致病因素。六气指风、寒、暑、湿、燥、火六种正常的自然界气候变化。六淫为病，除了气候因素外，还包括了生物（如细菌、病毒等）、物理、化学等多种致病因素作用于机体所引起的病理反应。故“六淫”译作“six pathogenic-Qi”[1]，意为“六种致病之气”。其包括的风、寒、暑、湿、燥、火六种外感病邪，分别译作“windy-Qi evil”“cold-Qi evil”“summer heat-Qi evil”“damp-Qi evil”“dry-Qi evil”“fiery-Qi evil”，意思分别为“风性之邪”“寒性之邪”“暑性之邪”“湿性之邪”“燥性之邪”和“火性之邪”。这种译法中，前缀表达了六淫以原有的自然气候因素为基础，后缀“-Qi evil”既表达了作为中医病因的邪气称呼，又表达了中医辨证求因观点下的病因概念，即通过人体的整体性反应来取象六气特性认识病因，亦即具有某种自然气候属性之邪气（中药气味学说中 Qi 有“属性”之意）。其中“windy-Qi evil”和“damp-Qi evil”尤能反映各自病邪的致病特点，因风邪“善行数变”，“为百病之长”，而“windy”兼有“易变的”“匆促的”“有力的”之意。湿邪致病，临床症状有沉重的特性，而“damp”兼有“不起劲的”“沮丧的”之意。

2. 七情与疠气的英译

七情指喜、怒、忧、思、悲、恐、惊七种正常的情绪反应，故“七情”译作“seven emotions”，意为“七种情绪”，其中的喜、怒、忧、思、悲、恐、惊分别译作“joy”“anger”“anxiety”“depression”“grief”“fear”“fright”，至于将“思”译作“depression”，意为“抑郁”，是因为中医学理论中“思”导致的典型病理变化——“伤脾”与“气结”，符合现代抑郁症的诊断，而且符合“思”属于情绪范畴的观点[2]。

疠气是一类具有强烈传染性的病邪，又称“毒气”“瘟疫”等，故将其译作

"pestiferous-Qi"，因"pestiferous"有"传染性的""有毒的""引起瘟疫的""邪恶的"之意。

3. 痰饮与瘀血的英译

痰饮在中医病因学说中指人体水液代谢障碍而形成的一种致病因子，乃水湿停聚而成。湿聚为水，积水成饮，饮凝成痰。故"痰饮"译作"endodamp-Qi-gregation"，意为"内湿性聚集物"；"饮"译作"aquigregation"，意为"水液聚集物"。而痰有狭义与广义之分，狭义之痰译作"phlegm"，为呼吸道分泌物；广义之痰译作"phlegm-Qi evil"，意为"痰性病邪"，属于辨证求因观念下的"痰"。至于瘀血，指因血行失度，使机体某一局部的血液凝聚而形成的一种病理产物。瘀乃血液停积、不能活动之意，故"瘀血"译作"stasis"。因"stasis"指医学上流血等的"郁滞""瘀血""郁积""停滞"。

参考文献

[1] 袁洪仁．谈中医术语"气"的英译．中国中西医结合杂志，1997，17（2）：108.
[2] 杜文东．论"思"的实质及其临床意义．中医杂志，2001；42（3）：187.

[原载《中国中西医结合杂志》，2002，22（5）：358.]

中医“神明”的英语翻译

李　展

“神明”（或“神”）原是中国传统文化的一个哲学概念，中医学根植于中国传统文化，故而潜移默化地借用一些传统文化的概念来诠释生命的现象及人与自然的关系。中医学的经典著作《黄帝内经》在先秦哲学思想的基础上，在探索生命本质的过程中，借用这个“神明”的概念，并将它重新包装，赋予新的元素，将其内涵进一步丰富与完善。从《黄帝内经》至今，在中医学领域里对“神明”的理解至少有三个方面是达成共识的：一是指自然界的运动规律；二是指生命原动力，是人的一切生命活动规律及其外在表现；三是指人的精神意识思维活动。这就是中医学“神明”概念的基本内涵。且“神明”这几个方面的内涵具有相关性，并非独立或截然分开的。虽然在某个场合有所特指，但更多是以整体状态出现。

综合目前相关期刊、工具书和专著等文献，中医“神明”一词的相关英语翻译有以下几种。

1. The mental faulty of a person reveals his or her vitality as well as mental and spiritual state. In a broad sense，it refers to life，but in a narrow sense，it refers to mental activity or spirit，神指一个人的生命力、心理和精神状态。狭义的神指精神活动或精神[1]。

2. The body can't live without the mind. 无神则形不可活[1]。

3. Combine mental activities and the movements in one. 心神合一[1]。

4. The heart houses the mind；或 The heart stores the spirt. 心藏神[1]。

5. The unity of physique and vitality；或 The unity of physique and mentality. 形神合一[1]。

6. House of the original spirit. 元神之府[2]。

7. Mental activity；或 Bright spirit. 神明[2]。

8.《WHO 西太区与世界中医药学会联合会中医名词术语国际标准比较研究：精、神、气、血、津、液部分》一文则总结“神”根据不同的意境可译作 spirit、mind、vitality 等。作为 spirit 的“神”，指人的精神活动，在“精、气、神”中“神”就可译作 spirit；作为 mind 的“神”是指人的思维活动，如在“安神”中“神”则可译作 mind，所以，“安神”译为 tranquilizing the mind；如指人的精神状态，也可译作 vitality[3]。

综上所述，目前对“神明”的英语翻译主要有 spirit、mind、vitality、mentality。我们再来看看这几个词汇的原意。

（1）spirit：①精神，心灵，灵魂。②幽灵，鬼怪，妖精。③活力，锐气，气魄。④具有某种精神、性情的人。⑤体质，精神实质，中心力量，本旨。⑥心情，情绪，兴致，态度，气度，胸怀[4]。

（2）mind：①思想，精神，头脑，思路，心情，心境。②记忆。③注意力。④意向，意愿。⑤看法。⑥有才智的人。⑦反对，介意。⑧注意，小心，当心。⑨照料，照顾，关心[4]。

（3）vitality：活力，生命力，生机，元气[4]。

（4）mentality：①智力，脑力。②心态，思想习惯[4]。

将 spirit、mind、vitality、mentality 这四个词的原意与中医学“神明”的内涵逐一对比，显而易见，这四个英文单词没有一个能完全表达“神明”的含义。而将“神明”译作 bright spirit 更是望文生义。何谓神明之明？“神”有名而无形，看不见、摸不着，但客观存在，我们可以通过它的各种征象去认识、理解它，神明具有客观性与可知性，此谓明。

除此之外，还有 life activity、magic、cereal nutrient 等译法。从某个角度来说，根据不同的语境进行对应翻译，这无可非议。但对中医“神明”这一概念来说，上述翻译总有一种几乎没有尽得其意之感。首先，“神明”是一个概念，对“神明”的理解要从整体观出发；其次，“神明”一词除上述意义外，还有一种只能意会、不可言传的内涵。

中国传统医学历史悠久、博大精深，随着我国加入 WTO，中医学逐渐为国际医药界认同、接受与重视，对国际医药学产生越来越重要的影响。把中医学翻译成英语推向世界是当务之急，这也是一项十分艰巨的任务。如何恰如其分、准确体现中医内涵的原意，又易为国外学者理解和接受，这是中医英语翻译的基本要求。但是，由于文化上的差异，要做到这一点确非易事。

信息的发展使不同国家、民族之间的文化、信息的交流日趋紧密，文化、信息的交流必须以语言作为桥梁和媒介，所以，不同语言之间的翻译工作甚为重要。翻译并非两种文字之间简单的转换，而是信息的传递，是一种跨文化的沟通。世界上没有一个民族的语言能完全解释另一个民族的语言，其主要瓶颈在于不同文化之间的差异。李照国老师则把中医翻译的难点概括为“对应语的缺乏和理解的偏差”，可谓一矢中的。

中医学富有中国传统文化特质，有着独特的理论体系，在其发展过程中受到中国古代哲学、天文学、气象学及宗教文化等因素的影响，其理论深奥，概念抽象，内涵及外延丰富，如果没有一定的传统文化功底，则不易掌握。其中有些表述连现代语言都无法阐述，更何况是用英语来翻译。再加上汉语文字的特殊性，大大增加了中医英语翻译的难度。

要不失本意地将中医进行英语翻译，特别是对一些重要的概念、定义，单靠直译，甚至望文生义的翻译，其效果会适得其反。不但我们自己看不懂，别人对中医学也只能进行片面、断章取义的理解，甚至会产生歧义，这大大有悖于我们的初衷。

其实，在中医英语翻译的众多方法中有一种音译法，可以作出弥补。1982年WHO委托西太区研究制定针灸经穴名称国际标准化方案时，采用了穴位的汉语拼音音译法，此法在针灸的国际化进程中得到了广泛的采用，效果显著。

中医基础理论中的一些概念，如阴阳、气、三焦、命门等，因其内涵丰富，且在自己的学术领域仍有争议，在英语中缺乏对应语，根据“语言国情学”的基本要求，一般应采用音译法译之。如将“阴阳”音译为Yin and Yang或Yin-Yang，把“气”音译为Qi等。这样就避免了理解上的偏差。其实，在我们现代汉语中也有许多词语是音译的外来语，如吉普车（jeep）、卡片（card）、啤酒（beer）等[5]。所以，我们不妨采用音译方法，将中医学“神明”一词音译为Shenming，将“神”译为Shen，这对于英语或其他国家的语言来说是外来语。他们可以从头开始，从其原意出发去认识、理解而掌握，最后接受它，犹如我们接受上述外来语一样。

语言是知识的载体，也是交流的工具，成功的沟通必须有“共同的语言”（并非同一种语言）。中医英语翻译的根本目的是让其他国家认识、接受中医。中医英语翻译的首要原则是必须在充分理解中医学相关知识的基础上进行翻译。根据翻译的信息性原则，当中医理论中有一些特有的核心名词术语在英语中根本没有对应词，或无论直译或意译都无法准确再现其内涵时，就应利用汉语拼音来代替，使之转化为一个统一的符号，代表某个特殊的概念，从而成为一种规范化的译名，以避免原文信息扭曲或丢失[6]。这对于保持中医特色，弘扬中国传统医学十分重要，而且目前国内外的实践证明，采用音译法翻译中医学某些特有概念是切实可行的。

参考文献

[1] 刘毅，徐江．中医英语．2版．天津：天津科技翻译出版公司，2007：28－286.

[2] 李照国．WHO西太区与世界中医药学会联合会中医名词术语国际标准比较研究：脏腑部分．中西医结合学报，2008，6（11）：1200－1204.

[3] 李照国．WHO西太区与世界中医药学会联合会中医名词术语国际标准比较研究：精、神、气、血、津、液部分．中西医结合学报，2008，6（10）：1090－1093.

[4] 陆国强．朗文袖珍英汉双解精选词典．上海：上海译文出版社，1994：442－837.

[5] 李照国，李相敏．言不过其辞，动不过其则——谈谈中医英语翻译中的音译问题．中西医结合学报，2007，5（6）：712－714.

[6] 丁雪光．中医核心词汇和经典语句翻译策略分析．中华中医药杂志，2006，21（8）：500－501.

[原载《中国中西医结合杂志》，2010，30（6）：656－657.]

谈“脏象”与“脏腑”术语的英译

袁洪仁

脏象学说是中医学的核心理论，其中含有许多脏腑术语，对其进行英译时必须忠实地表达其原意。

1. “脏象”与“脏腑”的英译

所谓脏象，“脏”指藏于体内的内脏，包括五脏六腑和奇恒之腑；象指“脏”的外在反映，其义有二：一是指内脏表现于外的生理病理现象，二是指内脏的解剖形态。故“脏”或“脏腑”可译作 viscera，因 viscera 意为“机体的内部器官”。脏象可译作 visceral-graph，意为“用特殊方式对脏腑记录的结果”。

2. “五脏”的英译

从形象上看，五脏属于实体性器官；从功能上看，“藏精气而不泻也，故满而不能实”（《黄帝内经》）。故“脏”可译为 fillessencery，意为“充满精气的场所”。五脏本从五行而来，故心、肝、脾、肺、肾分别可译作 cardiofire-Qi、hepatowood-Qi、splenosoil-Qi、pulmogold-Qi、nephrowater-Qi，意思分别为火性心、木性肝、土性脾、金性肺、水性肾[1]。这种译法中，五行之前的词根反映了五脏原有解剖学基础之事实，后缀五行强调了中医五脏的特殊性，其中后缀 Qi 尤能体现中医五脏是功能性概念。因为中医五脏是先贤用“视其外应，以知其内脏”的认识方法，以已有的解剖观察获得的认识为基础，按五行模式取类比象而作出的机体功能划分。

3. “六腑”的英译

从形象上看，六腑是中空性器官；从功能看，六腑“传化物而不藏，故实而不能满也”（《黄帝内经》）。故“腑”可译作“sitodigested duct”，意为“化物的引导结构”，既表达了六腑的功能特性，又表达了六腑作为引导化物之结构必然的中空形象。六腑中胃、小肠、大肠、膀胱、胆可分别译为 stomach、small intestine、large intestine、urinary bladder、gallbladder，符合中医名词术语英译中“仿照西医，求同存异”的原则[2]。但六腑中三焦是中医学特有的概念，翻译时应尽量符合其原意。中医学认为，“三焦者，确有一腑，盖脏腑之外，躯壳之内，包罗诸脏，一腔之大腑也”（《类经》），其功能为通行元气和运行水谷。故

“三焦”可译作 general sitodigested duct，意为“总腑”，表达了三焦能运行水谷，是“包罗诸脏，一腔之大腑”的特点，而饮食水谷的转化有赖于元气的激发和推动，即作为运行水谷的“总腑”三焦，必然有元气的通行，因此，general sitodigested duct 能确切地表达腑名三焦之原意。三焦在中医学中还表示人体分部，可译作“tri-Jiao”，包括上焦（upper-Jiao）、中焦（mid-Jiao）和下焦（lower-Jiao）。

4. “奇恒之腑”的英译

奇恒之腑形多中空，与腑相近；内藏精气，又类于脏。奇者异也，恒者常也。故奇恒之腑可译为 extra-ordinary viscera，因 viscera 既可表示脏，又可表示腑。奇恒之腑中脑、髓、骨、脉、胆、女子胞可分别译为 brain、marrow、bone、vessel、gall-bladder、uterus。

参考文献

[1] 袁洪仁. 有关中医五行学说术语的英译. 中国中西医结合杂志，1998，18（2）：110.
[2] 王朝辉，林岩，陈淑芬，等. 中医名词术语的分类及其英译的标准化. 中国中西医结合杂志，1997，17（2）：107－108.

[原载《中国中西医结合杂志》，2000，20（3）：164.]

谈中医名词术语“辨证论治”的英译

王得奎

正确英译中医名词术语，首先应准确地掌握名词术语的真实内涵，然后才能将其原意准确而完全地译出。目前从有关的杂志和辞典中可以见到，各种出版物对“证”有各种的理解，译法也各异。例如，有的将“证”理解为“症状”，译为symptom；有的理解为综合症状，译为symptom-complex、symptom-group，或symptom complex groups；有的理解为症状与体征，译为symptoms and signs；有的将“证”等同于疾病而把“表证”和“里证”分别译为outer-disease和inner-disease；也有的理解为综合征（征候群）而译为syndrome，不一而足。因此，“辨证论治”也就出现了各种译法，例如：①differential symptomatic treatment；②treatment according to differentiation of symptoms and signs；③traditional Chinese medicine treatment according to an overall differentiation of symptoms and signs；④selection of treatment based on the differential diagnosis；⑤diagnosis and treatment based on an overall analysis of symptoms and signs等。

关于如何理解“证”的真实内涵并准确地英译“辨证论治”的原意，首先应尊重古代各医家的不同理解和描述，也应结合现代的认识，以便找出“证”的真实内涵和“辨证论治”的确切含义，因此，笔者认为“证”的内涵应是中医通过四诊而获取的患者全部临床表现或全部症状和体征，按八纲、脏腑、六经、三焦、卫气营血和病因等中医理论进行分析归纳而得出的一组征候群或综合征。它体现了病因、病机、病位和疾病性质的综合概念。而症状是疾病对人们所引起的主观不舒适、不正常的感觉或一些较明显的病态改变。将“证”译为symptoms或symptom-complex或symptom-group或disease都是不准确的[1]，而译成clinical manifestation或symptoms and signs也尚欠妥，若译成syndrome则近于原意。

“辨证论治”是使用较多的名词术语，它说明了中医治疗是以辨证为前提，而辨证是治疗的根据。治疗就是根据辨证的结果按中医的立法、方药拟出适宜而具体的治疗方法，因此，“辨证论治”应译为：treatment according to differentiation of syndrome，从其语法结构上既突出了中心思想——治疗（treatment），又以介词短语according to differentiation of syndrome作为修饰它的定语以说明治疗是根据辨证的结果做出的。这样的译法既道出了“证”的真实内涵，也摆正了辨证与论治的逻辑关系，并突出了中医的治疗特点。

参考文献

[1] 邓家栋，张安. 诊断学基础. 北京：人民出版社，1964.

[原载《中国中西医结合杂志》，1996，26（4）：251.]

“证”的新译

李　雷　蒋俊明

辨证论治是中医学基本特色之一，其中证居于核心地位。对于“证”这一中医学基本概念的英译，本文提出新的见解，认为可将其译为 zhengery。

1. “证”的含义及其与有关概念的不同

证是机体在疾病过程中某一阶段的病理概括，是人体在疾病过程中典型的反应状态。同一种疾病，由于发病的时间、地区及患者机体反应性的不同，或处于不同的发展阶段，可表现出不同的证；不同的疾病在各自的发展过程中可表现出相同的证。辨证论治的结果，即产生了“同病异治，异病同治”的现象。症状（symptom）是患者主观感觉到的异常感觉或不适感觉；体征（sign）是客观检查到的病态表现。证由一系列相关的症状和体征构成，但用“症状和体征”绝不能说明证的阶段性、状态性和本质性。综合征（syndrome）是指构成某种病理情况而其特征尚未完全确定、其原因不明或原因多种多样的症状和体征的集合。同一综合征因时、因地、因人、因阶段的不同，可以辨为不同的证。显然，现代医学中具有特定含义的综合征与充满中医特色的证是两个不同的概念。

2. “证”的英译现状及其评价

对“证”这一中医术语的英译现尚不统一。较为常见的是 syndrome，代表性著作有《汉英医学大词典》（人民卫生出版社，1987）、《英汉对照实用中医文库·中医诊断学》（上海中医学院出版社，1990）、《英汉实用中医药大全·中医学基础》（高等教育出版社，1991）、《汉语主题词表》（科学技术文献出版社，1993）、《汉英双解实用中医词汇》（科学出版社，1993）、《汉英中医药分类词典》（新世界出版社，1994）等。其中《汉英医学大词典》《汉英中医药分类词典》还将“证”译为 symptom complex（即症状集合体）。此外，《汉英医学大词典》《中医药主题词表》（北京科技出版社，1987）、《汉语主题词表》将“辨证”翻译成 differentiation of symptoms and signs，即将“证”等同于 symptoms and signs。

关于“证”与 syndrome、symptom、sign 的区别已如前述，我们可以认为这些词汇在现代医学英语中找对等词的译法均不能正确表达“证”的含义，且易于导致误解。

3. “证”的新译

本文采用音意共译的方法，将“证”翻译为 zhengery，即由音译部分 zheng 和意译后缀-ery 共同组成。对于中医学中极少数现代医学中无法替代的重要概念，采用音译的方法是必要的。英语中大量外来词、新创词的存在使之更具有可行性。证作为联系基础理论和临床各科的桥梁和纽带，在中医学中占有重要的地位。在无满意翻译的情况下，将“证”音译为 zheng 是必要的、可行的。根据《牛津现代高级英汉双解辞典》（第 3 版），后缀“-ery”的含义为 state、quality、character，即状态、性质、特征。音译部分 zheng 与-ery 连接，增加了意译成分，反映了证的状态性、本质性。在现阶段，对辨证、辨证论治的翻译多为描述性、解释性，与其说是翻译，不如说是两个概念的英语解释。新译 zhengery 不仅可以避免一些不必要的误解，而且可使辨证、辨证论治的翻译得到简化。应用科技英语构词法中的转化法，可将“辨证”译为 zhengerify（及物动词和不及物动词）或 zhengerification（名词），相应地将“辨证论治”译为 zhengerify and treat 或 zhengerification and treatment。中医基础理论的翻译工作尚属初起阶段。笔者希望此时对中医英译进行“百家争鸣”，因为有竞争才有发展，有淘汰才有优选。只要中医学能够放光华于世界，本文甘做铺路的沙石。

[原载《中国中西医结合杂志》，1988，18（11）：644.）

试论“证”及其相关词语的英译

成肇智

证，古写作“證”，后俗写作“症”。在中医学中的本义，证是指医生通过四诊获得并用作诊断证据的一切临床信息，包括今人所说的症状、体征、病史及各种现代检测结果在内的一切可用作诊断凭据的资料。可见，把“证”或“证候”译成 symptom and sign（症状和体征）或 clinical manifestations（临床表现）虽大体不错，但欠完整、准确，因为中医的“证”（证候）不仅以症状、体征在内的临床表现为主要内容，而且涵括了病史、年龄、性别、职业、时令、气候、地理环境等一切对中医诊断有帮助的信息。所以，若把“证”或“证候”译成 clinical evidence（临床证据）似乎更能表达出此词的中医学本义及其完整的内涵。

临床上，证候并非一个一个地单独出现或杂乱无章地涌现，而都是由病机引起的多个证候常相伴出现，于是就产生了证候类型（简称证型）的概念。一个证型就是某一病机引起的一组证候或证候群。近年来，多把“证型”译作syndrome 或 symptom complex，前者乃西医学的综合征，而后者即症候群，其内涵比证型狭窄。按前述证候的英译，“证型”应译作 type of clinical evidences，“脾气虚证(型)”则可译为 spleen-Qi deficiency type of clinical evidences。主证、次证和兼证在证型中的地位各不相同，可分别译作 chief clinical evidence、subordinate clinical evidence 和 concurrent clinical evidence。

中医文献常用主证给疾病命名，而对每一种疾病又分若干证型给予诊治，因此，出现了“病证”这一与“疾病”概念基本一致的术语，并且病和证有时又混用而不分开，如中医学的痹病也可叫做痹证，而《伤寒论》则把“太阳证”称作“太阳病”。然而英译时却不能如此模棱两可，即“痹”只能译成病名而不能译成证型，“太阳”应译成证型而不宜译成病名。同时，“病证”一词也可简称为“证”。这样，一个“证”字在中医文献及口语中便可能有证候、证型和病证三种内涵，从而分别译为 clinical evidences、type of clinical evidences 和 disease（或 disorder)。至于某一句子中的“证”字究竟应如何英译，则需要先根据上下文正确判断其中文的具体内涵，然后再选用相应的英语表达。

“辨证论治”是当前中医学界使用频率最高的术语之一，可是它的英语表达却是一个老大难问题，长期得不到满意的解决。问题的症结主要不在英译方面，而是来自对“辨证”的中文解释有较大的分歧。归纳有关教科书和词典所载，“辨证”不外乎有四种解释：一是释为辨别、分析证候（症状和体征)；二是释为通过辨析证候以找出“病理症结”；三是释为探求和识别证型；四是释为辨清病因（实指病邪）、病位、病性和邪正关系等某一特定阶段的病理变化实质，即审察病机之意。与此相应，对“辨证论治”的英译也就五花八门。上述四种解释的分歧焦点是对“证”的不同理解，而且都欠妥当。第一种释“证”为证候，虽符合“证”的本义，但“辨证”和“论治”之间如何联系却成了悬念。为弥补此不足，后三种解释便有意识地“扩充”了“证”的内涵。第二种所谓“病理症结”，其内涵不清，且有增字足义之嫌。第三种释“证”为证型虽通，但证型作为及物动词“辨”的对象则欠妥，因为“辨”的对象只能是从四诊收集到的证候，而证型则要通过“辨证”得出病机结论后才能确定并命名，因此，把“辨证论治”的“证”释作证型不可取。第四种实际上把“辨证”释为辨别病机了，这不仅混淆了“辨”的对象和结果，而且也混淆了疾病的现象（证候）和疾病的本质（病机），势必造成这些重要概念及其相关词语使用上更严重的混乱局面。

显而易见，“辨证论治”一词先天不足，即它的文字构成决定了它表述不出需要它表述的学术内容。然而，若将其改为“辨证识机定治”或“审机定治”，则义明理顺，其英译也随之变得简易而流畅。较权威的《汉英医学大词典》（人民卫生出版社，1987）把“辨证论治”英译为“diagnosis and treatment based on overall analysis of symptoms and signs，the cause，nature and location of the illness and the patient's physical condition according to the basic theories of traditional Chinese medicine.”此译文既未把中医学的基本诊疗规律和学术特点表达清楚、准确，句子又冗长，且逻辑混乱。建议英译成 treatment according to the pathogenesis ascertained by overall analysis of clinical evidences，意即：辨证以识机，据机以定治。此译法能够简明扼要地表述出中医学的基本诊疗规律和学术特点。当然，像“辨证论治”这样内涵比较复杂的专业性术语出现在文章中时，有时为求句式简洁，也可采用音译（汉语拼音）的形式加以处理。

[原载《中国中西医结合杂志》，1999，19（9）：561－562.]

有关中医五行学说术语的英译

袁洪仁

中医五行学说认为，世界上一切事物均由木、火、土、金、水五类基本物质间的运动变化而生成的，并用五行之间的生、克、乘、侮关系来阐释事物之间的相互关系。现今中医学中，木、火、土、金、水又表示五种物质的属性，因而它们可分别译为 wood-Qi、fire-Qi、soil-Qi、gold-Qi、water-Qi。因中医学中气（Qi）既可表示物质概念（气血津液学说），又可表示属性概念（中药气味理论）。故用“Qi”搭配成复合词表达木、火、土、金、水的中医学内涵是较恰当的。至于生、克、乘、侮，可分别译作 foster（助长，促进，养育）、restrain（克制，抑制）、over-restrain（过度克制）、counter-restrain（反向克制）。其中 foster 的“养育”之意，尤能表达五行相生间的“母子关系”。

总之，中医英译准确性的前提是把握中医名词术语的真实内涵，它也可作为中医名词术语英译标准化的原则。

[原载《中国中西医结合杂志》，1998，18（2）：110.]

谈中医术语“气”的英译

袁洪仁

中医术语“气”的内涵较多，在中医及中西医结合等文献中有多种英译：①Qi；②vital energy；③vital-Qi；④healthy energy；⑤healthy Qi 等。按双语术语学的一般研究方法，要将一种语言的术语译成另一种语言的术语，首先要弄清前者的概念特性和使用范围，再从后者寻找前者的对等（equivalent）词或对应（correspondent）词或创造新词。要对“气”作出正确的英译，必须把握“气”的真实内涵。现对“气”的英译进行如下分析。

1. 气的含义

“气”在中医学中是一个重要术语，在气血津液学说中是一个物质概念，指构成人体和维持人体生命活动的最基本物质，具有运动着的活力很强的特性；在脏象学说中是一个功能概念，指脏腑或经脉的功能；在病因学说中是指气候或致病因素；在温病学说中是指外感热病发展中的某个病理阶段。而在英语中找不到一个词义符合中医术语“气”之内涵的对等词或对应词，单词“energy”意为“活力、精力、能量”，不能表达中医术语“气”的“物质”或“功能”等含义，故用译音“Qi”显得较恰当，既能反映中医特色，又能表达中医术语“气”的诸多内涵。而且科技英语中使用外来词也很常见，如 shock（休克）、Ameba（阿米巴）等。国外也常把“气”译作“Qi”，表明“Qi”的英译得到了外国人的认可而乐意加以使用。

2. 为了表达“气”在不同场合的含义，可加用英语搭配词

在气血津液学说中可将“气”译作“vital-Qi”，因“vital”有“与生命有关的”之意。相应地，“vital-Qi”可分成 prime vital-Qi（元气）、intra-thorax vital-Qi（宗气）、intrahemoced vital-Qi（营气）、peri-defense vital-Qi（卫气）等译法；在脏象学说中可译作 visceral Qi（脏气）、heart-Qi（心气）等；在病因学说中可译成 climate-Qi（气候之气）或 pathogenic-Qi（致病之气）；在温病学说中可译作 Qi-phase（气分）。相应地，就有 peri-defense-phase（卫分）、intrahemoced phase（营分）和 blood-phase（血分）的译法。

另外，关于中医术语“正气”的译法，应注意“正气”的双重含义：一是指真气。《灵枢·刺节真邪篇》曰：“真气者，所受于天，与谷气併而充身（者）

也”。二是相对于邪气而言，正气指机体的抗病能力，因此，“正气”可译作 healthy-Qi，因 healthy 有“有益于健康的”之意，能表达“正气”的“充身”和“抗病”之功用，而“邪气”可译作 evil-Qi（邪恶之气，有害之气）。

总之，中医术语的英译应规范、统一，才能使中医成为世界性医学，加速它在国外的传播。学术界应大力研究中医术语的英译问题。

[原载《中国中西医结合杂志》，1997，17（2）：108－109.]

谈谈中医学中“虚实”的翻译

兰凤利

阴、阳、表、里、寒、热、虚、实统称“八纲”，是辨证论治的理论基础之一。八纲辨证就是通过四诊，掌握辨证资料之后，根据病位的深浅、病邪的性质和盛衰，以及人体正气的强弱等，加以综合分析，归纳为八类证候的过程。疾病的表现尽管极其复杂，但基本上都可用八纲加以归纳。如疾病的类别，可分阴证与阳证；病位的深浅，可分表证与里证；疾病的性质，可分寒证与热证；邪正的盛衰，邪盛为实证，正虚为虚证。

“八纲”可直译为 eight principles，或根据其具体内容和所指，采用释义法译为 eight principal patterns；“阴、阳、表、里、寒、热”一般译为 Yin、Yang、exterior、interior、cold、heat，基本没有任何异议。

“虚实”的翻译却颇为混乱，主要有 deficiency and excess、emptiness and fullness、vacuity and repletion、asthenia and sthenia、depletion and repletion 等。

下面基于“虚实”的本义——“虚”指正气不足，“实”指邪气盛实，分析一下这几组译语。

1. deficiency and excess：deficiency 的意思是 state of lacking something essential，excess 的意思是 going beyond the normal limits，二者表示的都是异常状态，又没有走向极端[1]。而且，这对译语已为大多数作者所接受。WHO 颁布的《传统医学术语国际标准化方案》（2007）亦选用 deficiency and excess 作为“虚实”的标准化译语[2]。

2. vacuity and repletion：vacuity 有 absence or lack of something specified，absence of thought or intelligence 等含义，这个意义与“虚”的本义没有任何关系[3]；vacuity 的另外一个含义是 the state of being vacuous or without contents，vacancy，emptiness[4]。但是，我们知道，如果正气“虚”到这个程度，即正气完全失去，生命也就不复存在了。repletion 的意思是 the state of being fully provided or filled，esp. with food[5]，也不恰当。

3. emptiness and fullness：其含义与 vacuity and repletion 基本相同，不再赘述

4. asthenia and sthenia：asthenia 的意思是 being weak，not having any strength[6]，从词义来看，仅适于描述“气虚”的情况，却不适于描述阴虚、血虚、精虚及其他虚证；而 sthenia 的词义与 asthenia 相反，指“强壮、健康”的

状态，不符合“实”的本义——邪气盛。

5．depletion and repletion：deplete 的意思是 to lessen greatly in amount，contents，etc.[5]，因而用 depletion 表达“虚”，有点趋向极端了——即大部分“虚证”没有虚到这个程度。由此可见，无论是从“虚实”的本义出发，还是从 deficiency and excess 的出现频率来看，还是遵循 WHO 的建议，“虚实”均宜译为 deficiency and excess。

参考文献

[1] Xie ZF. On the standard nomenclature of traditional Chinese medicine. Beijing：Foreign Languages Press，2003：158.

[2] 世界卫生组织 . WHO 西太区传统医学名词术语国际标准．北京：北京大学医学出版社，2007：115.

[3] Wiseman N，Feng Y. A practical dictionary of Chinese medicine. 2nd ed. Beijing：People's Medical Publishing House，2002：645.

[4] Webster's encyclopedic unabridged dictionary of the English language（new revised edition）. New York：Gramercy Books，1994：1577.

[5] Addison Wesley Longman Limited. Longman dictionary of contemporary English. Beijing：The Commercial Press，1998：1277，395.

[6] Collin，PH. Dictionary of medicine. Beijing：Foreign Language Teaching and Research Press，2001：43.

[原载《中国中西医结合杂志》，2010，30（6）：655－656.]

中医诊断学中常用辨证证名英译探讨

李永安

目前中医诊断学中常用辨证证名的英译形式较为混乱，比较突出的问题是由于缺乏科学的翻译原则和方法，使得有些译名的形式不符合科技术语的要求，有些释义性名词译文较长，甚至出现不定式短语、分词短语和介词短语等。例如："肾不纳气"和"肠虚滑泻证"分别被译为：failure of the kidney to maintain normal inspiration 和 lingering diarrhea due to asthenia of the large intestine。现仅就中医辨证证名的英译谈一些个人看法。

1. 翻译的原则

个人认为，对辨证证名翻译时，应掌握以下原则：①科学性原则：所谓科学性原则是指标准化的辨证证名的英译形式要语义准确（semantically precise）、词形简明（morphologically concise）、符合现代科技术语的构成机制（structurally consistent with the formation and usage of modern scientific and technological terminology）。②简洁性原则：中医用语的突出特点之一就是简明扼要，用字少而表意深刻，辨证证名亦是如此，因此，译名时应尽量达到简洁性这一原则。③信息性原则：辨证证名一般都承载一定的信息，即对该名词的内涵具有直接或间接的说明作用。这样的名词能使人见词明意，很有实用性，因此，翻译时也应使译名同样具有信息性。

2. 翻译的方法

具体的翻译方法有：①直译：根据其证名，直接译出所对应的英文。例如：表证、寒证、虚证等可分别直译为 exterior syndrome、cold syndrome、asthenia syndrome。直译主要适用于八纲辨证类证名。②意译：根据其证名含义，译出证名。例如，血分证是温热病邪由表已深入血分较为深重的危急阶段，因此，可意译为 hemophase syndrome。意译主要适用于卫气营血辨证类证名。③音译：主要适用于六经辨证类病名。例如，太阳病、少阴病等可分别音译为 Taiyang disease和 Shaoyin disease。④词素仿造译法：词素仿造译法是综合体现以上翻译方法三原则最有效的译法，可广泛地应用在中医名词英译之中，它将使中医名词英译最终走向标准化之路。例如，有人将"肝火上炎"和"心气虚"等证分别译为 flaming-up of liver fire、insufficiency of the heart-Qi，如用词素仿造可将其简化为 hyperhepatopyrosis 和 hypocardioqi 这样两个词。读者从这两个词的构成词素（hyper：过多；hepato：肝；pyrosis：热病理状态；hypo：不足；cardio：心；Qi：气）上，完全可以猜出其证名含义。这样的译名能使人见词明意，完全符合科学性、简洁性和信息性翻译原则。

3. 辨证证名译文

3.1 八纲辨证类证名

表证：exterior syndrome；里证：interior syndrome；寒证：cold syndrome；热证：heat syndrome；寒热真假证：false manifestations of cold or heat syndrome；虚证：asthenia syndrome；实证：sthenia syndrome；阴证：Yin syndrome；阳证：Yang syndrome；阴虚证：asthenic Yin；阳虚证：asthenic Yang；亡阴证：Yin depletion；亡阳证：Yang depletion。

3.2 气血辨证类证名

气虚证：asthenic Qi syndrome；气陷证：collapsed Qi syndrome；气逆证：reversed flow of Qi；气滞证：Qi stagnation syndrome；血虚证：hemopenia syndrome；血瘀证：blood stasis syndrome；血热证：hemopyrosis syndrome；血寒证：hemocryosis syndrome；气滞血瘀证：Qi-stagnated blood stasis；气血两虚证：deficiency of both blood and Qi；气虚失血证：Qi deficiency hemorrhage；气随血脱证：hemorrhagic exhaustion of Qi。

3.3 脏腑辨证类证名

心气虚证：hypocardio-Qi；心阳虚证：hypocardio-Yang；心血虚证：cardio-hemopenia；心阴虚证：hypocardio-Yin；心火亢盛证：hypercardiopyrosis；心脉痹阻证：obstruction of cardiac vessel；痰迷心窍证：phlegm-stagnated；痰火扰心证：cardiac disturbance by pyretic phlegm；肺气虚证：hypopulmono-Qi；肺阴虚证：hypopulmono-Yin；风寒束肺证：anemocryosis-obstructed lung；风热犯肺证：anemopyretic invasion of lung；热邪壅肺证：retention of pulmonary pyrosis；痰湿阻肺证：accumulation of hygrosic phlegm of lung；脾气虚证：hypospleno-Qi；脾阳虚证：hypospleno-Yang；中气下陷证：sinking of splenogastric-Qi；脾不统血证：splenic failure for intravascular blood circulation；寒湿困脾证：cryohygrosis-obstructed spleen；湿热蕴脾证：hygropyrosis retention of spleen；肝气郁结证：stagnation of hepato-Qi；肝火上炎证：hyperhepatopyrosis；肝血虚证：hepatic hemopenia；肝阴虚证：hypohepato-Yin；肝阳上亢证：hyperhepato-Yang；肝风内动证：upstirring of hepatanemia；寒滞肝脉证：accumulation of hepatocryosis；肝经湿热证：hygropyrosis of hepatic meridian；肾阳虚证：hyponephro-Yang；肾阴虚证：hyponephro-Yin；肾精不足证：insufficiency of kidney essence；肾气不

固证：unconsolidation of nephro-Qi；肾不纳气证：nephric failure for normal inspiration；胃阴虚证：hypogastro-Yin；食滞胃脘证：retention of indigested food in stomach；胃寒证：gastrocryosis；胃热证：gastropyrosis；胆郁痰扰证：gallbladder stagnated disturbance of phlegm；大肠湿热证：colihygropyrosis；大肠液亏证：coliliquopenia；肠虚滑泻证：prolonged colipenic diarrhea；小肠实热证：sthenic enteropyrosis；膀胱湿热证 cystohygropyrosis。

3.4　六经辨证类证名

太阳病：Taiyang disease；阳明病：Yangming disease；少阳病：Shaoyang disease；太阴病：Taiyin disease；少阴病：Shaoyin disease；厥阴病：Jueyin disease。

3.5　卫气营血辨证类证名

卫分证：defending phase syndrome；气分证：Qi phase syndrome；营分证：trophophase syndrome；血分证：hemophase syndrome。

[原载《中国中西医结合杂志》，1995，15（8）：499－500.]

谈谈中医“实”和“虚”的英译

卢文超

“实”和“虚”在中医中出现广泛，如实证、虚证、实热、实寒、虚热、虚寒、气虚、血虚、脾虚、肾虚等，不仅在病名中，而且在其他的句子里也经常出现。目前，“实”和“虚”主要有如下几种英译法：①把“实”译为 sthenia，把“虚”译为 asthenia；②把“实”译为 excess，把“虚”译为 deficiency；③把“实”译为 Shi，把“虚”译为 Xu。上述译法中又以第 2 种译法最为常用。第 1、2 种译法基本上是根据“实”和“虚”的意义进行对译，第 3 种译法为音译。

古人由于科学条件的限制，不可能认识到发生疾病时机体的各种病理变化，只能从整体上观察，当患者有抵抗力时，称为“实”；当患者缺乏抵抗力时，称为“虚”，因此，“实”和“虚”的命名，对古人来说其含义是恰当的。但是在翻译时，我们应该考虑到，读者的对象是习惯于现代医学概念的外国人，他们注重实验观察到的病理改变，而这种病理改变是复杂的。例如实热和实寒时，虽同为实证，机体的功能有可能是亢进的，也可能是低下的。实热时交感-肾上腺髓质功能偏亢进，而实寒时则降低；又如阴虚和阳虚，虽同为虚证，阴虚时核酸和能量代谢亢进，阳虚时则低下，因此，把“实”和“虚”分别用含义“亢进”和“缺乏”与英语对译，外国人会难以接受。

实际上，把“实”和“虚”按词义翻译时，由于在英文中找不到意义相同的对应词，因此，只能用含有亢进、过度、虚弱、缺乏等意义的英文词来对译，这实际上和“实”与“虚”的原意有了不小的出入，外国人看到这些英文词后，往往理解为“功能亢进”和“功能减退”。例如，当我们把“肾虚”翻译为 deficiency of kidney 时，外国人就很容易把它理解为“肾功能不全”；又如阴虚型甲状腺功能亢进，把“阴虚”译为 deficiency of Yin 时，外国人会感到莫名其妙，一个功能亢进的疾病怎么能和“功能减退”联系起来呢？

现代研究已经发现，实证与快调节有关，虚证与慢调节有关[1]。由于“实”和“虚”本身的词义与快调节和慢调节的意义并无联系，因此，当我们采用第 1、2 种译法时，外国人必须要从“亢进”和“缺乏”再转个弯，理解为“快调节”和“慢调节”。而采用音译就既简单又方便，由于“Shi”和“Xu”本身没有实质性的英文含义，通过注释，外国人就可以把“Shi”和“Xu”直接和快、慢调节功能失调这一本质联系起来。

中医学中，还有虚多实少、虚实并见、由实致虚等提法，如果把“实”和

“虚”采用第1、2种译法代入上述句子中，就会很不自然，而把“实”和“虚”的音译（即第3种译法）代入上述句子中，就显得灵活得多了，因此，笔者认为，翻译“实”和“虚”最好采用音译的方法。

参考文献

[1] 刘亚光．分子生物学与中西医结合．浙江中医学院学报，1979，(增刊)：26.

[原载《中国中西医结合杂志》，1999，19（6）：366.]

“整体观念”翻译之浅见

何成诗

中医学的基本特点有两个，一是整体观念，二是辨证施治。“整体观念”这个术语在中医学中具有独特含义，对其正确理解至关重要，只有准确翻译才能使外国人体会到其实质。但要想在英语中找到合适的对等词是比较困难的。关于“整体观念”，在《汉英常用中医词汇》及新出版的《中医基础理论》上册中，或译为“as a whole”，或译为“unity”，或译为“entirety”。在此愚意认为值得商榷，提出来谨供参考。

“整体”就是完整性、统一性。“整体观念”作为中医术语有两层基本含义。从结构上来说，人体各个组成部分之间是不可分割的，在生理上是相互联系、相互资助、相互制约的，在病理上也是相互影响的。同时，人又生活在自然界中，自然界的运动变化又可直接或间接影响人体，人体也必然相应地产生生理或病理上的反应。重要的是人体绝不是由组成它的各个组织器官的简单相加。

汉语中“整体”二字，英语中表达的词较多，常见的有 whole、unity、entirety、complete 和 holistic。现对这些词汇进行分析。

（1）whole：《牛津现代高级英汉双解辞典》（以下简称《牛津辞典》）的解释为“not injured or damaged；unbroken”。《英汉辞海》认为 whole 来自中古英语的“hool healthy”，意思为 unhurt。综合其他工具书得出其确切含义为“完整体的，齐全的，未受损的”，可见其表示的是“没有受损的完整性”。这显然与中医学认为人体是一个有机整体的观念不相符。

（2）unity：《牛津辞典》解释道：“the state of being united，an arrangement of parts to form a complete whole”，“联合、结合、统一、协调”。《英汉辞海》认为 unity 指“相关部分的总和。复杂的整体或整个系统由不同部分、因素组成一体的完整性”。显然 unity 表示的“整体”重点在与组成整体的“单位”（unit）相对，指的是从 unit 到 unity 的联合状态。而 unit 在医学上主要用来表示“单元、单位、遗传单位”。如果用在中医学中易让人误以为“人是由一些组织器官组合而成”。

（3）至于 entirety、complete，大都解释为 whole、unbroken，即与 whole 大致相同。从词义角度看这几个词用来表示中医整体观均欠准确。中医整体观本身也是一个确定的重要术语，英语中也应用一个固定的词对译。

（4）holistic：日常用得少，在古印欧语中亦有“全部的、完整的、未受损的”含义，后来被用作指一种哲学理论（holism）。这种观点认为自然界起决定作用的因素是一些不能归结为部分的总和的整体（如有机体）；整体不是各个部分的总和或可被分解为彼此分立而无联系的单个元素，这样，holistic 的含义也有了一些变化，即有“强调部分与整体之间的有机联系或功能关系的含义”。如果用 holistic 翻译中医整体观，也就具有一定的哲学渊源，可见，从词源学角度上看，holistic 比其他几个词更准确一些。

从以上分析可以看出，在 whole、unity、entirety、complete、holistic 几个词中，以 holistic 之含义最接近中医“整体观”。

中医较传统西医更加重视精神、情志和环境对人体的影响。当前关于新的医学模式的讨论也正是为了吸取中西医之所长创造出新的医学。医学的“整体化与技术化是当今医学的两大主要发展趋势”。所谓整体化即整体医学。J. Smuts（1870—1950）首先把 holistic 引入医学，创用整体医学——“holistic medicine”一词。其观点认为精神和生命都是由单位结构组成的，它们综合产生自然的总体或有机体，一个整体总是大于它的部分的总和。整体医学更重视人的心理、环境、工作、经济状况对人健康的影响。由于对传统西方医学的不满，近十多年来，整体医学一直是西方医学界的热门话题。如 1973 年 G. Westberg 在美国伊利诺尹州创建了第一所整体健康中心（Holistic Health Center），让患者既能得到生理上的治疗，又能获得精神上的满足。1978 年 5 月美国整体医学学会（American Holistic Medical Association）在丹佛尔市成立。以后，“整体健康学会”（Association for Holistic Health）以及整体健康和营养研究所（Holistic Health and Nutrition Institute）陆续成立。不论整体医学的哪一个学派，实际上都与中医学有许多相同之处，从某种意义上说整体医学就是西方医学吸收东方医学的一个尝试。国外的“中医热”与整体医学运动的高潮密切相关。所以，用与整体医学相同的词“holistic”翻译中医术语“整体观念”，实际上是把中医学放在世界医学发展趋势上来考虑，使外国人能结合他们自己的历史更深刻地理解中医学的整体观。

总之，无论从词源学角度，还是从医学发展方向上考虑，holistic 比其他几个词更能准确地反映出中医学整体观的含义，同时也更有助于外国人理解中医学的优势。

[原载《中国中西医结合杂志》，2001，21（9）：714.]

中医反治法英译评析

蒋基　昌文娟　柳江帆

反治法是中医防治原则的重要内容之一，包括“寒因寒用”“热因热用”“塞因塞用”和“通因通用”等。随着中医药在世界的传播，反治法的英译也有各种不同的译法。本文就这些译法，特别是与 2007 年 10 月 16 日 WHO 颁布的《传统医学国际标准名词术语》中的译法进行比较分析，辨别优劣，旨在进一步规范统一这些中医术语的英译。

1. 反治法的常见译法

“寒因寒用”“热因热用”“塞因塞用”和“通因通用”的常见英译有：

1.1　treating coldness with the cold, treating hotness with the heat, treating obstruction with tonics, treating openness with purgatives[1]。

1.2　using medicines of cold nature to treat pseudo-cold syndrome, using medicines of hot nature to treat pseudo-heat syndrome, to block up for a blockage, to drain for a drain[2]。

1.3　using medicines of cold nature to treat pseudo-cold syndrome, using drug of hot nature to treat pseudo-heat syndrome, treating obstructive diseases by tonification, treating disease with profuse fluid discharge by increasing fluid discharge[3]。

1.4　treating cold with cold, treating heat with heat, treating the unstopped by unstopping, treating the stopped by stopping[4]。

1.5　using cold for cold, using heat for heat, filling for the stuffed, opening for the opened[5]。

1.6　treating pseudo-cold diseases with drugs of cold nature, treating pseudo-heat diseases with drugs of hot nature, treating the obstruction syndrome with tonics, treating diarrhea with cathartics[6]。

1.7　treating cold with cold, treating heat with heat, treating obstruction with obstructing, treating diarrhea with purgatives[7]。

1.8　treating cold with cold, treating heat with heat, treating the stopped by stopping, treating the unstopped by unstopping[8]。

2. 反治法的英译评析

2.1 “寒因寒用”和“热因热用”

用寒凉性质的药物来治疗具有假寒征象的病症，称为“寒因寒用”；用温热性质的药物来治疗具有假热征象的病症，称为“热因热用”。把“寒因寒用”和“热因热用”翻译成 using medicines of cold nature to treat pseudo-cold syndrome, using medicines of hot nature to treat pseudo-heat syndrome[2]；using medicine of cold nature to treat pseudo-cold syndrome, using drug of hot nature to treat pseudo-heat syndrome[3]；treating pseudo-cold diseases with drugs of cold nature, treating pseudo-heat diseases with drugs of hot nature[6]，只是解析说明了这两个术语的含义，并不是标准的术语翻译，有悖于中医术语翻译的简洁性原则和回译性原则。中医术语的一大突出特点就是简明扼要，用字少而表意深刻，因此，在翻译时一定要强调简洁。只有这样才能保证译名的信息密度，以便于读者记忆和表达。把“寒因寒用”和“热因热用”翻译成 treating coldness with the cold 和 treating hotness with the heat[1]比上述译法要简洁得多，基本上符合简洁性原则。但在同一个术语中，把“寒”分别译成 coldness 和 the cold，把“热”分别译成 hotness 和 the heat，前后不统一，英语语感上也不习惯。可能译者的目的是为了让读者明白 coldness 是指假寒征象的病症，the cold 是指寒凉性质的药物；hotness是指假热征象的病症，the heat 是指温热性质的药物。但作为读者，当他们阅读时会有这样的感觉吗？实际上这就是中文语言模糊性的特点：“寒”可以指假寒征象的病症，也可以指寒凉性质的药物；“热”可以指假热征象的病症，也可以指温热性质的药物，因此，还是把“寒”和“热”，分别译成 cold 和 heat 比较简练。把“寒因寒用”和“热因热用”翻译成 using cold for cold 和 using heat for heat[5]或者 treating cold with cold 和 treating heat with heat[7,8]，非常符合中医术语翻译的简洁性原则和回译性原则，应该说这两种译法都非常出色。在第一种译法中，using 与“用”相对应，介词 for 用来表示目的对象，相比第二种译法更符合回译性原则。但作为一个中医术语，使用 using 来翻译，显得太通俗化，而 treating 要比 using 专业性更强一些，也许这就是 treating cold with cold 和 treating heat with heat 被列入《传统医学国际标准名词术语》的原因之一。

2.2 “塞因塞用”

“塞因塞用”是指用补益药治疗具有闭塞不通症状的病症，适用于因虚而闭阻的真虚假实证。把“塞因塞用”译为 treating obstruction with tonics[1]，treating obstructive diseases by tonification[3]基本上表达了原文的意思，但不太符合回译性原则。把“塞因塞用”译为 filling for the stuffed[5]，treating the stopped by stopping[8]，to block up for a blockage[2]，则非常有创造性，译文简练，便于

记忆。不难看出，译者在翻译这个术语时是经过苦思冥想、反复推敲的。难怪鲁迅先生谈到翻译工作的甘苦时曾说过，写作时若写不出一个词语，可以回避，翻译却不行，也还得想，一直弄得头昏眼花，好像在脑子里摸一个急于要开箱子的钥匙，却没有。在 filling for the stuffed 的译文中，把“塞”译成 filling 和 the stuffed，与原文的意思有较大出入。filling 是“填充”的意思，the stuffed 是“被填满”的意思，尤其是指空的东西被填满。比如：The child stuffed his pockets with candy（小孩口袋里装满了糖果）或 He stuffed himself with turkey（他大吃了一顿火鸡）[9]。用 filling 来指“用补益药治疗”，用 the stuffed 来指“闭塞不通症状的病症”，译文欠妥。treating the stopped by stopping 和 to block up for a blockage 是两个不错的译文。但“闭塞不通”不完全等于停止，用 stop 这个动词来翻译值得商榷，by stopping 也不能反映“用补益药治疗”这个含义。与 stop 相比，block 这个动词更能反映“闭塞不通”的含义。为了与 treating cold with cold 和 treating heat with heat 形式相统一，不妨将 to block up for a blockage 改成 treating blockage with blocking。由于两种语言的差异，在不能对应翻译的情况下，将“塞因塞用”翻译成 treating blockage with blocking 或 treating obstruction with obstructing[7] 不失为一种比较恰当的译文。

2.3 “通因通用”

“通因通用”是指使用具有通利作用的药物来治疗具有通泻症状的实证。不知道什么原因，《英汉汉英中医辞典》把“塞因塞用”和“通因通用”都翻译成了 treating the stopped by stopping，使人费解。Treating disease with profuse fluid discharge by increasing fluid discharge[3] 回译成中文为“用增加液体排泄的方法来治疗具有大量液体排泄的疾病”，与原文的概念相比，真是牛头不对马嘴。可以说这是一种拙劣的译文，有悖于中医术语翻译的科学性和简洁性原则。在 treating openness with purgatives [1]、opening for the opened[5]、treating diarrhea with cathartics[6] 和 treating diarrhea with purgatives[7] 的译文中，用 open 来翻译“通”是欠妥的。open 是“打开”的意思，放在这个中医术语里面根本无法体现“通”的含义。diarrhea（腹泻）和 purgatives（泻剂）、cathartics（泻药）这三个词也未能完全表达“通泻症状的实证”和“通利作用的药物”。其实，通因通用是以通治通，适用于食积腹痛、泻下不畅、瘀血所致的崩漏，膀胱湿热所致的尿频、尿急、尿痛等。治法上也有发汗法治汗出、通下法治下痢、涌吐法治呕吐、破血法治下血等，因此，可以说这三种译文基本上是不正确的。把“通因通用”译为 to drain for a drain[2] 和 treating the unstopped by unstopping[8]，则非常简练，符合中医术语翻译的简洁性原则和回译性原则。但 drain 是“排水”的意思，用它来表达“通”的含义明显欠妥。用 unstop 来翻译“通”这个字也值得商榷。首先，英文词典中没有 unstop 这个单词，是译者把它生造出来的；其次，

“不停止”并不等同于“通”，unstop 并不能完全表达“通”的含义。就人体而言，气机升降出入是体内新陈代谢活动的基本过程，“通”与“不通”关系到脏腑经络、气血阴阳等各方面的功能。就中文语言而言，“通”的含义很广，可以指气机通畅，通利作用的药物、通泻症状的实证等。在这种情况下，不妨把“通因通用”译为 treating flow with flow，也许更为准确贴切。

3. 讨论

通过对前述反治法英译的分析，其译文的正误优劣一目了然。《传统医学国际标准名词术语》把“寒因寒用”和“热因热用”分别翻译成 treating cold with cold 和 treating heat with heat，非常简洁明了；把“塞因塞用”和“通因通用”分别翻译成 treating the stopped by stopping 和 treating the unstopped by unstopping 值得商榷，也许把“塞因塞用”和“通因通用”分别翻译成 treating blockage with blocking 和 treating flow with flow 更为准确，更符合中医术语翻译的简洁性原则和回译性原则。

中医术语英译是一项艰巨并富有挑战性的工作，它要求译者既要精通英语，又要熟悉中医基础理论，也只有这样才能正确翻译中医术语，更好、更快地促进中医的对外传播与发展。

参考文献

[1] 柴可夫，张庆荣．中医基础理论．北京：人民卫生出版社，2007：300.
[2] 刘燕池，刘占文．中医基础理论．北京：学苑出版社，1998：279－280.
[3] 金魁和．汉英医学大辞典．北京：人民卫生出版社，2004：1789，1858，1862，1898.
[4] 魏迺杰、英汉汉英中医辞典．长沙：湖南科学技术出版社，1996：489，603，609，666.
[5] 谢竹藩．新编汉英中医药分类辞典．北京：外文出版社，2002：213.
[6] 欧明．汉英中医辞典．广州：广东科技出版社，1986：503，389，535，425.
[7] WHO International Standard Terminologies on Traditional Medicine in the Western Pacific Region.（2007－10－16） [2010－12－5] http：// www. wpro. who. int/NR/rdonlyres/14B298C6－518D－4C00－BE02－FC31EADE3791/0/WHOIST－26JUNE－FINAL. pdf.
[8] 彭勃，谢建群．中医内科学．北京：人民卫生出版社，2007：217.
[9] Mish FC. Webster's ninth new collegiate dictionary. Massachusetts：Merriam-Webster Inc，1987：1171.

[原载《中国中西医结合杂志》，2011，31（8）：1143－1145.]

浅析活血化瘀的英译

赵瑞安

“活血化瘀”这一术语在中医及中西医结合等文献中出现的频率很高，而其英译也各异。在近 4 年的《中国中西医结合杂志》中大概有以下几种译法：①promoting blood circulation and removing blood stasis；②promoting blood circulation to remove stasis；③promoting blood circulation and relieving stasis；④activating blood circulation to dissipate blood stasis；⑤activating blood circulation to remove stasis；⑥blood stasis removing；⑦HuoXue Hua-Yu。《汉英医学大词典》（人民卫生出版社，1987）中则译成：promoting blood circulation by removing blood stasis。从以上几种英译来看，虽形式多样，却能看出对“活血化瘀”的英译已略具雏形，但需进一步完善，加以统一。笔者试作以下分析。

1. 活血化瘀的含义

活血化瘀是中医的重要治则之一，是祛除瘀血、疏通血脉的方法。血液由于阻滞而变为瘀血，必须祛除才能使血脉流通，消除病变。曾应用“活血祛瘀”“祛瘀活血”等术语，而现在基本上以“活血化瘀”取而代之。因为“活血化瘀”中的“化”字既能表达“祛”之去除之意，又能生动地描述化瘀的微观变化。活血的目的是消除瘀血，显然，“活血”在“化瘀”之前较合理。

2. promote 与 activate 辨析

两词均为及物动词，promote 意为 help the progress of something（促进，助长），如：The organization works to promote friendship between nations。activate 意为 make something active（使活化，活化，激活），如：antigen activates B lymphocyte。活血之意除有促进和改善微循环外，还有血液流变学方面的改善，促进多种巨噬细胞和淋巴细胞的活化及促进细胞因子的分泌等作用，故“活血”之活的对应词应以 activate 较为理想。

3. 介词的应用

中医名词术语中应注意介词的应用。介词短语有多种作用，如作状语、形容修饰语、宾语补足语等，称为语法歧义（grammatical ambiguity），故要注意其用法。“活血化瘀”中的“化瘀”可用介词短语表达，作 activate 的宾语补足语，可译作 activating blood circulation against stasis，活血的目的就是为了抵抗、消除瘀血，而 against 可以表示这层意思，使翻译更能达到信息密度的要求。至于用 stasis 还是 blood stasis，因前已有 blood，后可省略，以免累赘。

中医经历了 2000 多年的临床实践，形成了独特的医学理论体系，尤其是近代中西医结合的深入研究，完善了中医的基础理论。但要使中医成为世界性医学，除了高质量的研究外，也要重视中医术语的英译。翻译是工具，是通向各国的桥梁，将中医名词术语的英译规范化，有利于将我国的传统医学准确地传遍世界，为人类造福。

[原载《中国中西医结合杂志》，1996，16（4）：250－251.]

中医脉象翻译的原则和方法

李永安

脉诊是中医学中一种特殊的、重要的诊断疾病的方法。它在中医临床诊断中占有非常重要的地位。然而，由于缺乏科学的翻译原则和方法，目前，中医脉象名称的英译形式较为混乱。尽快实现它们的英译的标准化是一个亟待解决的问题。本文谨就这一问题进行一些探讨。

1. 翻译的原则

1.1 科学性原则

所谓科学性原则，是指标准化的中医名词术语的英译要语义准确，词形简明，符合现代科技名词术语的规则。

1.2 回译性原则

所谓回译性原则，就是英译的脉名在形式和结构上要尽量与其中文接近，这样中文读者或听众在读到或听到某一脉象名称的英译时，头脑里能够反映出相应的中文，能够使读者根据其译名而得知其原名词。这样才能实现信息的双向传递作用，达到真正的双向信息交流。

2. 翻译的方法

2.1 直译

直译就是根据脉象的字面含义直接译成英文。例如，细脉、迟脉、散脉等可分别直译为 thready pulse、slow pulse 和 scattered pulse。直译适用于大多数带有一个形容词命名的脉象。

2.2 意译

意译就是译出脉象名的深层含义，而不拘泥于表面文字。例如，釜沸脉和屋漏脉等可根据其含义意译为 ebullient pulse 和 dripping pulse 等。意译适用于一些以取象类比法命名的脉象名。

2.3 仿造词译法

仿造词译法是利用已知词和词素创造新词的译法。这种方法包括词层仿造和词素层仿造两种方法。词层仿造法适用于大多数以取象类比命名的脉象名。例如，弹石脉和鱼翔脉可分别译为 stone -flicking pulse 和 fish-swimming pulse。词素层仿造法适用于某些虽带有一个形容词命名但脉象特征含义丰富的脉象。例如，濡脉和长脉可分别译为 leptosuperficial pulse 和 ortholong pulse。

3. 中医脉象的命名特点及其翻译的关键

绝大多数中医脉象的命名是以一个形容词加“脉”构成，例如，疾脉、促脉、洪脉等，因此，翻译的关键是选择一个恰当的形容词或类形容词的词。

4. 中医脉象的特征及其翻译

4.1　脉位异常为主的脉象

脉位异常指脉位发生浮、沉、长、短等异常变化。这类脉象翻译的关键是选择一个能恰当体现脉位变化的形容词。这类脉象包括：①浮脉：脉位表浅，轻触即应，稍重按则感觉脉搏力量减弱，但无空虚感。古人以“如水漂木”来形容。拟译为 floating pulse。②濡脉：脉居浮位，脉搏无力，浮中并见细象，概之可谓浮而细软。拟译为 leptosuperficial pulse（lepto-：细、小，例如，leptocephalic：头盖骨狭小的；leptodactyly：脚趾细长）。③芤脉：脉位表浅，轻取即得，脉体大而应指有力，稍按则有空虚感，并且脉管有一定硬度，如按葱管之状。拟译为 hollow pulse。④革脉：脉位在深部，浮取即得，脉形弦大，中空外坚，如按鼓皮之状。拟译为 tympanic pulse。⑤沉脉：脉搏位置较深，用轻指力按触察觉不到，用中指力按触，脉搏也不明显，只有用重指力按触，才能感觉到脉搏明显的搏动。拟译为 deep pulse。⑥牢脉：脉位在深部，轻取重取均不应。其脉形大而且长，脉势微弦而有力。拟译为 firm pulse。⑦伏脉：脉象较沉，部位更深，需重按至筋骨才能触及。脉象极细，微弱无力，甚至触摸不到脉搏的跳动。拟译为 hidden pulse。⑧短脉：脉位很短，仅在关部脉搏跳动较为明显。寸、尺二部脉搏模糊不清，似有似无。拟译为 short pulse。⑨长脉：长脉是脉管搏动范围超过本位的状态。其特点是长而且直。拟译为 ortholong pulse（ortho -：直，例如，orthostichy：直列线，orthopteran：直翅目，orthotropism：直生性）。

4.2　脉率异常为主的脉象

脉搏的频率发生异常改变称为脉率异常，包括脉率过速和脉率过缓两类。①数脉：脉搏来去快速，脉率在 90～139 次/分钟，脉率基本规整。拟译为 rapid pulse。②疾脉：脉来急速，脉率快于数脉，在 140～180 次/分钟。脉率基本规整。拟译为 swift pulse。③迟脉：脉搏来去迟缓，在 40～59 次/分钟，形似屋漏水之状，脉率规整或不规整。拟译为 slow pulse。

4.3　脉律异常为主的脉象

脉搏节奏不规整的脉象称为脉律异常。这类脉象名称的翻译应尽量用能体现脉律变化的形容词。它们包括：①促脉：脉来急数而有不规则间歇的现象。拟译为 rush pulse。②结脉：脉来缓慢而有不规则歇止的现象。拟译为 discontinuous pulse。③代脉：脉来中止，止有规律。拟译为 intermittent pulse。

4.4 脉形异常为主的脉象

脉形异常是指脉搏形态的改变。主要表现是脉搏幅度和升降速度的异常。翻译时应尽量选择能体现脉形变化的形容词。①洪脉：脉体阔大，状如洪水，来势很强，去势较缓。拟译为 floody pulse。②细脉：脉体细小，但应指分明，故前人以“状若线丝”作比喻。拟译为 thready pulse。③滑脉：脉搏来去流利圆滑，如触圆珠盘中滚动一般。拟译为 smooth pulse。④涩脉：脉搏来去艰难，应指涩滞，无滑润之感。拟译为 unsmooth pulse。⑤弦脉：脉来搏指有力，形直体长，如按琴弦。拟译为 taut pulse。⑥紧脉：脉来急紧，绷紧有力，状如牵绳转索。拟译为 tense pulse。⑦缓脉：脉来一息四至，稍快于迟脉。拟译为 moderate pulse。

4.5 脉势异常为主的脉象

脉势异常指脉搏力量强弱的改变。翻译时应能用体现脉势变化的形容词。该类脉象包括：①实脉：在寸、关、尺三部脉搏无论轻取、重按均有力，而且体长形大，有充实感。拟译为 sthenic pulse。②虚脉：与实脉相反，在寸、关、尺三部无论轻取、重取皆无力，甚至有空虚感。拟译为 asthenic pulse。③弱脉：脉位较深，重按始得，脉形细小，脉搏无力。拟译为 weak pulse。④微脉：脉象极度细弱无力，若有若无，按之模糊，至数不清。拟译为 feeble pulse。⑤散脉：浮散无根，轻触可得，重按则无；至数不清，脉率不齐，但无歇止之象。拟译为 scattered pulse。

4.6 十怪脉

中医临床诊断上还有所谓的“十怪脉”，表示生命出现垂危现象的极其异常的脉象。它们包括：①偃刀脉：脉象弦细而紧急，有如用手指摸刀刃之感觉。拟译为 knife-edge-feeling pulse。②转豆脉：脉来捉摸不定，如豆之旋转状。拟译为 bean-rolling pulse。③麻促脉：脉象急促而不规则。拟译为 irregular running pulse。④雀啄脉：脉象急数，节律不调，止而复作，如雀啄食。拟译为 sparrow-pecking pulse。⑤屋漏脉：脉搏很久跳动一次，且间歇不均，如屋漏滴水之状。拟译为 dripping pulse。⑥弹石脉：脉象无神，如以指弹石之感。拟译为 stone-flicking pulse。⑦解索脉：脉来快慢不等，脉力强弱不均，脉率在 90～130 次/分钟，有手解绳索之感。拟译为 cord-unfastening pulse。⑧鱼翔脉：脉来似有似无，如鱼翔之状。拟译为 fish-swimming pulse。⑨虾游脉：脉来隐隐约约，去时一跃而逝，如虾游之状。拟译为 shrimp - darting pulse。⑩釜沸脉：脉象浮数之极，有出无入，如锅中水沸，绝无跟脚。拟译为 ebullient pulse。

中医脉象英译标准化只是中医名词术语英译标准化的一个微小部分。笔者希望通过这次探讨与译界同仁进行交流，为中医名词术语英译标准化的早日实现尽自己的微薄之力。

[原载《中国中西医结合杂志》，2004，24（12）：1130 - 1131.]

基于隐喻认知的脉象术语英译研究

梁杏　兰凤利

无论在中国还是在西方，隐喻研究都有着悠久而连续的传统，早已超越了诗学、修辞学、语言学的局限，成为语言哲学、科学哲学、认知哲学所关注的重要命题。G. Lakoff 和 N. Johnson 在 1980 年出版的《我们赖以生存的隐喻》（*Metaphors We Live by*）一书中，将隐喻定义为“用一种事物来理解另一种事物”（understanding one thing in terms of another），首次提出了概念隐喻理论（conceptual metaphor theory），用源域（source domain）与目的域（target domain）之间的映射（mapping）以及意象图示（image schema）来解释隐喻现象，从而得出隐喻是一种“跨域映射”（cross-domain mapping）。跨域映射是一种思维方式，是人们参照已知的、熟悉的、具体的概念去认识和思考未知的、陌生的、抽象的概念的认知方式，从而开辟了从认知角度研究隐喻的新途径[1]。隐喻本质上是一种认知现象，是人们认识世界的根本方法之一，是科学思维的一个重要途径[2]。Lakoff 以来的学者们大体概括了概念隐喻具有如下几个基本特点：普遍性、认知性和系统性[3]。中医学中的概念隐喻同样具备这几个特点：第一，普遍性：隐喻在中医学中无处不在——中医学，从术语到语篇乃至整个医学体系都是隐喻[4]；第二，认知性：取象比类是中医学中隐喻形成的过程和方法，中医学中的隐喻反映着中医学特有的取象比类的思维模式和方法论[5]；第三，系统性：中医学中的概念隐喻广及自然、社会、政治、军事等现象，共同构建起中医学的文化预设前提——“天人合一”。这些特点为中医学概念隐喻翻译策略取舍提供了内在依据，为评价中医概念隐喻翻译提供了合理标准。鉴于隐喻、取象比类不仅陈述、建构了中医学理论体系，而且也是中医学发展的重要方法之一，因此，中医概念隐喻英译应遵循唯一标准——即反映中医学隐喻、取象比类思维模式的翻译策略和标准，这对于继承、发展、传播中医学至关重要[6]。本文基于隐喻认知和自建中医脉学汉英双语语料库，通过探寻常见脉象术语命名源流，对比分析同一脉象的不同英译，正本清源，为常见脉象术语确定佳译。

1. 常见脉象概念隐喻的英译与解读

王叔和《脉经》言“脉理精微，其体难辨。弦、紧、浮、芤，展转相类，在心易了，指下难明”。那么，如何描述脉象，并为脉象定名？常见脉象术语基本都是概念隐喻，大多数脉象概念隐喻通过显性隐喻描述和界定。“所谓显性隐喻，即一般人们所说的明喻（simile）。明喻的特点是明确说明两者是一种对比关系，英语中典型的明喻形式是 A is like（or as）B，而汉语中的典型形式是‘A 像 B’。许多词典和教科书把隐喻作为明喻的一种浓缩形式”[2]。绝大多数中医脉学概念隐喻正是其明喻（显性隐喻）描述的浓缩形式，如“浮脉，‘如水漂木’（木浮在水中）”。有的脉象通过“‘经脉是河流’，河流中的水呈现出何种状态，经脉中的水也呈现出何种状态”[7]这一隐喻描述加以界定。古代医家通过目标域（本体）形象地描述、界定始源域（喻体）——脉象。久而久之，喻体的特征被转移到本体脉象上，使用这类转移的表达形象、清晰、简洁，这些隐喻的语义特征最终固化为术语，成为脉象术语概念本身。文树德教授（Paul U. Unschuld）提出决定隐喻存亡的理性原则：既然中医学至今仍然宣称以《黄帝内经》所建立的概念系统为圭臬，因此，在《黄帝内经》时代就存在的隐喻就应在翻译时予以保留[8]，因此，本文认为确定脉象术语佳译应以“基于隐喻认知，体现译语意象与其隐喻描述意象一致”为原则。

1.1 常见脉象的隐喻描述

古籍中同一脉象常有多种显性隐喻（即明喻）描述，其中一些隐喻描述生动、形象、易懂，沿用至今并被收入现代中医教科书。这些广为流传的显性隐喻描述为基于隐喻认知的脉象术语翻译提供了依据（表 1）。

表 1 常见脉象的显性隐喻描述及其译文

常见脉象（始源域/本体）	经典显性隐喻描述原文（目标域/喻体）	经典显性隐喻描述译文
浮	“如水漂木”	“like wood floating on top of water”[9]
沉	“如石投水，必极其底”	“like a stone dropped in water，must sink to the extreme”[9]
芤	“中空外实，状如慈葱”	“center is empty，external is replete，its shape is like an onion stalk”[9]
散	“涣散不收，如杨花散漫之象”	“scattered and not restrained，like the image of willow flowers scattered all over the place”[9]
紧	“如转索无常”	“like a tightly stretched rope”[10]
细	“若丝线之应指”	“feels like a fine thread”[10]
弦	“如张弓弦”；“状若筝弦”	“like a drawn bowstring”[9]； “its shape is like the strings of a zither”[9]
革	“如按鼓皮”	“like pressing the skin of a drum”[9]
滑	“往来流利，如盘走珠”《诊家枢要》	“move backward and forward very quickly，being smooth and slippery”[11]； “like pebbles rolling in basin”[12]

续表

常见脉象（始源域/本体）	经典显性隐喻描述原文（目标域/喻体）	经典显性隐喻描述译文
濡	“极软而浮细，如绵在水中”	“extremely soft as well as floating and fine, like a thread in water”[9]
长	“如揭长竿末梢”	“like raising a long rod (with) a thin tip”[9]
数	“脉流薄疾”（“薄疾”：“急迫”）	“the pulse flows, nearly racing”[9]
洪	“来盛去衰”	“comes with force but recedes calmly”[10]
涩	“如轻刀刮竹”	“like a light knife scraping bamboo”[9]
缓	“应指缓和，往来甚匀，如初春杨柳舞风之象”	“responds to the fingers harmonious and moderate, going and coming very evenly, like the image of willows dancing in the wind at the beginning of spring”[9]
动	“动无头尾，其动如豆”《诊家正眼》	“moves without head and tail, like stirring beans”[9]

注：表1中经典隐喻描述原文除滑脉、动脉外，均来自《濒湖脉学》。

1.2　常见脉象术语英译现状

众所周知，中医名词术语一词多译的现象由来已久。表2所收集的译语来自8本具有代表性的英译中医读物，并且译者的学术背景、知识结构也各不相同。

表2　8本具有代表性的英译中医读物中常见脉象术语英译

脉象	P·H[11]	王吉民、伍连德[12]	黄焕松[10]	Flaws B[9]	魏迺杰[13]	李照国、鲍白[14]	谢竹藩[15]	WHO[16]
浮	superficial	superficial	floating	floating	floating	floating	floating/superficial	floating
沉	deep/sunk	deep	sinking	sunken	sunken	sunken	sunken/deep	sunken
芤	—	hollow	hollow	scallion-stalk	scallion-stalk	hollow	hollow	hollow

续表

脉象	P·H[11]	王吉民、伍连德[12]	黄焕松[10]	Flaws B[9]	魏迺杰[13]	李照国、鲍白[14]	谢竹藩[15]	WHO[16]
散	—	scattered	scattered	scattered	dissipated	scattered	scattered	dissipated
紧	short-tremulous	tense	tight	tight	tight	tense	tense/tight	tight
细	slender	slender	thin	fine	fine	thin	thready/thin/fine	fine
弦	long-tremulous	taut	wiry	bow-string	string-like	taut	wiry	string-like
革	hard	hard	leather	drum-skin	skin	—	tympanic	drumskin
滑	slippery	slippery	slippery	slippery	slippery	slippery	slippery	slippery
濡	soft/fluid	soft	soft	soggy	soggy	soggy	soft	soggy
长	long	long	long	long	long	long	long	long
数	—	quick	rapid	rapid	rapid	fast	rapid	rapid
洪	over-flowing	over-flowing	flooding	surging	surging	full	surging	surging
涩	sharp	small	choppy	choppy	rough	astringent	choppy	rough
缓	slow	tardy	leisurely	moderate/relaxed	moderate	moderate	moderate/relaxed	moderate/relaxed
动	movedble	tremulous	moving	stirring	stirred	—	throbbing	stirred

1.3 基于隐喻认知的英译分析

1.3.1 浮脉 floating pulse 为浮脉基于隐喻认知的译语。因“浮”直译为 float，floating 与“如水漂木”的漂浮意象一致。superficial 为早期译语，用以表达脉位浮浅，而 floating 可反映浮脉来源和隐喻认知，这一译语近 30 年来被越来越多的译者使用。

1.3.2　沉脉　sunken pulse 为沉脉基于隐喻认知的译语。因“沉”直译为 sink，与投石入水后，石沉水中（“如石投水，必极其底”）的意象一致。“必极其底”说明石头已沉入水底，所以 sunken 比 sinking 要好。sunk 多用作 sink 的过去式和过去分词，《柯林斯英语词典》（*Collins English Dictionary*，下文中英英解释均来自该词典）中 sunk 为形容词，解释为 with all hopes dashed/ruined，与沉脉隐喻描述意象不符，故不宜采用。deep 为早期译语，仅说明沉脉的脉位深，无法表达沉脉的隐喻意象，故不如 sunken 准确。

1.3.3　芤脉　scallion-stalk pulse 为芤脉基于隐喻认知的译语。《本草纲目》言：“葱一名芤”。scallion-stalk pulse 回译成中文为葱秆脉，与芤脉来源相符，scallion-stalk 又可表达脉体如葱管般中空而软的意象。此译法虽不如 hollow pulse 常用，却是基于隐喻认知和芤脉本源的直译，比 hollow pulse 更能揭示其隐喻文化特征。

1.3.4　散脉　scattered pulse 为散脉基于隐喻认知的译语。形容词 scattered 意为 spread or dispersed in an untidy or irregular way，英语中常有 scattered cloud 等描述，用 scattered 表现“杨花散漫之象”栩栩如生，意象相符且富有文化气息。在《柯林斯英语词典》中 dissipated 可与 scattered 互解，但 dissipated 另一释义为 indulging without restraint in the pursuit of pleasure 偏贬义，又与杨花散漫之象相去甚远。

1.3.5　紧脉　tight pulse 为紧脉基于隐喻认知的译语。因“紧”直译为 tight，与“如转索无常”的紧态意象一致。在英语中形容紧紧拧转的绳索，tense 不如 tight 常用。tremulous 多用以形容声音或人的神情胆怯、战栗，与原文对紧脉描述的意象不一致，且与紧脉隐喻内涵相去甚远，故抛弃不用。

1.3.6　细脉　fine pulse 为细脉基于隐喻认知的译语。“细”直译为 fine，形容词 fine 解释为 very thin or slender，与细脉“细来累累细如丝”的意象一致。英语中形容线、绳、丝等的细更常用 fine 而非 thin、slender。西医中有 thready pulse，“thready”意为“（medicine）（of the pulse）barely perceptible；weak；fine”，即细弱且几乎不能感觉到。而细脉的特点是脉体细软且重按应指连连，thready 词义太过。

1.3.7　弦脉　bowstring pulse 为弦脉基于隐喻认知的译语。因 bowstring 回译为“弓弦”，与“如张弓弦”的隐喻描述一致。string 是多义词，语义不够明确。虽词典中 string 有琴弦之意，但其常用义为细绳、线、带子，故不宜采用。long-tremulous 为早期译语，译语冗长，内涵不够准确，现已不再使用。

1.3.8　革脉　drumskin pulse 为革脉基于隐喻认知的译语。因 drumskin 表

达目标域“鼓皮”的隐喻意象比 hard、leather、skin、tympanic 要形象、准确。虽为新造之词，但用词浅显易懂，也是 WHO 支持的术语。

1.3.9 滑脉 slippery pulse 为滑脉基于隐喻认知的译语。“滑”直译为 slippery，且与滑脉“往来流利”的意象相符，由表 2 知，译语 slippery pulse 深入人心。

1.3.10 濡脉 soggy pulse 为濡脉基于隐喻认知的译语。《柯林斯英语辞典》中形容词 soggy 有如下解释：“①soaked with liquid；②（of bread，pastry，etc.）moist and heavy”，这与海绵吸水后软而光滑的意象十分相似。soggy 和 soft 相比较，仍优于词义宽泛的 soft。

1.3.11 长脉 long pulse 为长脉基于隐喻认知的译语。“长”直译为 long，与其形容脉体如长杆般“端直以长”的隐喻意象一致。从表 2 知长脉译语高度统一，实属难得的佳译。

1.3.12 数脉 rapid pulse 为数脉基于隐喻认知的译语。因数脉的隐喻源于古人“经脉是河水”的认知，rapid 用以形容脉势如水势急速、险峻，与“脉流薄疾”的隐性隐喻描述意象一致，优于“quick”和“fast”。

1.3.13 洪脉 surging pulse 为洪脉基于隐喻认知的译语。因洪脉的隐喻亦源于古人“经脉是河水”的认知，surging 用以形容脉势如洪水势般“来盛去衰”，优于词义宽泛的 full。overflowing 与 flooding 所表现的意象有河水已溢出河道之感，若采用则易引起误解，误以为经血溢出脉外。

1.3.14 涩脉 “rough pulse”为涩脉基于隐喻认知的译语。《说文解字》曰：“濇，不滑也”，涩脉形容指下感觉如同“轻刀刮竹”般涩滞，rough 与“涩”的意象一致。choppy 所描绘的意象是不断变化、改变方向的汹涌波涛，astringent 多指收敛剂、止血药，两者都与涩脉涩滞不滑的意象有出入。

1.3.15 缓脉 leisurely pulse 为缓脉基于隐喻认知的译语。《广韵》曰：“缓，舒也”，英文中 leisurely 可形容舞步悠闲从容，此处可以表达缓脉如“初春杨柳舞风”般缓和舒展的意象。slow、tardy 为早期译语，易与迟脉混淆，不宜采用。

1.3.16 动脉 stirring pulse 为动脉基于隐喻认知的译语。stir 表达搅动豆子后四处滚动的意象，与“动无头尾，其动如豆”的意象一致，而 move 所描述的移动多有确定的方向。stirring 表达一个进行中的动态，比 stirred 要好。throbbing 多用以形容心中悸动的感觉，无法体现“动无头尾，其动如豆”的隐喻含义。

2. 结语

2.1 基于隐喻认知翻译脉象术语，可在一定程度上体现中医学独特的思维方式。在英译的过程中不重视理解隐喻，可能会导致译文偏离原文隐喻意象和原文化语境，丢失中医学隐喻的文化内涵。体现隐喻认知的脉象术语翻译能够保留中医学取象比类思维过程和方法论，保留源语所蕴含的脉象意象。“中医术语的英译应遵从同一标准，即采用保留该术语原始比喻内涵的英译作为该术语的唯一标准化译语，通过定义或注释解释说明术语的源流及其史学价值、文化价值和医学价值，使中医学及其负载的文化独立而完整地传入西方。这样我们传播出去的不仅仅是中医药学知识和技术，还有中国传统科学独特的哲学内涵和方法论——天人合一、取象比类，以及中医文化”[17]。

2.2　基于隐喻认知翻译脉象术语，应体现译语意象与隐喻描述意象一致的翻译原则。对同一脉象有诸多不同的隐喻描述，翻译时应依据广为流传的显性隐喻描述意象作为择定译语的依据，同时应仔细挑选译语用词，尽量避免汉语与英语之间的意象表达存在偏差。当今我们仍遵循古籍中的隐喻描述认识、理解、体悟脉象，那么在翻译的过程中选择与隐喻描述意象一致的译语，可以使英语读者经历和我们一样的学习感悟过程，即通过了解脉象术语的隐喻涵义进而理解、体悟具体的脉象。基于隐喻认知的脉象术语翻译有助于英语读者揭开心目中脉诊神秘奥妙、变幻莫测的面纱，使脉诊学习逐步变得“在心易了，指下渐明”。

2.3　基于隐喻认知翻译脉象术语，能实现译语的回译性，便于实现信息的双向交流。体现隐喻认知的直译译语具有很强的回译性，便于实现信息的双向交流。张海红认为，“术语翻译与术语内涵解释是翻译的两个不同阶段，应区别对待”[18]。基于隐喻认知的脉象术语英译简洁、准确，可以有效地避免将“翻译”（translation）变成“阐释”（interpretation）。由于概念隐喻具有系统性，那么基于隐喻认知的脉象翻译也具有系统性。一些脉象术语源于“经脉是河水”的隐性隐喻，描述水流状态的词可以用于描述脉势，如洪脉 surging pulse、数脉 rapid pulse 选词均为描述水流特征的词，提示我们基于隐喻认知的翻译可使传达的信息内在逻辑更紧密。

参考文献

[1] Lakoff G，Johnson M. Metaphors we live by. Chicago：University of Chicago Press，1980：112，246，253-254.

[2] 束定芳．隐喻学研究．上海：上海外语教育出版社，2008：99-100，51-52.

[3] 蓝纯．认知语言学与隐喻研究．北京：外语教学与研究出版社，2008：112-115.

[4] Lan FL. Culture，philosophy，and Chinese medicine：Viennese lectures. Frankfurtam Main：Peter Lang，2012：279-296.

[5] 兰凤利，Wallner FG. 取象比类——中医学隐喻形成的过程与方法．自然辩证法通讯，2014，36（2）：87-93.

[6] 兰凤利．中医名词术语英译：唯一还是多重标准？中国中西医结合杂志，2010，30（2）：

188－192.
[7] 贾春华．一个以水为始源域的中医概念认知系统．北京中医药大学学报，2012，35(3)：165.
[8] 魏迺杰．中医名词术语翻译探讨．英汉汉英中医词典．长沙：湖南科学技术出版社，1996：63.
[9] Li Shizhen. The Lakeside Master's study of the pulse. Flaws B translated. Boulder：Blue Poppy Press，1998：33－53.
[10] Huynh HK，Seifert GM. Pulse diagnosis. Sydney：Paradigm Publications，1981：61－95.
[11] Du Halde JB. The secret of the pulse. The general history of China. Volume Three. London：John Watts，1674：384－390.
[12] Wong CK，Wu LT. History of Chinese medicine. Shanghai：Mercury Press，1932：60－61.
[13] Wiseman N，Feng Ye. A practical dictionary of Chinese medicine. Brookline：Paradigm Publications，1998：471－472.
[14] 王鲁芬．中医诊断学．李照国，鲍白译．上海：上海中医药大学出版社，2002：125－129.
[15] 谢竹藩．新编汉英中医药词典．北京：外文出版社，2002：138－141.
[16] World Health Organization. WHO international standard terminologies on traditional medicine in the Western Pacific Region. Western Pacific Region，A WPRO Publication（WHO Regional Office for the Western Pacific），2007：100－106.
[17] Unschuld PU，Hermann T，Zheng JSH. Huang Di Nei Jing Su Wen：annotated translation of Huang Di's inner classic-basic questions. Berkeley，Los Angeles and London：University of California Press，2011：345，717.
[18] 张海红，施蕴中．论中医术语脉象的翻译．中国中西医结合杂志，2006，26(7)：655.

[原载《中国中西医结合杂志》，2014，34(6)：760－763.]

论中医脉象术语的翻译

张海红　施蕴中

脉诊是中医学最基本、也是最重要的一种诊断方法，是中医学的一大特色[1]。要想让国际医坛能全面深刻地认识中医，了解中医脉诊是非常必要的。中医脉象术语是几千年来脉学各家理论经验积累的结晶，其内容丰富、珍贵而又复杂多样，这无疑给翻译工作带来了一定的难度。近年来翻译工作者们多方探索脉象术语的翻译，努力使脉象术语翻译得体、简单，从而易于广大学者及群众理解和接受。不同的中医英文书籍中脉象有不同译法（表1）。

表1　不同中医英文书籍中脉象的不同译法

脉名	《中医英语翻译技巧》[2]	《中医诊断学》[3]	《常用脉象英译探讨》[4]
滑脉	slippery pulse	rolling pulse	smooth pulse
涩脉	unsmooth pulse	sluggish pulse	—
实脉	sthenic pulse	strong pulse	forceful pulse
微脉	indistinct pulse	—	faint pulse
虚脉	asthenic pulse	faint pulse	feeble pulse
洪脉	full pulse	—	flood pulse
缓脉	regular pulse	sluggish pulse	moderate pulse
弦脉	stringy pulse	taut pulse	wiry pulse
濡脉	soft pulse	soggy pulse	leptosuperficial pulse
促脉	abrupt pulse	running pulse	rush pulse
沉脉	sunken pulse	deep pulse	deep pulse

虽然这说明了中医翻译界积极探索而使脉诊翻译出现大好局面，为脉诊译名标准化打下了群众基础，但同时，同一脉象的多种译法又会造成概念混乱，大大影响脉诊被国际医坛理解和接受的进程，因此，亟须翻译原则来约束规范，使其通俗明了，从而更容易在国际上被认同。翻译原则是我们进行脉诊翻译的前提和基础，有不少翻译工作者都对中医术语翻译原则进行了阐述，综合他们的知识理论，笔者谈谈自己的一些观点。

1. 中医术语翻译原则

1.1 区分术语命名和术语内涵解释

术语翻译与术语内涵解释是翻译的两个不同阶段，应区别对待。纵观现今脉象术语翻译，有的命名语言啰嗦，使术语成为内涵解释，例如有人将“结脉”译成 slow pulse with irregular intervals，这一翻译就混进了太多冗余信息，不是定义脉名，而是解释其内涵，显然这不符合术语需要简明扼要的原则。术语翻译只有言简意赅、简洁明了才便于使用，丰富而深刻的内涵应放到术语解释中去。区分开术语命名及内涵解释，做到术语简洁化，内涵深刻化，应该是术语翻译的重要原则。

1.2 尽可能使用常用词

有人喜欢使用 leptosuperficial pulse（濡脉）这样的偏词进行翻译，以显示中医术语的与众不同。为什么要尽量使用英语常用词进行中医翻译？首先，中医翻译的主要目的是为了沟通，如果使用偏词、怪词，让人不知所云，就达不到沟通的目的。其次，常用词是英语的核心部分，英语现在实际上已成为国际性语言，用英语学习研究中医的人母语并非都是英语。使用语言的共性部分比较容易突破语言障碍，顺利地进行沟通。在词汇层面上，英语共性部分就是常用词。

怎样确定常用词的范围，这是语言学家多年来力求解决的问题。为了解决这一问题，语料库语言学的工作为常用词的确定打下了良好的基础。例如，“Bank of English”建立了近 20 亿英语语料的语料库，通过计算机分析找出最常用的词汇，编纂出了《柯林斯 Cobuild 英语词典》《*Collins Cobuild English Dictionary*》这样的英语常用词词典，这类常用词字典的产生防止了不同方言间信息交流的不便。常用词包括普通常用词和专业常用词。普通常用词指公众常使用的词汇，专业常用词指在某个领域经常使用的术语。中医学常用词应包括传统医学和现代医学领域的常用词。使用常用词可以让中医翻译更通俗易懂。本着尽可能使用常用词的原则，恰当地运用通俗明了的医学术语进行翻译，则可以既便于中外交流沟通，也不失医学的严谨性。

1.3 根据常用词缀进行翻译

为了保证术语简明扼要，有时不得不使用造词的手段。魏迺杰[5]曾主张根据西医词汇的造词模式，以拉丁文或希腊文的字根创造新词作为中医用语的译词。但是如果造出的词中国人不认识，外国人也不认识，这种词就很难有生命力，因此，笔者认为构造词这一手段可以使用，但应尽量限制在常用词构词法内。例如洪脉，《中华脉诊》这样形容：“壮如水之洪流，波之涌起，脉洪大也”[6]，由此我们翻译该脉时会很自然地想到 flood 的波涛汹涌之势。此时“洪脉”需要一个形容词来命名，凭着常用构词法，可选用 floody pulse 来定义洪脉。虽然 floody

这一词在常用词英语字典里并不存在，但是名词后面加一个“y”后缀变成形容词这一构词法在一般常用词字典中是常见的，属于常用后缀。所以 floody 能够很容易被大众理解和接受。由此可见，用构词法造词是可行的，但要看是什么样的构词法则，用一个大家都熟悉的常用词缀和用一个生疏的拉丁文词根构词，结果是截然不同的。将“濡脉”翻译为 leptosuperficialpulse[4]之所以没有生命力，主要是因为这是一个由罕见的拉丁文词缀构造的词。

1.4 翻译术语选择要有区分性

有些相似脉象的术语译名使用了相同的词，如 faint，有人用来翻译“微脉”，有人用来翻译“虚脉”，这很容易造成混乱，因此，要注意选词的区分性，通过译名区分不同的脉象。

2. 脉诊翻译

一套术语名词的翻译要实用，其多对应率要尽可能低，这样才经得起“反译测验”（back translation test）[5]。本文重点讨论一脉多译的几种脉象的翻译。

2.1 滑脉

《中华脉诊》[1]对滑脉这样定义：“流利为滑，速度较快，即脉管迅速扩张又迅速缩小的状态”，往来流利，如盘走珠。《诊家枢要》载有：“滑，不涩也，往来流利，如盘走珠，不进不退”[6]。孙思邈也说过：“按之如珠子动，曰滑”。《脉诀启悟注释》记载：“滑脉应指替替然，往来之势流利圆滑，如盘中之走珠，如荷叶之承露”[6]。这些都说明了滑脉往来流利、如盘走珠的特点。滑脉的翻译有 slippery pulse、smooth pulse、rolling pulse 等。现分析一下这几种翻译方式：① slippery的意思是 difficult to hold，stand on，or move on，because it is smooth[7]（滑的，光滑的）。②smooth 的意思是 having an even surface without points[7]（平坦的，光滑的）。③rolling 在字典中并没有太符合滑脉的意思，但是由于其对应的动词 roll 是滚动的意思，所以 rolling 的意思也是“滚动的、滑动的”。

分析以上三词的含义可以看出 slippery 和 smooth 都体现出了“滑”的特点，而 rolling 则体现了“滚”的特点，smooth 和 slippery 的光滑是 without points（没有滚珠的感觉），但滑脉的最大特点恰恰是“按之如珠子动”[6]，所以用 smooth 和 slippery 翻译滑脉不如 rolling 贴切。rolling 既能体现出如珠般滚动的意思，同时也蕴涵了“流利圆滑“的意思，更能准确地表达滑脉的特点。

2.2 涩脉

《中华脉诊》中对涩脉这样定义：“艰滞为涩，脉搏升降速度徐缓，即血管的扩张和收缩表现徐慢的状态”[6]，其形状为“往来滞涩，如雨沾砂”[3]。《素问·脉要精微论》滑伯仁说：“涩，不滑也，虚细而往来难，三五不调，如雨沾砂，如倾倒刮竹”[6]。涩脉的翻译有：unsmooth pulse、sluggish pulse、uneven pulse、 rough pulse 等。unsmooth、uneven 在《牛津高阶英汉双解词典》[8]中是“不平滑”的意思（not even，not smooth）；sluggish 则表示：it moves，works or reacts much slower than normal[7]（缓慢的，迟钝的）；rough 的意思为：having an uneven or irregular surface，not smooth[7]（不平的，粗糙的）。unsmooth、uneven 和 rough 都表达了涩脉“往来滞涩，如轻刀刮竹”[3]的特点，而且也可以感觉到该脉象往来缓慢，比 sluggish 单单强调“缓”要准确、简单又通俗易懂。sluggish 的外延太广，好几个相似脉都有“缓慢”的意思，如缓脉、迟脉等脉象，用 sluggish 易产生误解，造成概念混乱，所以 sluggish 不如其他三个译法好。

2.3 实脉

《中华脉诊》[1]中对实脉的定义是：“脉管内的血液充实度增强，呈紧张状态”[6]。形状“大而且有力，不疾不迟”[3]，对于该脉有 sthenic pulse、strong pulse、forceful pulse、excess pulse 等多种译法。strong 的含义是：having great power[7]（强有力的[8]）；excess 为名词，意思为：more than reasonable，expected or moderate[7]（过度的，过分的[8]）；forceful 的意思为：strong and powerful[7]（强有力的[8]）。forceful、strong、sthenic 都表达了实脉“动而有力”[6]的特点。excess 是名词，而且为“过度的，过分的”，描述实脉也不准确，不可取。在上面三种译法中如果 sthenic 译为实脉的话，那么它的反义词 asthenic 便是虚脉的意思了。一对反义词用起来比较容易理解记忆，也可以把虚脉跟其相似脉象的译名区分开来有助于读者分辨理解，所以笔者认为 sthenic pulse 是实脉的最佳译法。

2.4 微脉

《中华脉诊》中指出：“微脉，细弱，不显，指脉幅小，为动脉血量减少而波动无力的状态”[6]，形状极细而软，似有似无[3]，如《脉经》中说“极细而软，或欲绝，若有若无。”微脉的译法有：indistinct pulse 和 faint pulse。现介绍一下这两种译法。① indistinct：not easily seen or felt，vague[7]（不清楚的，模糊的[8]）。②faint：means that cannot be clearly perceived by the sense[7]（微弱的，模糊的[8]）。这两个词无太大区别，问题在于 faint 这个词使用率过高，好几个脉象都能用它来命名，要想与其相似脉区分开来，最好用 indistinct pulse 来代替。

2.5 虚脉

虚脉是一种浮大力薄、举按空虚[5]的脉象。崔氏《脉诀》中说：“形大力薄，其虚可知”[6]。《灵枢·始终》载“虚者，脉大如其故而不坚也”[6]。虚脉的英译有 asthenic pulse、faint pulse 和 feeble pulse 等译法。这三个词的区分度很小，都可以定义虚脉，但为了更好地与其相似脉区分，正如在实脉中讲到的，用 asthenic比较好。

2.6　弱脉

弱脉是一个很容易与虚脉相混的脉象，指脉细小、沉伏、搏动无力[6]的状态，形状沉而细软。如《脉经》载："弱脉极软而沉细，按之欲绝于指下。"常用weak pulse和feeble pulse来翻译弱脉。由于使用feeble pulse，既可以理解为弱脉，也可以理解为虚脉，容易造成概念混乱产生误解。而weak pulse则既清楚又贴切地形容出了弱脉的虚弱无力的指下感觉，建议译为weak pulse。

2.7　濡脉

濡脉蕴涵了一种浮软无力的状态。《中华脉诊》中这样描述其形态："浮细无力，气势软逊"[6]。《脉经》中则说："软脉，极软而浮细"；滑伯仁说："濡无力也，虚软无力，应手散细，如棉絮之浮水中，轻手乍来，重手即去"[6]。现有soft pulse、soggy pulse和eptosuperficial pulse等译词。现介绍一下这三种译法：①soft：changing shape easily when pressed；not hard or firm to touch[7]（软的，柔的）；②soggy：very wet[7]（湿的）；③leptosuperficial（细、小、薄的）。从上述分析我们可以看出，leptosuperficial是一个较为生僻的单词，用它来定义濡脉不符合简洁明了的原则，不可取。濡脉有一种"如棉絮浮于水面"[6]的指下感觉，给人一种湿漉漉、不顺畅、不干爽的感觉。soft虽然有细软的意思，但表现不出它的"涩、湿"的特点来；soggy本身指"湿的"，并有湿之不爽、晦涩的内涵，用来翻译濡脉比较合适。

2.8　促脉

促脉指脉搏的搏动时快时慢或时有中止的参差不齐的状态。《中华脉诊》中说到它的形状时指出："数而一止，止后能回"[6]；《濒湖脉学》载："来去数，时止复来，如蹶之趣，徐疾不常"[6]，说明了促脉"脉率数快，数中有止，好像急遽行走之人突然停止似的"[6]特点。对这个脉象有abrupt pulse、running pulse、rush pulse几种译法。这几种译法的特点为：①abrupt：sudden and unexpected；not smooth；disconnected[7]（突然的，不连续的[8]）；②running、rush都是匆忙的意思，反映不出促脉"突然停止，开始"的转变特点，而abrupt包含两种意思，既能反映出促脉不连续的特点，又能表现出其"突然"的指下感觉，用该词命名促脉最合适。

2.9　结脉

《中华脉诊》[1]中这样描述结脉，"迟缓一止，止后能回"。《脉经》则载有："结脉往来缓，时一复来"[6]。《诊家正眼》述有："迟滞中时见一止。"另有定义"脉搏在迟缓中时而一止的状态，且止无定数"[6]。结脉的译法也很多，如irregular intermittent pulse、knotted pulse等。irregular intermittent pulse指不规则的停顿中止的脉象[8]。knotted pulse指像绳结一样，断断续续，不连续的脉象[8]。此外，还有一种译法为slow pulse with irregular intervals，这个译法十分准确地把结脉的指下感觉表示了出来，但违背了“简洁”的原则，可用于解释内涵，但不可为术语。比较 irregular intermittent pulse 和 knotted pulse 两个译法，knotted 把结脉断续、不连贯的特点全部表达了出来，既明了又简单，还不乏形象生动，比 irregular intermittent 更易接受。

2.10 沉脉

《中医诊断学》描述：“沉脉轻取不应，中取应指，中按则跳动有力”[3]。《中华脉诊》则讲“深下为沉，具有潜藏与内的特点，行于筋骨，如石投水”[6]。《濒湖脉学》也说：“沉脉，如棉裹纱，内刚外柔。如石投水，必极其底”，因此，有 sunken pulse 和 deep pulse 等译法。①sunken：something that has gone to the bottom of the water[7]（沉入水底的）；②deep：extending a long way from top to bottom[7]（深的，沉的）。这两个词都可以形容沉脉“深入筋骨，不易被捕捉”[6]的特点。但是 deep 这个词常易联想到伏脉这个相似脉，根据翻译要有区分度的原则应予回避。sunken 比 deep 更能代表沉脉这种“如石投水，必极其底”的特点，形象简单，更适合用来翻译沉脉。

2.11 弦脉

《中医诊断学》中说“脉来端直而长，按之如弦状，挺然指下”[3]。《脉经》也说：“按之如弓弦”，这都说明了弦脉“平直有力”[6]的特点，stringy pulse、taut pulse、wiry pulse 等都可以译为弦脉。①stringy：like string[7]（像细绳的、线状的[8]）；② taut：something is stretched very tightly[7]（拉紧的，不松弛的[8]）；③wiry：thin but is very strong[7]（硬而坚韧的[8]）。比较上述译法，wiry 来形容弦脉“直而有力”的特点最好，因为它包含了 stringy 和 taut 中“细和直”的含义，同时也说明了弦脉“有力坚韧”的特点，比其他单词翻译得更准确。

准确贴切地把脉诊的相关术语翻译出来，是促进中西医文化交流的必要途径，同时也是弘扬祖国文化遗产，将中医推向世界的“东风”之力。笔者衷心希望能为中医学走向世界尽绵薄之力。

参考文献

[1] 赵恩俭．中医脉诊．天津：天津科技出版社，2001：78-79.

[2] 李照国．中医英语翻译技巧．北京：人民卫生出版社，1997：124-125.

[3] 龙致贤．中医诊断学．北京：学苑出版社，1998：150-167.

[4] 李永．中医常用脉象英译探讨．中国科技翻译，1994，26（4）：32-34.

[5] 魏迺杰．中医西传与翻译问题．医学与哲学，2001，22（7）：51-54.

[6] 刘芳，刘冠军．中华脉诊．北京：中国中医药出版社，2001：89，120，114，148，154，161，171，198，210，216.

[7] 柯林斯 Cobuild 英语词典．上海：上海外语教育出版社，2000：5，427，597，667，859，1569，1576，1585-1587，1655-1657，1675，1710，1922.

[8] 霍恩比．牛津高阶英汉双解词典．4 版．李北达译．香港：牛津大学出版社（中国）有限公司，1997：5，518，574，758，825，1433－1434，1517，1566，1744.

［原载《中国中西医结合杂志》，2006，26（7）：655－658.］

《黄帝内经》英译中美学价值的损失与补偿

沈晓华

在浩瀚如烟的中国古代文库中，《黄帝内经》（以下简称《黄帝内经》）作为一本医学典籍被归入“经史子集”的“经”书之列，足见其在中国古代社会的重要价值。如同《诗经》的成书境遇一样，《黄帝内经》分为《素问》和《灵枢》两部分，在西汉末期由众多医家编纂而成，而古时的医家多数是抱有“不为良相，便为良医”思想的来自“士”阶层的文人，因而其语言风格继承了先秦诸子百家的神韵，文字精练畅达，温婉含蓄，诗意盎然，俊雅悠长，其美学价值与博大精深的医理一道随着历史的长河绵延至今，成为中华民族文明中的一颗璀璨之星。正是由于《黄帝内经》的重要医学和美学价值，海内外学者多次将其译成英文。迄今为止的英译本已有十余种之多，但将这些译本与《黄帝内经》原本进行比照之后，人们发现，某些文本在翻译成译语之后损失了原本中美学层面的价值，作为典籍文本应有的“形意”和“神韵”在英译中流失。然而，现有的《黄帝内经》英译研究却将目光局限于医学价值的传译，而忽略了美学层面的价值损失。

1.《黄帝内经》的美学价值

中医文献学家钱超尘对《黄帝内经》语言层面，尤其是训诂和音韵方面的研究，为人们拨开了《黄帝内经》神秘的面纱，展现出清新淡雅的医学典籍之美。他认为：“《黄帝内经》通体观之，系一部散文著作”[1]。《黄帝内经》原本具有散文美的基本特质，即语言美和意境美。译者作为原本的读者，也是体悟原本文学艺术价值的审美主体，译者与原本作者在情感上产生审美共识，体悟文本中的语言美和意境美，是其通过翻译风格和翻译手法尽力补偿美学层面损失的前提。作为中国古代医学散文的代表，《黄帝内经》的语言美体现在形式、韵律和修辞三个方面。①形式：《黄帝内经》行文工整对称，用词简洁凝练，例如：“昔在黄帝，生而神灵，弱而能言，幼而徇齐，长而敦敏，成而登天”，六个四字格仅二十四个字便把黄帝从出生到登基的成长历程完整地展现出来，语言精妙绝伦，恰到好处。②韵律：尾词押韵，多用叹词，例如：“夫四时阴阳者，万物之根本也，所以圣人春夏养阳，秋冬养阴，以从其根，故与万物沉浮于生长之门。逆其根，则伐其本，坏其真矣。”“阴、根、门、本、真”都是尾词的押运，读来朗朗上口，加上“夫、者、也、矣”这些叹词辅助，富有极强的音律感和节奏感，吟诵起来更为舒畅婉约。③修辞：频用排比、对偶、互文、比喻等修辞格，例如："是以志闲而少欲，心安而不惧，形劳而不倦……是以嗜欲不能劳其目，淫邪不能惑其心。"五个整齐划一的句式结构运用了排比和对偶的修辞，将上古之人的生活状态淋漓尽致地表现出来，富有极其浓厚的古代诗歌意味，又如"圣人春夏养阳，秋冬养阴"则是诗词互文手法的典型代表，体现了其行文的整体性和逻辑性。

《黄帝内经》的意境美在于其行文将医理之"意"融于养生之"境"，例如："中古之时，有至人者，淳德全道，和于阴阳，调于四时，去世离俗，积精全神，游行天地之间，视听八达之外，此盖益其寿命而强者也。"诗性的语言将人与自然天地的物我合一、彼此关照如磅礴的中国山水画一般描绘出来，"至人"的养身调息、内外兼修在"游行天地之间，视听八达之外"的感悟中融于超凡脱俗的玄妙之境。

2.《黄帝内经》英译中美学价值的损失

医学典籍英译在语言转换过程中往往只顾及医学含义的传达，而忽视了典籍作为文学著作本身的美学价值。《黄帝内经》之所以能够成为古时文人所青睐的一本著作，原因之一就在于编撰者将精深的医理置于优美的文学语境之中，让语言之美和意境之美浸润在文字之间，吸引和感染读者，因而，在译文中呈现出原文之"美"是英译《黄帝内经》必然要考虑的因素，也是判断英译质量的标准之一。但要在译语中完全保留原文之"美"却是很难做到的，因为源语和目标语之间存在着不可避免的语言文化差异。英国翻译家卡特福德甚至认为，翻译由于语言和文化上的困难存在不可译性[2]。就《黄帝内经》英译而言，医古文与现代英语存在着诸多差异：医古文语言精练，结构对称，一般单字成意，内涵丰富，行文间多有押韵，节奏感强，而现代英语若要表达与医古文源语相同的意思，是很难做到单字成意且结构对称的；同时，因受限于意义的传达及特定翻译目的的实现，英语单词的选用也很难实现与医古文同样的音韵效果。如《素问·生气通天论篇》中"溃溃乎若坏都，汩汩乎不可止"在译成英文后变为"This disease occurs suddenly like the overflow of a river that is impossible to be brought under control"[3]。译者为实现意义的传递，采用了整合源语句式的方法，译文通达流畅，但也由于这样的处理而未能将"溃溃乎"和"汩汩乎"译出，失去了源语中叠词的音韵效果。由此可见，医古文中存在显著的不可译性，而正是由于这种不可译性所导致的语言效果的损失使得医古文翻译补偿的研究具有了重要的现实意义。

3.《黄帝内经》英译中美学价值的补偿

国内外学者对翻译补偿的定义有所不同，但普遍认为翻译补偿是一种技巧，是对翻译过程中难以避免的损失进行的修复，其中较为学界认可的是 K. Harvey

的定义："Compensation is a technique which involves making up for the loss of a source text effect by recreating a similar effect in the target text through means that are specific to the target language and/or text."（补偿是通过使用译语或译语文本特有的方法，在译语文本中再造一种类似的效果，从而对源语文本效果的损失进行弥补的一种技巧）[4]。《黄帝内经》文本英译时所产生的美学价值损失是由于文本意义传递和美学形式传递之间的不一致造成的，在英译时如何忠实地传达文本意义，同时再现其语言美和意境美是横亘在译者面前的难题。虽然东西方读者在美的理解层面有所不同，但对于美的追求是一致的，丢失了美学价值的《黄帝内经》译文便丧失了这部著作作为散文的文学特性。除非万不得已，原文的审美价值和文化信息都应尽量保留[5]，因而，译者有必要通过翻译补偿技巧减少这部分损失，尽力复现原文的美学价值。在实际翻译操作中，译者可以采用的具体翻译补偿技巧有：整合补偿（具体为：整合并划一句式结构，仿效并再造音韵结构，调整并转换修辞格），以及替代补偿、增益补偿、概念具体化、文中加注等。笔者以李照国教授所译《素问》和 Maoshing Ni 博士所译《素问》两个版本为语料，同时结合笔者的试译，对《黄帝内经》美学价值的英译问题做一尝试性分析。

3.1 语言美的补偿

例句一：上古有真人者，提挈天地，把握阴阳，呼吸精气，独立守神，肌肉若一。（出自《素问·上古天真论篇》）译文一：The immortals, who knew the secrets of the universe and held Yin and Yang, the world, in the palms of their hands. They extracted essence from nature and practiced various disciplines such as Dao-in and Qi Gong, and breathing and visualization exercises, to integrate the body, mind and spirit[6]. 译文二：There were so-called Zhenren (immortal beings) in ancient times [who could] grasp the law of nature. They followed the principles of Yin and Yang, inhaling fresh air, cultivating their spirit and keeping their muscles integrated[3]. 译文一中，译者为了使不了解中医的非专业人士理解原文的意思，侧重取意而舍形，并应用了增益的补偿技巧，译文产生了科普的效果，但原文中四字格的句式被完全打乱，失去了工整对称的形式美。译文二在句式表达上似乎与译文一近似，但在形式美的处理上明显优于前者。译者在第二句通过三个结构工整的动名词短语作状语，部分体现了原文的对称性。笔者在两位译者的基础上，通过整合句式，统一译文结构，在译文的形式美方面做了如下尝试：In ancient times was there the true men, mastering the rules of heaven and earth, following the principles of Yin and Yang, breathing the essence of Qi from the universe, concentrating the mind of body inside, and integrating the muscles with physical efforts. 这里，笔者试将译文结构统一成"现在分词＋名词＋介词＋名

词”的形式，尽力实现对称工整的原文效果。同时，为实现句式结构的整齐划一，试译开头用倒装结构，将 true men 放在后面，以便于直接引出其后做修饰成分的动名词结构。《黄帝内经》全篇音韵丰富，韵式多样，其韵律美主要体现在韵脚（即一个句式句末押韵词的韵母）的频繁使用，如例句一中，“地、气、一”押的都是“i”这个韵母。然而，要在译文中也用“i”作为韵脚来押韵，难度是非常大的，甚至不可能实现。从音韵结构看，例句一呈现出 ARARAR 的特点（A 为无韵结构，R 为有韵结构），因此，在英译时译者可以仿效这样的韵式结构，利用其他可能的韵脚在译文中再造类似的音韵效果，以实现韵律美的补偿。如试译在第 2、4、6 三个名词短语的句末分别使用了 earth、universe、efforts三个词，分别以元音“ə”加辅音“θ、s、ts”构成韵脚，产生 ARARAR 的音韵效果。

例句二：夫四时阴阳者，万物之根本也，所以圣人春夏养阳，秋冬养阴，以从其根，故与万物沉浮于生长之门。逆其根，则伐其本，坏其真矣。（出自《素问・四气调神大论篇》）译文一：The transformation of Yin and Yang in the four seasons is the basis of the growth and the destruction of life. The sages were able to cultivate the Yang energy in spring and summer and conserve the Yin energy in autumn and winter. By following the universal order, growth can occur naturally. If this natural order is disregarded, the root of one's life will be damaged and one's true energy will wane[6]. 译文二：[The changes of] Yin and Yang in the four seasons are the roots of all the things [in nature]. So the sages cultivate yang in spring and summer, while nourish Yin in autumn and winter in order to follow such roots (the changes of Yin and Yang in different seasons). Violation of these roots means destruction of the Ben (primordial base) and impairment of the body[3]. 若以标点符号为分界考察每一个词组，例句二中的押韵词为“阴、根、门、本、真”，韵脚为“en”，音韵结构可以记为：ARARRRRRR。两段译文的处理方法相似，均以直译为主。在古汉语形式和语音的保留方面，译文二的选词和句式结构更胜一筹。译者在处理原文最后三个并列结构时，使用了三个名词化短语，行文紧凑，精练达意。但两段译文都忽略了韵律的英译问题，失去了原文的节奏感。笔者仿效原文的音韵结构，试译如下：The alternation of Yin and Yang in the four seasons is the basis of all the organisms in the nature, thus the sages nourish Yang in spring and summer, and support yin in autumn and winter, to comply with the natural rules and order. Therefore, they live as per the principles with pleasure. Violation of the natural rules and order, leads to the collapse of one's basic health structure, and the destruction of his original energy from nature.

此外，关于叠音词的英译，译者也可效仿原本的音韵结构。例如，上文所提到的“溃溃乎若坏都，汩汩乎不可止”的叠词音韵效果可以通过选用两个开头辅音相同的英文单词以构成头韵，实现补偿目的。笔者根据这一策略，试译如下：It happens on the patient suddenly as if the damaged cities corrupt and collapse, and the floods burst with bubbles out of control.

作为一本医学散文著作，《黄帝内经》也大量使用了丰富多彩的修辞格。若能在英译时结合译语读者的文化背景，适当调整并转换修辞格的类型，便能在准确传达意义的同时保留修辞效果。

例句三：六经为川，肠胃为海，九窍为水注之气。（出自《素问·阴阳应象大论篇》）译文一：The movement and traveling of Qi and blood in the six channels is like a river flowing; and the stomach and large intestine, which contain the fluids and food, are like the ocean. The nine orifices are like the spring where water gushes in and out[6]. 译文二：The six-channels act as mountains and valleys, the intestines and the stomach act as the seas, the nine orifices are the regions where Shuiqi (Water-Qi) infuse[3]. 例句三将六经喻为河流，肠胃比作大海，九窍形容成水气灌注的地方，描述生动形象。例句中未使用比喻词，是典型的暗喻手法，在英译时可增加比喻词，将暗喻修辞显性处理成明喻修辞，使意义更加明确。译文一将暗喻转换成明喻，同时进行了适当的增益，如“the stomach and large intestine, which contain the fluids and food,”使译文更具可读性，但译者将“六经”处理成“The movement and traveling of Qi and blood in the six channels”显然偏离了原文的意思。译文二保留了暗喻修辞，句式结构上也更加忠实于原文，但意义更为隐含，容易使译语读者望文生义，同时译者将“六经为川”译为“The six-channels act as mountains and valleys”是一个明显的误译。笔者在两段译文的基础上试译如下：The six channels are similar to flowing river, the stomach and intestines are similar to grand ocean, and the nine orifices are similar to places where water Qi infuse.

例句四：五藏有腧，六府有合。（出自《素问·痹论篇》）译文一：For the five Zang, access the Shu points; for the six Fu, access the He/sea points[6]. 译文二：The five Zang-organs have their acupoints and the six Fu-organs have their He-Sea[3]. 例句四中出现的是古汉语中常用的互文修辞，即上下文各说一半内容而省略掉另一半的内容，但两部分相互交错和补充，合而为一构成完整的意思。上文“五藏有腧”只说一半内容，而省略了“五藏有合”，下文“六府有合”则省略了“六府有腧”，上下文合在一起的完整意思应是：五脏和六腑都有腧穴和合穴。两段译文都按照原文句式结构直译，由于英文中不存在互文修辞，这样的处理方式不仅失去了修辞效果，更使得译文与原句含义产生了偏差。然而，若将例句译为：Both five Zang-organs and six Fu-organs have Shu acupoints and He acupoints。译文虽含义到位，却无半点修辞意味。此时，应适当调整和转换修辞格。基于这一补偿技巧，笔者在英译时将互文修辞格转换成了对照修辞格。试译如下：Both five Zang-organs and six fu-organs have acupoints. They have acupoints of Shu；they possess acupoints of He.

3.2　意境美的补偿

《黄帝内经》虽不是诗歌，却蕴藏着诗歌般的韵律和修辞。更为重要的是，其行文间透露出的意境美以诗化的语言将中医养生和治疗理念与人的内心感悟联系起来，使看似无法触摸的医理变得生动且富于感染力，而《黄帝内经》的意境美又是透过中医和中国传统文化意象传达出来的，因而，其文化意境之美在译成英文时让译语读者产生同样的感悟在于文化意象的英译处理。

例句五：太虚寥廓，五运迴薄。（出自《素问·五常政大论篇》）译文：The heavens is boundless. The Wuyun（Five-Motions）moves fast and continuously[3]。例句五中，“太虚”“五运”都是中国道家文化中的意象概念。在英译时，若能较为恰当地传达原文中这两个文化意象，便能较为理想地传达原文的意境。然而，当中西方文化意象之间出现语义缺省，甚至产生价值冲突时，译者便需要采用替代、增益、概念具体化、文中加注等英译补偿技巧，以消除因文化差异因素带来的意境美的损失。西方文化中并无“太虚”和“五运”这些概念，因而译文当保留其术语，同时在文中加注以解释其意。李照国教授的译文遵循“译古如古，文不加饰”的原则[3]，充分保留了《黄帝内经》的文化意境之美（由于 Maoshing Ni 博士未在其译本中翻译该句，故不作考查）。他在处理“五运”时采用了文中加注的补偿手段，使读者能够对照源语和译语概念，体悟原文的思想境界。但在“太虚”一词的处理上，笔者认为还应做一定的训诂研究。该词在古汉语中为多义词，可解释为道、气、天空、宇宙等。在《素问·五运行大论》中，岐伯曰：“地为人之下，太虚之中者也。帝曰：凭乎？岐伯曰：大气举之也。”可见，“太虚”在《黄帝内经》中应解释为宇宙：地球因大气托举而悬浮于宇宙之中。因而该词可译为：Taixu（universe），而译为 heavens（天空）则不符合原文意境。同时，原句中“廓”“薄”为押韵词，音韵结构为 RR。结合音韵美的补偿翻译，笔者试译如下：The domain of Taixu（universe）is boundless，the circulation of Wuyun（Five -Motions）is endless.

例句六：如临深渊者，不敢堕也。手如握虎者，欲其壮也。（出自《素问·针解篇》译文一：When acupuncturing，one should be prepared and careful，as if one is facing a deep abyss. Move carefully so as not to fall. In handling the needle，hold it as if holding the tiger——firmly grasped and in control[6]. 译文二：［The attitude toward needling is］just like approaching to the abyss［means that one］must be very careful［in performing needling therapy］.［The figure of speech that one holds the needle] as if grasping the tail of a tiger means to hold [and manipulate the needle] with strength[3]. 这两段译文均采用了增益的补偿技巧，译文一补出 When acupuncturing，译文二补出 The attitude toward needling，使主旨义更为明晰。译文二 approaching 这一动态动词的使用比译文一“facing”这一静态动词的使用更能显示出用针者的小心谨慎、如履薄冰。译文二在翻译“手如卧虎”时采用了“概念具体化”的补偿技巧，译者将手握住虎的具体部位译出：the tail of a tiger，使读者更易体会用针时应掌握的力度和方法。

例句七：黄帝乃择吉日良兆而藏灵兰之室，以传保焉。（出自《素问・灵兰秘典论篇》）译文一：I must pick the best day and time to receive and store this knowledge. I must put this in my secret chamber and preserve it and pass it down to future generations[6]. 译文二：The Huangdi selected an auspicious day and stored these cannons* in the royal fragrant room for passing on to the later generations[3]. 例句中有两个重要的文化意象：“吉日良辰”和“灵兰之室”。从文化意境的传达来看，译文二更为传神和贴切：译者用 auspicious 将古文中的“吉”译出，从中体现了古人对于风水运程的敬畏以及黄帝本人对于“灵兰秘典”的格外重视。相比之下，译文一中 best day and time 符合第一人称的叙述方式和口语化的表达内容，未能传译出中国传统文化语境。关于“灵兰之室”，明代吴昆注《黄帝内经・素问》云：“灵台兰室，黄帝藏书之所”[7]。可见，“灵兰”实为“灵台”和“兰室”两个地名。两则译文均采用了替代的补偿技巧，以弥补因地名直译而造成的语义缺省。两相比较，译文二以 royal fragrant room 替代地名，暗含了藏书地点的皇家气息，同时 fragrant 一词也较符合“兰”的特点，其源语文化语境得以彰显。译文一的 secret chamber 则较为直白，对源语文化语境未做保留，语言形式更倾向于译语文化。

4. 结语

《黄帝内经》作为一本散文体的医学典籍，其蕴含的美学价值不容忽视。译者在处理译文时，应当考虑原文的形式美、韵律美、修辞美和意境美。为保留英译过程中可能流失的这部分美学要素，译者可采用的翻译补偿技巧有：整合补偿（具体分为：整合并划一句式结构，仿效并再造音韵结构，调整并转换修辞格）、替代补偿、增益补偿、概念具体化和文中加注等。虽然中医英译研究经历了数十年的发展历程，受到翻译学界的广泛关注和重视，但中医补偿翻译研究却相对滞后，系统的专门性论述鲜有所见。希望笔者关于《黄帝内经》美学价值的英译补偿观点能够为这一领域的深入研究提供一定启示。

注释：* 原译文中为 cannons（大炮），显然与《黄帝内经》原本语义不符，应改为 canons。

参考文献

[1] 钱超尘．内经语言研究．北京：人民卫生出版社，1990：228.

[2] Catford JC. 翻译的语言学理论．穆雷译，北京：旅游教育出版社，1991：109.

[3] 李照国．黄帝内经·素问．西安：世界图书出版公司，2005：9，19，23，31，75，113，519，825，599.

[4] Baker M. Routledge encyclopedia of translation studies. London：Routledge（Taylor & Francis Group），2001：37.

[5] 夏廷德．翻译补偿研究．武汉：湖北教育出版社，2005：243.

[6] Maoshing Ni. The Yellow Emperor's classic of medicine. Boston：Shambhala Publications，Inc.，1995：3，7，23，35，162，193.

[7] 吴昆．黄帝内经素问吴注．北京：学苑出版社，2001：43.

[原载《中国中西医结合杂志》，2012，32（5）：704－708.]

《黄帝内经》常用文化负载词英译

张　璇　施蕴中

中医学是受中国古代哲学思想影响建立起来的一门传统医学，其丰富的文化色彩和人文内涵是现代医学所不能比拟的。《黄帝内经》是一部重要的中医典籍，其医学价值和人文色彩必须在英译中给予同等程度的重视。文化负载词是标志民族文化的突出代表，《黄帝内经》中的文化负载词往往是体现中医对人体生理病理独特认识的重要词汇，因此，文化负载词的英译是《黄帝内经》英译的重点和难点，对其处理的好坏关系到整个文本的翻译质量。本文选取《黄帝内经·素问》的第一章及李照国和威斯的两个英译本作为语料，分析《黄帝内经》中文化负载词的特点及两个译本不同的处理手段。

1. 文化负载词及其研究意义

1.1　文化负载词（culture-specific lexicon）

有的学者借用包惠南和包昂先生对词汇空缺（zero of equivalent word）的定义“源语词汇所承载的文化信息在译语中没有对应语”[1]作为负载词的定义。彭智蓉认为文化负载词是“标志某种文化中特有事物的词、词组和习语。这些词汇反映了特定民族在漫长的历史进程中逐渐积累的、有别于其他民族的独特的生活方式”[2]。每个国家或民族都有自己独特的发展历史，有自己独特的生活环境，形成不同于其他国家或民族的独特词汇——文化负载词。文化负载词是民族文化的标志，具有鲜明的民族特征。

邓炎昌等[3]根据源语和译语的对应情况，将文化负载词分为四类：第一，源语词在目标语中没有对应语，如阴阳、五行、八卦等。第二，词汇在两种语言中表面意义相同而内涵不同。例如，在中国，龙被看做中华民族的象征，是炎黄子孙不屈不挠、英勇无畏的精神支柱，象征着高贵和成功。在封建社会，龙用来指代帝王，皇族的后代被称为“龙子龙孙”，皇帝穿的衣服叫“龙袍”。而“龙”在英文中的对应词“dragon”却是有尾巴、有翅膀，又能吐火的邪恶象征。第三，一种语言中的词语在另一种语言中有多个对应词，但没有一个词能与之完全对等。如，“干部”一词与 official functionary administrator 在意思上均有重叠，但不能完全对等。第四，词语的基本含义大致对等，而第二层含义或附加义不同。张敬丰认为对文化负载词的分类应该以奈达对文化的分类为标准，将其分为经济文化负载词、物质文化负载词、社会文化负载词、概念文化负载词和语言文化负载词五类[4]。

1.2　研究意义

"翻译不仅是跨语言的交际活动，更是跨文化的交际活动，处理的是不同文化背景下的两种语言系统"[5]，"每个民族都有各自的文化焦点，而词汇总是朝着特定文化的焦点方向发展变化得日益详尽和复杂。如果文化间的焦点相似，不同语言词汇间语义对应和交叉的情况就很普遍。相反，不同语言的词汇间语义冲突甚至空缺的现象就十分突出"[6]。汉语和英语分别代表了东西方两种不同的文化，文化焦点差异大，词义空缺现象明显，文化负载词翻译的好坏关系到译语读者是否能够正确理解原文，是翻译的重点和难点。

2.《黄帝内经》及英译本简介

《黄帝内经》分《素问》和《灵枢》两部分，成书于战国时期，是中医理论的奠基之作，被列为中医四大经典著作之首。《黄帝内经》语言精练，文化色彩浓厚，具有很高的医学价值和文学价值，至今依然是中医学专业学生的必读之作。《素问》主要阐述中医基础理论，为后世中医学的发展打下了坚实的基础。1925—2005 年，《素问》正式出版过 11 个英译本。"这些译本产生于不同的历史时期，由不同背景的译者翻译，译本之间差异巨大，反映了中医古籍英译事业的发展进程"[7]。本文将主要选取两部译作，研究其中文化负载词英译的处理。一部是《黄帝内经》的首部英译本，由 Ilza Veith 于 1945—1946 年翻译（*The Yellow Emperor's Classic of Internal Medicine*）。另一部是 1997 年出版的入选《大中华文库》的李照国英译本（*Yellow Emperor's Canon of Medicine Plain Conversation*），以期比较中外两种文化背景下，不同时期的两位著名译者对文化负载词的处理方式。本文重点将《素问》第一篇《上古天真论篇第一》中的重要中医文化负载词的翻译做简要分析，以期找出《黄帝内经》中文化负载词翻译的一般规律。

3.《黄帝内经》中文化负载词的英译

3.1　《黄帝内经》中文化负载词的选择标准

通过对多个学者给出的文化负载词定义的比较以及对《黄帝内经》原文的仔细阅读和分析，笔者认为需要将包惠南和包昂先生的定义适当扩大，将文化负载词定义为"源语词汇所承载的文化信息在译语中没有对应语的现象，或两种语言中文化意义不完全重合的词语"。比如，"昔在黄帝，生而神灵，弱而能言，幼而徇齐，长而敦敏，成而登天。"登天"一词，汉语表示登天子之位"。中国古代，受"君权神授"思想的影响，君王被称作"天子"，朝廷被称作"天朝"。而在英语中，受宗教文化的影响，“登天”的对应语为 ascend to heaven，表示上天堂，即“去世、死亡（pass away）”。“登天”和 ascend to heaven 形式上虽然对应，但在文化意义上不重合。如果将“登天”译为 ascend to heaven，会给译语读者造成文化误读。

3.2　《黄帝内经》中文化负载词的分类

经过手动检索，《黄帝内经》第一篇《上古天真论篇第一》中共出现文化负载词 101 处（包括重复）。根据词性可分为三类：

3.2.1　名词类文化负载词　此类占大多数。名词类文化负载词又可分为三类：第一，人名类，如“黄帝”“岐伯”等；第二类，中医常用解剖及生理病理术语，如“阴阳”“精”“气”“任脉”“天癸”等，这类文化负载词占名词类文化负载词的大多数；第三类，其他，是除以上两类外，易造成文化误读的词语，如“春秋”（指年龄）、“百岁”（虚指，并不是指 100 岁）。

3.2.2　动宾类文化负载词　如“登天”（登天子之位）、“入房”（男女之事）等。动宾类文化负载词虽然占的比重较小，但是却常因理解不正确而误译。

3.2.3　形容词类文化负载词　形容词类文化负载词是占比例最小的一类。比如“神灵”表聪明的意思。

3.3　两译本文化负载词翻译策略比较

李照国先生和 Ilza Veith 女士两位译者在翻译《黄帝内经》时都采取了适度异化的原则，但异化程度及表现方法有所不同。异化与归化使用的多少往往受母语文化及对原文理解程度的影响。两位译者有完全不同的文化教育背景，有完全不同的工作条件。李照国先生的母语为汉语，曾获英语语言文学学士学位和中医学博士学位；该译本依靠了中医专家翻译好的白话文；译者在上海中医药大学工作，有相对较丰富的汉语参考资源。Ilza Veith 女士的母语为英语，专业为医学史；她完全不懂中医，并且缺乏懂汉语和中医的人协助她开展翻译工作；她的汉语工具书严重缺乏，主要依靠法语、德语等其他语种的工具书。两位译者对《黄帝内经》原文意思的理解自然大不相同，相比之下，李照国先生本更胜一筹。但在译文的遣词行文上，母语为英语的 Ilza Veith 女士自然比李照国先生运用得更加得心应手。

3.3.1　名词类文化负载词翻译策略比较

3.3.1.1　人名类文化负载词：两位译者在人名翻译的处理上是基本一致的，即音译为主，或辅以字对字解释。如李照国本将“黄帝”译为“Huangdi”或“Yellow Emperor”，Ilza Veith 女士本用威妥玛拼音音译为“Huang Ti”或“the yellow emperor”。李照国本将“岐伯”译为“Qibo”，Ilza Veith 女士本将“岐伯”用威妥玛拼音音译为“Chi Po”。

3.3.1.2　中医常用解剖生理病理术语：对此类词语，李照国先生主要采取音译加括号夹注的方法。如“神”，他译为“the Shen (mind or spirit)”，“精气”被译为“Jingqi (Essence-Qi)”等；而 Ilza Veith 女士则不同，有时是字对字翻译，有时是夹注。比如“神”被译为“soul”或“mind”，“精”被译为“true (essence)”。再如，“天癸”是中医特有的生理词汇，天，是指先天，癸，是指癸水。天癸就是藏于肾中具有促进生殖功能的一种先天而生的物质”[8]。这一词汇反映了我们的祖先对男女生殖功能的产生以及衰退的认识，在英语中属于“文化空缺”，给翻译造成了很大的局限性。李照国采取的是音译“tiangui”附尾注加以解释的方法。Ilza Veith 女士则是采取根据文义将其意译的方法，于是在她的译文中就出现了如下众多的英文“天癸”表达方式。二七而天癸至（女子）：When she reaches her fourteenth year she begins to menstruate；二八肾气盛，天癸至（男子）：When he is sixteen years of age the emanations of his testicles become abundant and he begins to secrete semen；七七任脉虚，太冲脉衰少，天癸竭，地道不通，故形坏而无子也（女子）：When she reaches the age of forty-nine she can no longer become pregnant and the circulation of the great thoroughfare pulse is decreased. Her menstruation is exhausted, and the gates of menstruation are no longer open；her body deteriorates and she is no longer able to bear children；七八肝气衰，筋不能动，天癸竭，精少，肾藏衰，形体皆极（男子）：At fifty-six the force of his liver (肝气) deteriorates, his muscles can no longer function properly, his secretion of semen is exhausted, his vitality diminishes, his testicles (kidneys) deteriorate, and his physical strength reaches its end。

李照国先生以异化为主的译法完整地保留了中医术语，有利于英译读者了解“天癸”一词以及中医思维方式，但其接受程度如何还有待进一步的考证；而 ILza Veith 女士以归化为主的译法更有利于译语读者理解原文的含义，但却不利于中医术语英译词的标准化以及中医术语在英语读者中的推广。

3.3.1.3　其他名词性文化负载词：两位译者对名词性文化负载词的翻译都是以结合语义意译为主。如：“余闻上古之人，春秋皆度百岁，而动作不衰”，李照国先生译为：I am told that people in ancient times all could live for one hundred years without any signs of senility。威斯女士译为：I have heard that in ancient times the people lived (through the years) to be over a hundred years, and yet they remained active and did not become decrepit in their activities。再如，“以欲竭其精，以耗散其真”，这里的“耗”是名词，是通假字。通假字是中国古书的用字现象之一，“通假”就是“通用、借代”的意思，就是用读音相同或者相近的字代替本字。“耗”在这里通“好”，是“嗜好”的意思。“以欲竭其精，以耗散其真”行文对仗，“欲”和“耗”乃近义词。李照国先生将其译为：(As a result) Their Jingqi (Essence-Qi) is exhausted and Zhenqi (Genuine-Qi) is wasted。译文

舍其形求其意。Ilza Veith 女士将其译为：Their passions exhaust their vital forces；their cravings dissipate their true（essence）。译文既保留了对仗的形式，又准确传达了原文的意义，语句更加生动，用词更加灵活，不失为意、形均与原作贴合的佳作。

3.3.2 动宾类文化负载词翻译策略比较 李照国先生对此类文化负载词采取的是结合语境意译的方法。如对“今对时之人不然也，以酒为浆，以妄为常，醉以入房”中“入房”，他译为 seek sexual pleasure；对“昔在黄帝，生而神灵，弱而能言，幼而徇齐，长而敦敏，成而登天”中的“登天”，他译为 become the Emperor。Ilza Veith 女士则采取字对字或加脚注的翻译策略，但未免显得过于拘泥于原文，不利于译语读者理解甚至会造成误解。比如将“入房”直接译为 enter the chamber（of love），将“登天”译为 ascend to heaven 等。

3.3.3 形容词类文化负载词翻译策略比较 李照国先生和 Ilza Veith 女士都采取了结合语义意译的方法。如“愚智贤不肖不惧于物”，李照国本译为：Neither the ignorant nor the intelligent and neither the virtuous nor the unworthy feared anything。Ilza Veith 本译为：（In such a society）no matter whether men are wise or foolish，virtuous or bad，they are without fear of anything。再如“昔在黄帝，生而神灵”，李照国版译为：Huangdi or Yellow Emperor，was born intelligent。Ilza Veith 本译为：In ancient times when the Yellow Emperor was born he was endowed with divine talents。两位译者均有时能保持形容词的词性，有时词性则有所变化。

文化的差异性和复杂性决定了文化负载词翻译在策略上的灵活和变通的特点。由于翻译的目的是促进两种文化的交流，所以适度的异化是十分必要的。

比较不同文化背景下的译者在不同时期的译本中文化负载词的翻译，对中医经典著作的翻译具有重要而现实的意义。作为语料试分析，本文只选取了《黄帝内经》第一篇《上古天真论篇第一》中的文化负载词的翻译进行了比较研究，还有待进一步拓展和深入。

参考文献

[1] 包惠南，包昂．中国文化与汉英翻译．北京：外文出版社，2004：10.

[2] 彭智蓉．试论文化负载词汇的翻译．疯狂英语．教师版，2006（6）：43-46.

[3] 邓炎昌，刘润清．语言与文化——英汉语言文化对比．北京：外语教学与研究出版社，1989：9-10.

[4] 张敬丰．文化负载词与词组研究及其翻译．福建：福建师范大学出版社，2003：6-10.

[5] Bandia PF. Translation as cultural transfer：evidence from African creative writing. Traduction，Terminologie，Tedaltion，1993，6（2）：55-78.

[6] 潘利锋．从英译鲁迅小说看文化负载词汇的翻译．天津外国语学院学报，2004，11（4）：

12－14.
[7] 兰凤利.《黄帝内经素问》英译事业的描写性研究（1）. 中国中西医结合杂志，2004，24（10）：947－950.
[8] 王洪图. 内经选读. 上海：上海科学技术出版社，2001：35.

[原载《中国中西医结合杂志》，2008，28（10）：941－944.]

《黄帝内经·素问》英译事业的描写性研究

兰凤利

《黄帝内经》分为《素问》和《灵枢》两部分，为我国现存最早的较为系统和完整的医学典籍。《黄帝内经·素问》（以下简称《素问》）是《黄帝内经》的重要组成部分，它不但是中医学基本理论的渊薮，也是我国优秀文化遗产的重要组成部分，2000多年来一直指导着中医学的发展。直到今天，《黄帝内经》仍列“四大经典”之首，为学习中医者的必读之书，也是世界各国研究我国古代文明史、医学史的重要著作。

1925—2003年，出现了9种《素问》英译本，成为中医古籍英译史上一道独特而灿烂的风景。这些译本产生于不同历史时期，具有鲜明的时代烙印，体现了中医学名词术语英译在国内外的发展进程。这些译本之间差异很大，有些是由于译者对原文的理解不同，有些是由于特定历史因素对译者的意图和倾向造成的不同影响。显然，如果今天只用某一翻译标准对这些译本进行规定性的褒贬，那么，有些译本的历史价值则会被一笔抹杀，因此，我们引入多元系统理论，对每种译本的特征及其产生的原因、背景进行全面历时性描述，以真正了解《素问》英译事业的伟大意义。

1. 翻译研究新视角：多元系统理论与描写性翻译研究

多元系统理论（polysystem theory）是以色列特拉维夫大学学者I. Even-Zohar在20世纪70年代初攻读博士学位（研究范围为文学翻译理论）时提出的一种理论。多元系统理论“绝不以价值判断为准则来预先选择研究对象”，并且强调“批评”（criticism）与“研究”（research）之间的差别[1]。从我国翻译研究的历史及现状来看，我们所关注的焦点多为个人翻译经验的总结和交流，以及具体译作的分析和点评等，即Even-Zohar所说的“批评”，却忽视了翻译研究中的另外一个天地，即“研究”。“批评”属于应用性研究，偏重于对翻译实践的指导；而“研究”则更着重于对翻译实践活动的描述、揭示和认识。20世纪80—90年代，Even-Zohar的年轻同事G. Toury又发展了其理论，提出描写性的翻译研究方法论。该方法论是将翻译结果视为既成事实，追寻影响翻译过程的社会历史因素以及翻译作品在译语文化多元系统中的功能和地位，并对此进行“全面历时性描述”（comprehensive diachronic description）。这一描写性方法适用于对多年以前产生的翻译作品或是不同历史条件下产生的同一作品的不同译本进行研究。由于它能有效地避免评论者自身所处历史时期的审美期望的干扰，能真正昭示每一种翻译作品的特征和价值，因此，对于跨越了近80年、在不同历史时期产生了9种译本的《黄帝内经·素问》，英译事业十分适合这种描写性研究。从另一个意义上来说，这一翻译事业也为描写性翻译批评方法论提供了珍贵的个案。

2.《素问》英译事业的描写性研究

《素问》英译事业的描写性研究分为3个部分。第一部分以表格形式简要介绍《素问》的9种英译版本。第二部分是对译本的全面历时性描述。本文将《素问》的英译历程分为3个历史时期，根据不同时期译本的特征，力图考证特定历史背景中译者的意图，不同历史时期《素问》英译本在英美文化（医学文化）多元系统中不同的地位及功能，以及特定历史条件之下中医古籍英译的规范与倾向。第三部分是作者在历时性描述的基础上总结出来的《素问》英译历程的发展脉络。

3.《黄帝内经·素问》9种英译本简介

见表1。

4.《黄帝内经·素问》英译历程的历时性描述

4.1　第一阶段：1925—1950年

这一历史时期有3种《素问》英译本：Dawson译本、Ilza Veith译本及黄雯译本。中医学对西方的交流与传播始自明代。最早是由来华传教士带着颇为好奇的心理或将自己的亲身经历介绍给西方的。意大利传教士利玛窦（Matteo Ricci，1552—1610）在《利玛窦中国札记》中第一个比较准确地向西方介绍了中国医学[12,13]。而真正全面介绍中医学的书是《医钥和中国脉理》（*Clavis Medica ad Chinarum Doctrinam de Pulsibus*）。此书分六大部分，译有王叔和的《脉经》、舌诊、气色诊病等医理及中药名289条。作者为卜弥格（Michel-Pierre Boym，1612—1659）。《医钥和中国脉理》1680年在德国法兰克福出版（拉丁文）[12,14]。

至于中医古籍的早期译介，则要至少推后100多年。1812年，法国学者勒牡萨发表了以《本草纲目》为主要对象来讨论中国医药的论文，并获医学博士学位[12]。1855年，香港出版了《洗冤录杂记》（*Notice of A Chinese Work on Medical Ju-risprudence Entitled Se Yuen Luh*，或"*Records of the Washing away Injuries*"）[14]。

最早译介中医学"四大经典"之首《素问》的，是1925年德国人Percy. M Dawson的一篇英文论文（表1）。当时正是"西方中心论"盛行的20世纪20年代，德国、英国和美国都属于世界强国。中医疗法尽管于17世纪就已传入欧美，但其应用范围基本上局限于华人及亚裔。而西医学，即现代医学，在西方仍然保持着强大自足的状态。英译中医学及中医经典只能在英美医学文化体系中处于非

表 1 《素问》9 种英译本简介

译本	1[2,3]	2[3]	3[4,5]	4[6]	5[7]	6[8]	7[9]	8[10]	9[11]
出版年代	1925	1949	1950	1978	1995	1997	1997	2001	2003 年开始
翻译历时*	不详	4～5 年	14 年	几年（<10 年）	历时较长，作者未明确注明具体时间	书中未提到	书中未提到	不详	11 年
译者	Percy. M. Dawson ②	Ilza Veith	黄雯	Henry C. Lu 组织	Maoshing Ni	未署名，编绘者为青年画家	吴连胜、吴奇父子	朱明	Paul U. Unschuld
译者身份	不详	医史学家，当时在约翰·霍普金斯大学医史研究所攻读博士学位	广州孙逸仙医学院院长、医师	加拿大人	哲学博士、医学博士，出生于中医世家，在美国从事中医临床和教学	不详，据推测为出版社策划翻译	在美从事中医临床工作	国内中医学院本科毕业，中医师	德国慕尼黑大学医史研究所所长、教授
译文标题	Su-wen, the Basis of Chinese Medicine	The Yellow Emperor's Classic of Internal Medicine	Nei Ching, the Chinese Canon of Medicine	《内、难全集》	The Yellow Emperor's Classic of Medicine: A New Translation of the Neijing Suwen with Commentary	The Illustrated Yellow Emperor's Canon of Medicine	The Yellow Emperor's Canon Internal Medicine	The Medical Classic of the Yellow Emperor	Huang Di Nei Jing Su Wen

续表

译本	1	2	3	4	5	6	7	8	9
译文内容	节译《素问》	1—34 章	选译《素问》的重要章节及评注	全译《黄帝内经》《难经》	全译《素问》,译者将对原文的阐释融入译文	选择《黄帝内经》中有关养生的章节,配以漫画、示例	全译《黄帝内经》,以汉英对照的形式出版	高等中医院校第5版教材《内经讲义》	参考相关论文3000余篇,全译《素问》及历代600多部相关著作中的注释
篇幅	6页	32开,共260页,译文占156页	33页	不详	32开,301页	16开,209页	16开,共831页,其中《素问》占487页	32开,302页	2003年出版首册介绍《素问》,共520页;译文三册尚未出版
发表形式	以论文形式发表在 *Annals of Medical History*	美国 Williams & Wikins 出版社出版	发表在 *Chinese Medical Journal*	不详	美国 Shambhala 出版社出版	海豚出版社出版	中国科学技术出版社出版	外文出版社出版	多册,由加利福尼亚大学出版社陆续出版

续表

译本	1	2	3	4	5	6	7	8	9
附加部分	不详	医史研究所所长之序，《黄帝内经》内容简介（76 页）、王冰注、林亿等新校正序及参考文献、索引，译文正文下有丰富的脚注	不详	不详	译者前言、翻译说明、致谢、发音说明、参考文献、译者简介及索引	《黄帝内经》十三方及“性情修养范例”——以恐胜喜、以怒胜思、以喜解忧、以愁解忧、以悲胜喜、以喜胜怒	无	不详	首册《素问——中国古代医学典籍中的自然、知识和意象》，为整个译本的概论，其中还附有五运六气学说的介绍
再版或重印	/	1966 年，加利福尼亚大学出版社修订再版	/	不详	不详	1997 年第 1 版，2001 年第 2 次印刷	1997 年 12 月第 1 版，2002 年 8 月第 4 次印刷	/	/

注：* 翻译历时指开始翻译时间与出版时间相隔的时间；** 在着手翻译《素问》前，Izza Veith 在 5 部著作中找到了《黄帝内经》的片段译文。其中，仅 Percy M. Dawson 的英文论文专论《素问》发表时间最早，且篇幅最长，翻译规模也最大，因此，作为最早译介《素问》的译文，而其他略而不提。这一点尚可与王吉民、傅维康编著的《中国医史外文文献索引（1682—1965）》互为证明。

常边缘的地位。而此时，在中国，一方面，西医学的传播如火如荼；另一方面，中医学的地位和作用因国民党政府的导向而处于历史低谷，且中西医之间的论争、交流、结合愈演愈烈。这一历史时期，美国公开出版《素问》英译本是具有开拓创新意义的。这一历史时期《素问》的3种英译本具有如下特征。

4.1.1 主要从医学史的角度译介《素问》

3位译者中，只有黄雯是医师（是否为西医师尚未可知），其历经10余载，翻译了《素问》的一些重要章节，并详加评注，1950年发表在《中华医学杂志》英文版上，使西方学者有机会看到成书于2000多年前的中国医学经典的概貌。其他两位西方学者都是从医学史的角度译介《素问》的。Percy M. Dawson介绍《素问》的论文发表在《医学史年鉴》（*Annals of Medical History*）上。Ilza Veith女士则是医史学家，她在序中说："这部典籍的翻译，代表了医史学家的方法，而非汉语言学家的方法。希望这一初步研究能成为对该书原文进行进一步研究的起点，尤其是在众多的语言学问题上给予特别关注[3]"。20世纪上半叶英译《素问》的主要目的表明，在西方世界中，这部伟大的中医学经典的地位十分卑微，只被医史学家关注，它对人民健康以及疾病防治方面的医学价值没有得到丝毫体现。

4.1.2 中医名词术语的英译以归化为主

1913年，美国医史学家F. Carrisen出版了近700页的《医学史》一书，有关中国医学的内容介绍不满一页，且有谬误。当时伍连德先生致函质询。F. Carrisen复函曰："中医或有所长，顾未见有以西文述之者，区区半页之资料，犹属外人之作，参考无从，遂难立说，简略而误，非余之咎"[15]。显然，中医学，包括《素问》这样的中医学经典，处于西方医学文化多元系统中的边缘位置。在Even-Zohar看来，当翻译文学处于文学多元系统的边缘位置时，"译者的主要工作，就是为外国的文本找来最佳的现成二级模式。结果是译本的充分性不足"[1]。

以Ilza Veith译本为例。Ilza Veith在翻译中医名词术语时所采用的翻译策略着重于译文在西方的"可接受性"。她多采用归化的方法，套用本国医学（西医学）现成的二级模式，大量地借用西医学术语表达中医学概念。如她将"经，经脉"译为"arteries (veins)（动脉，静脉）"，"经络系统"译为"the vascular system（血管系统）"，"天癸"译为"menstruation（月经）"等[3]。再如，中西医对脾的认识有极大的不同：西医认为脾是免疫器官，功能是清除死亡的细胞和对抗感染，而中医学认为脾的主要功能是"主运化（水谷精微）"。Ilza Veith为了使译文更能被西方读者接受，不惜明知误译，干脆将原文中的"脾"译为"stomach（胃）"。如"阴阳应象大论"一章中，Ilza Veith将"血生脾"译为"the blood enlivens the stomach"，"甘生脾"译为"the sweet flavor nourishes the stomach”，“在藏为脾”译为“of the viscera they create the stomach”，“思伤脾”译为“extreme sympathy is injurious to the stomach”等[3]。

4.1.3 为促进医学文化交流采取补偿措施

Ilza Veith 翻译《素问》，是希望能够达到医学文化交流的目的。为了使英语读者真正理解和欣赏《素问》，她采取了许多措施，比较突出的是撰写长篇引言介绍《素问》和中医学、使用附录及大量使用脚注，为读者提供必要的文化信息。Ilza Veith 译本的引言部分“《素问》之分析”长达 76 页，约占整个译本篇幅的 1/3，介绍了《素问》的成书年代及作者、哲学基础（包括道、阴阳、五行、天干等）、解剖学及生理学概念、诊断、《黄帝内经》中的疾病、治疗学概念、针灸等，并附图 24 幅。附录部分近 20 页，包括《四库全书总目提要》对《素问》的介绍、王冰注序、林亿等新校正序（均为英译文）及参考书目。译文中大量使用脚注，主要解释中国传统文化现象的词语、中医学独特的概念以及王冰注的译文。当时，《科学》（*Science*）、《内科学档案》（*Archives of Internal Medicine*）、《美国医学会会刊》（*Journal of the American Medical Association*，*JAMA*）、《加州医学》（*Galifornia Medicine*）等权威杂志均给予 Ilza Veith 译本很高的评价。

4.1.4 翻译及发表的形式不正规

由于这一历史时期译者的主要目的在于帮助西方学者了解《素问》而不在意其中所体现的中医学理论体系的完整性，因此，这一历史时期的翻译形式便只是片段翻译。Percy M. Dawson 的译文只有 6 页，黄雯的译文有 33 页。Ilza Veith 翻译了《素问》的 1—34 章，156 页。此外，这些译文出版的形式也不正规。除了 Ilza Veith 译本由出版社正式出版以外，Percy M. Dawson 和黄雯的译文只是登载在期刊上。

4.1.5 译本的社会功能较弱

20 世纪上半叶，《素问》英译本在英语文化多元系统中处于非常边缘的地位。如 Ilza Veith 本打算全译《素问》，但在英译了《素问》的 1—34 章之后，却确信，“1—34 章包含了《黄帝内经》几乎所有的基本观点[3]”。言外之意，读者如读了这前 34 章的译文，便基本上窥见了《黄帝内经》的“全貌”。当然，中医从业者都不会同意她的观点。另外，同一译本的社会功能也会随着社会环境的变化，如中医学在中国大陆的复苏及在西方的传播而悄悄地转变。Ilza Veith 译本修订再版本（1972 年）的封底这样写道，“自 1949 年《素问》英译本第 1 版问世后，中国的中医医疗实践呈现出生机勃勃的复兴景象，而且，它以惊人的速度传遍了西方，甚至传遍了美国。对中医学（包括针灸）这一历史悠久的治疗方法的科学研究提高了人们对其历史及哲学基础的兴趣。由于远东思想及其历史在当今的知识体系中越来越重要，《黄帝内经》也逐步超越了其医史界限”。

4.2 第二阶段：1978—1997年

这一历史时期产生了4种《素问》英译本：加拿大人Henry C. Lu的译本，Maoshing Ni的译本，吴连胜、吴奇的译本，以及周春才、韩亚洲编绘的题为《〈黄帝内经〉养生图典》的漫画版译本。

中华人民共和国成立后，党和政府特别重视中医药学的发展。1958年，毛泽东主席题词："中国医药学是一个伟大的宝库，应当努力发掘，加以提高"。1969年，周恩来总理也多次讲话，指出，"要提倡西医学中医，形成风气"。1971年7月17日，《人民日报》公布针刺麻醉获得成功，这一消息震惊了全世界。1976年上海、北京等地开始举办"外国医生针灸学习班"，并在WHO的协助下，在北京、上海、南京设立了"国际针灸培训中心"。随着美国前总统尼克松访华（1972年），中医药和针灸疗法再次叩开了美国的大门。1973年1月、3月，美国相继创刊出版了《美洲中医杂志》（*American Journal of Chinese Medicine*）和《美国针灸杂志》，极大地推动着针灸、中医事业在美国及西方世界的发展。中药、推拿、气功、食疗以及医古文、中医经典等中医药理论与技术也随之全面进入美国。这一时期，WHO组织专家对针灸学名词术语英译进行标准化，国内的欧明、谢竹藩、帅学忠等教授以及英国学者魏迺杰等均致力于中医名词术语的英译及工具书的编写，从而大大地促进了中医药及针灸学英译事业的发展以及英文书籍的出版。中医药和针灸疗法以前所未有的速度迅速传播海外。这一时期的译本具有如下特征。

4.2.1 翻译着眼于《素问》的医学（中医学）价值

这一时期出现的4种英译本都侧重于译介《素问》中所反映的中医学知识。Henry C. Lu在序中说，"本书对中国经典的翻译是依循中国历史上就已经形成的对原文的传统的解释。由于中国学者对经典有各种解释的版本或者持有不同的看法和观点，然而翻译时有两条原则必须遵循，即保持原文的连贯性以及使之与中国医学的现代理论保持一致"[6]。中医从业者都知道，所谓"中国医学的现代理论"都源于《黄帝内经》，那么从Henry C. Lu翻译时所遵循的两条原则可以看出，Henry C. Lu译介《素问》的着眼点是向西方传播《素问》中所反映的中医学知识。Maoshing Ni和吴氏父子都是在美国从事临床工作的中医师。Maoshing Ni在"翻译说明"中说，"这一译本，绝非是任何意义上的学术版本，因此，我确信汉学专家可以推出更完美的译本。而我是从一名临床医生的角度，从中医学及哲学学生的标准以及对中医感兴趣的外行人的角度来译释这一经典的"[7]。该译本封面将《素问》称为"中国保健疗法的奠基之作（The Essential Text of Chinese Health and Healing）"，版权页的图书分类栏明确将其归为"中医学"类：Ⅰ. Su Wen；Ⅱ. Medicine，Chinese—— Early Works to 1800。而《〈黄帝内经〉养生图典》编绘者的身份是"青年画家"，该书封面将《黄帝内经》称为

"中国古代延年益寿养生奇书"，版权页图书在版编目数据［"内经—养生（中医学）—……"］也明确表示该译本为中医学养生保健书籍。

这一时期英译《素问》的主要目的是将其作为中医学的经典之作来译介，着重体现它对人民健康、疾病防治等方面的医学价值，并对西方学习或从事中医临床工作的人以及对中医感兴趣的普通大众提供参考。英译《素问》，不再仅被医史学家作为医史资料关注，它在养生、疾病防治等方面的医学价值正在被以临床中医师为主体的译者日益彰显出来。英译《素问》在英美国家医学文化多元系统中的地位也正在由边缘向中心缓慢移动。

4.2.2　这一时期的译本基本上是编译者意图和出版商意愿折中的产物

Maoshing Ni 出生于中医世家，是一位在美国从事中医临床、教学的中医师、讲师。Maoshing Ni 曾接受过中、西方两种医学体系的教育，同时具有哲学博士、医学博士学位，在中医领域涉足甚广。Maoshing Ni 编译出版了多部中医学书籍。从译者的"翻译说明"（见前述）可以看出，译者为了迎合西方读者的兴趣，以对中医感兴趣的外行人及中医专业的学生为读者对象，以一种轻松的笔调，对《素问》进行了译释。实际上，我们可以将 Maoshing Ni 的译本看成《素问》英文版"白话解"或"今释"。出版商在该译本的封底是这样介绍的，"《黄帝内经》是道家最重要的经典之一，同时也是中医学的最高权威。……《黄帝内经》原文概念丰富，语言简洁，内容详细。译者将自己对原文的阐释融入译文，这不仅有助于阐明原文的意思，而且有助于创造出一个对学生以及所有对中医的基本原则好奇的人高度可读性的叙述本"[7]。吴氏父子的译本以汉英对照的形式在中国大陆出版，不仅迎合了大陆以汉英对照出版中医药著作的市场需求，而且还填补了国内《黄帝内经》英译领域的空白。该译本的重印次数也证明，该书的出版是译者与出版商意愿折中的产物，并迎合了时代发展和市场需求。

随着"美国针灸热、中医热"的兴起，西方人对中医养生保健越来越感兴趣。以此为契机，海豚出版社同时推出了《〈黄帝内经〉养生图典》一书的汉英对照本、德译本和法译本。该书选择有关养生的部分章节内容，配以生动形象的漫画，冠之以"中国古代延寿养生奇书"，满足了西方读者对《黄帝内经》中的中医养生保健方法的渴求。该书各种语译本均已重印，颇受欢迎。

4.2.3　中医名词术语的英译符合国内外中医英译的发展趋势，翻译策略以异化为主

这一时期，国内外出版了不少汉英英汉中医词典。在国内，以欧明、谢竹藩编写的工具书选用者较多，而国外以魏迺杰编写的工具书选用者较多。

近 10 年来中医药事业在美国发展迅速。在美国不但有独立的中医诊所，而且在西医的医疗中心、戒毒所、康复中心、老人院以及健康食品店、中药店等处都设有中医或针灸诊所。这些中医医疗单位，以前大多单纯用针灸，现在约有

60%以上兼用中药[16]。这一时期的情况表明，中医学已逐步进入英美国家的医疗系统。而英译《素问》在英美国家医学文化多元系统中也逐步缓慢向中心位置移动。在 Even-Zohar 看来，当翻译文学在译入语文学的多元系统中占据中心位置时，翻译活动就在参与创造译入语文学中新的、一级模式的过程，这时，“译者的主要任务就不单是在本国的文学形式中寻找现成的模式，把原文套进来；相反地，译者即使打破本国的传统规范，也在所不惜。在这种情况下，译文在‘充分性’（adequacy，即复制原文的主要文本关系）方面接近原文的可能性最大[1]”。

这一时期的《素问》英译就属于这种情况，译者基本上都不随便套用现成的西医学术语表达中医概念，而多采用异化的方法表达独特的中医概念，且符合国内外中医英译的发展趋势。如吴译本、Maoshing Ni 译本及漫画译本均采用国外通行的“channels and collaterals”表达“经络”。Maoshing Ni 译本还偶尔采用“meridians”（WHO）来对译“经脉”。再如，吴译本及 Maoshing Ni 译本均采用音译加解释的方法分别将“天癸”译为“Tiangui（the substance necessary for the promotion of growth，development and reproductive function of human body）”“tian kui，or fertility essence”。再如，这一时期的译者在面对中西医对脾的功能的认识的巨大差别时，能坦然将“脾”译为“spleen”。正如魏迺杰所说，“在西传的过程中，中医并不能为了配合西方人的需求而有所改变。而西方意欲学习中医的人也绝对无法经由一种‘以其本身较为熟悉的知识系统将中医学重新过滤’的学习方式获得成功，他们必须真正地进入中医的世界”[17]。Maoshing Ni、吴氏父子在翻译《素问》中的中医名词术语时，在译语的“充分性”方面比前一时期更接近原文。

4.2.4　吸收了当代《素问》的研究成果

20 世纪上半叶尚未有《素问》今译本问世，Elza Veith 等译者只能按自己的理解翻译《素问》的部分章节。《素问》文辞古奥，翻译中时常出现因理解不当而致的误译。Maoshing Ni 和吴氏父子则完全不同。新中国成立后，继各地中医学院纷纷成立之后，对《素问》的校释、研究工作全面开展，成果也层出不穷。这使得 Maoshing Ni 和吴氏父子在翻译过程中有机会应用当代《素问》的研究成果。事实也正是如此。Maoshing Ni 译本书后所列的参考书目中共有 17 部新中国成立后出版的《素问》，包括校勘、注释、今译（语译）、专题研究等。吴氏父子的译本虽未列出任何参考书目，但据笔者随机抽样，将其中的中文部分与郭霭春的《〈黄帝内经素问〉校注语译》的“校”进行比对，二者如同出一辙。从出版时间来看，郭霭春的著作于 1981 年出版，而吴氏父子的译本于 1997 年出版，显然，吴氏父子在翻译过程中大量地应用了郭霭春的研究成果。此外，吴氏父子译本“《素问》王冰注序”的英译与 Ilza Veith 的英译几乎完全相同，这说明吴氏父子也曾参阅 Ilza Veith 译本。

4.3 第三阶段：2001—2003 年

这一时期产生了 2 种《素问》英译本：朱明译本和文树德（Paul U. Unschuld）译本。朱明选择高等中医院校第 5 版教材《内经讲义》[18]为翻译底本。《内经讲义》在体例上采用了选节、选篇分类注释的方法（分阴阳五行学说、脏象学说、经络学说、病因病机学说、病证、诊法、治则治法、养生学说八类），并在“绪论”部分增加了《黄帝内经》的沿革、基本学术思想、主要内容和学习方法等内容。众所周知，《黄帝内经》包括《素问》和《灵枢》。那么，从严格意义上说，朱明译本不是《素问》译本。此外，朱明译本中某些术语的翻译也值得商榷，如将“岐伯”译为“Uncle Qi”。因此，这里主要讨论文树德译本的特点。中医、针灸的立法、教育及相关书籍的出版在西方，尤其是在美国，发展迅速。中医、针灸疗法已不再仅是“民间疗法”，在美国有了“合法身份和地位”。这一时期，文树德译本主要具有如下特征。

4.3.1 原文版本经过精心的选择

《素问》有多种不同的版本。普通读者一般不会注意到版本之间的差别，但这些差别确实给负责任的译者带来很大的麻烦。据有关文献记载，《素问》一书，在汉、魏、六朝、隋、唐各代出现了多种不同的传本。但这些传本大都亡佚，流传下来的主要是该书的注本。《素问》完整的注本，最早一种是六朝齐、梁间（6世纪）全元起注本。全氏的祖本是《素问》9 卷本（该注本在南宋以后即已失传）。此后，唐宝应元年（762 年），王冰在全氏注本的基础上，对该书进行了重新整理注解工作，并改为 24 卷本。该书流传到 11 世纪中叶嘉祐、治平年间（1057—1067 年），又由北宋政府的校正医书局，以林亿为首，在王冰注本的基础上，再次进行校勘，书名也改称为《重广补注黄帝内经素问》，共 24 卷。此后，各种《素问》刊本均以此刊本为据，该刊本同时也成为后世《素问》各种版本的祖本。此后，《素问》一书在版本方面的演变主要可分为 24 卷本、12 卷本、50 卷本、9 卷本系统以及明代以后的新注本系统。其中 24 卷本系统是根据王冰、林亿整理校注本（即嘉祐原本）直接刊刻的各种版本。如嘉靖二十九年（1550年）顾从德据宋本影刻本，即明刊本［由于该刻本刊刻精良，故此后又有据其再次影刻与影印的刊本，如日本安政三年（1856 年）占恒室影刻本、1922 年恽铁樵及 1956 年人民卫生出版社影印本等］[19]。

如果译者是《素问》研究的门外汉，那么他（她）可能完全意识不到《素问》不同版本之间的差异。最早的 Elza Veith 译本就只基于一种原文版本——京口文成堂摹刻宋本《黄帝内经》。很可能，她选择这一版本仅仅是因为它是最方便得到的一种版本而已。尽管 Maoshing Ni 译本的“参考书目”中列出了上起于隋朝（605 年）杨上善的《黄帝内经太素》至今（1990 年）的 31 部有关《素问》

的著作，但在其“翻译说明”中，却没有任何有关“版本选择”的只言片语。从吴译本封面标明的“（唐）王冰原注”以及原文又大量采用郭霭春的校勘成果来看，译者也没有对《素问》版本进行选择。与以前的译者不同，文树德极其注重《素问》各方面的价值，为此精心挑选合适的原文版本。从出版的首册来看，译者对《素问》的成书年代、版本流传、内容等均有比较深入的研究和把握。从该书书后“参考书目”中所列的首要资料（primary sources）来看，该书的英译及研究是以现藏于台北国立中医医药研究所的1550年顾从德据宋本的影刻本，即明刊本的复拍本为底本。对原文版本如此精心地选择充分说明文树德英译《素问》的态度极其严肃、认真、负责。这一常为过去的译者所忽略的步骤，却成为文树德研究、翻译准备过程中的重要环节。这种精心的准备工作也表明，新时期译者的翻译目的在于真正全面再现《素问》的价值。

4.3.2　大量吸收历代，包括当代《素问》的研究成果

文树德将20世纪中国作者发表的3000余篇论文以及过去中日两国作者的600多部专著作为次要资料加以引用。他说，“我们对原文的理解和阐释反映在英译文中，同时，我还非常谨慎地引用了尽可能多的且合理的赞同以及反对的中日两方的观点”[11]。可以说，他所主持的《素问》的翻译工作是迄今西方规模最大的中医典籍翻译工程。

4.3.3　翻译与研究紧密结合

在慕尼黑大学医史研究所，通过国际合作，文树德主持的《素问》英译课题历时10余年才得以完成。2003年出版的首册是多册课题成果中的第一册。文树德在“序”中说，“这项课题范围广泛。课题旨在产生出第一部语义正确的《素问》英文全译本以及一个有助于将来对原文研究工作的研究工具。……译文将分三册出版。此外，Hermann Tessenow还对构成《素问》的历史及结构层次的近350个不相连片段进行详细分析。这一研究结果也将分数册出版”[11]。可见，这一课题的系列成果，包括文树德英译本本身，都体现了翻译和研究的紧密结合。

4.3.4　医、史、文并重，力求全面反映《素问》的价值

译者文树德是一位医史学家。这项课题的中方主要协作者是中国中医研究院中国医史文献研究所的郑金生研究员，他也是一位医史学家。文树德教授几乎一生致力于中医学（史）的研究，仅加利福尼亚大学出版社就出版了他的两部专著［*Medicine in China*：*A History of Pharmaceutics*（1986年）和 *Medicine in China*：*A History of Ideas*（1988年）］、两部译著［《难经》（1986年），《银海精微》（与他人合译，1998年）］。在刚出版的首册的“序”中，他说，“《黄帝内经》，包括《素问》和《灵枢》，在中国医学史上所起的作用可以同希伯克拉底的著作在古欧洲的作用相比。各方面的进步、发展和显著变化使希伯克拉底沦落成为一个已经过时的传统的荣誉创始人。与之相反，在当代临床背景下，很多中医师仍然把

《素问》看成一个理论灵感和实践知识的有价值的源泉。……读《素问》不仅可以提高我们对作为中国文明不可或缺的一部分的中医学的起源的理解、认识，而且还为有关对现存威胁如疾病、夭亡危险的欧洲和中国处理方法的不同及相似之处的严肃而又广博的讨论提供了一个非常必要的起点。此类讨论对评判中国知识传统中的疾病和健康的文化概念是必要的。不管是出于竞争还是互相补充的考虑，在为人类健康的无休止探索中，当今使中、西医学共存的政治企图，使这类讨论看来是必需的。……我准备了一个初步的译本，把它作为与 Hermann Tessenow 广泛合作的起点。他的语文学知识为取得的成果——即将出版的三册译文，做出了决定性的贡献”[11]。

4.3.5　为促进医学文化交流采取补偿措施

为了使英语读者真正理解和欣赏《素问》，文树德采取了许多措施。从目前出版的首册来看，比较突出的是撰写单独的一册《黄帝内经素问——中国古代医学典籍中的自然、知识和意象》，即首册，全面介绍《素问》；在即将出版的译文中，除《素问》译文外，选译了历代 600 余种《素问》相关著作中有见解、合理的注解和阐释；Hermann Tessenow 对构成《素问》的历史及结构层次的近 350 个不相连片段进行了详细分析（数册）。

出版的首册长达 520 页，内容、体例酷似中国出版的高等中医院校使用的教材，其中夹杂有大量的《素问》引文，详尽地介绍了《素问》的源流、书名含义、历代相关著作、内容的全面评述（包括阴阳学说、五行学说、人体和脏腑、气血、经络、病因、疾病、诊法、各种疗法）、跋、注释、长达 110 页的附录——“《素问》中的五运六气学说”的介绍、参考书目和索引。在该册的“序”中，译者还对曾给予经济、组织及学术帮助的单位和个人表示诚挚的感谢。这说明《素问》的翻译不仅体现了译者的才能与辛劳，而且凝聚了许多人的智慧与努力。

4.3.6　中医名词术语的英译自成体系，别具一格

这一时期，中医名词术语的英译向标准化进程迈出了重要一步。在国内，谢竹藩教授受命于国家中医药管理局，进行“中医药名词术语英译标准化”的研究，并在该项研究的基础上编著出版了《新编汉英中医药分类词典》（2002 年）。在国外，魏迺杰与他人合作出版了《实用中医辞典》（英文版）（*A Practical Dictionary of Chinese Medicine*，第 2 版，1998 年由美国 Paradigm Publications 出版，2002 年由人民卫生出版社原版引进）。魏迺杰所提出的词汇“不但为许多翻译者所采用，更被美国三大中医文献出版社中的两家（Paradigm 出版社和 Blue Poppy 出版社）指定为其出版品之英文词汇标准”[20]。

然而，文树德教授并未采用国内外任何一套英译词汇表达中医概念。文树德教授可以说是魏迺杰的学术前辈，在他为魏迺杰的《英汉汉英中医词典》所作之

序中说，“中、西方学者无法就中医学充分交流的一个主要障碍就是意欲将中医学的概念和术语名词传达与西方读者的中、西作者，他们所译定的中医英文词汇都是令人遗憾的不充分、不恰当，过于频繁地滥用现代西医学专业术语来意译中医书籍，已经混淆了中医学思想的独立性。同样，尝试由希腊文、拉丁文去创造新字以建立一个做作的术语词汇系统也蒙蔽了传统中医词汇与中文日常用语极为相近的特性。……深望此本辞典不但能在中国早日被广为接受，更能成为西方国家用以翻译中医学有关用书的指导原则”[17]。显然，译者没有选用现成的中医术语词汇系统表达中医概念的主要原因是译者想使译文在“充分性”方面更接近原文。

早在1986年，文树德就出版了英译《难经》。他曾经提出“比喻”存亡的理性原则，即既然中医至今仍然以《黄帝内经》所建立的概念系统为圭臬，因此，在《黄帝内经》时代便存在的比喻就应该予以译出[17]。当时，他就将“经脉”译为“conduits”，“脏腑”译为“depotsand palaces”，等等。再比如，在刚出版的首册中，除了继续采用以前的译语外，他还将“五行学说”译为“the five-agents doctrine”（目前，the five-elements theory 和 the five-phases theory 分别是国内外最为流行的译语），“经络学说”译为“vessel theory”，“经脉”译为“conduit vessel”等。译者不惜打破常规，术语翻译自成体系，显然是和中医学在英美国家（尤其是美国）医学文化多元系统中的地位提升密切相关。在这一社会背景下，译者不惜一再打破本国的传统规范，力求译文在“充分性”方面尽可能接近原文。

4.3.7　译本具有较强的社会功能

文树德译本力求全方面反映《素问》的价值。他说，课题旨在产生出第一部语义正确的《素问》英文全译本以及一个有助于将来对原文研究工作的研究工具，“这部著作不能也没有声称有关《素问》的一切已尽在其中。相反地，我们应该只把它看成一个起点，一个能引起更多学者对原文的学术关注的起点，而不是只愿意注意到《素问》以及相关的古代中国著作”[11]。我们可以把文树德译本看成是第一部“真正学术意义上”的全译本。

由此，我们可以得出以下结论：第一，文树德译本将成为西方对《素问》进行广泛研究的基点并提供参考；第二，正如芝加哥大学 Donald Harper 的评价“… the essential reference for ancient Chinese medicine and a valuable tool to research on early Chinese civilization.”（……是中国古代医学的重要参考资料和对中国早期文明研究具有价值的工具。）《素问》将不仅被视为“中医学经典”，而且将成为研究中国医学的起源以及中国早期文明的重要而又有价值的参考。

5.《素问》英译事业的发展脉络

对不同历史时期《素问》英译本的全面描述已将《素问》英译事业的发展脉

络清晰地展现在我们面前。这一历程跨越近 80 年，包括 9 种不同译本，其发展脉络可以概括为表 2 所示的 6 个方面。

表 2 《素问》英译事业的发展脉络

	第一阶段	第二阶段	第三阶段
翻译目的	主要是帮助西方人了解《素问》的概貌	主要译介传达《素问》中的中医学知识	全面再现《素问》的价值
翻译方法	片段翻译	全译，编译，选译	真正学术意义上的全译
翻译形式	多采用西医学术语（归化）表达中医概念	迎合时代发展，多采用“异化”方法表达中医概念	对原著风格、内容各方面的忠实再现，独具一格
译者身份	主要为对《素问》及中医学知之甚少的西方医学史学家	主要为在美国从事临床工作的中医师	主要为医史学家，重要合作者中有语文学家
对原文版本的选择	任意选择	任意选择	精心选择明顾从德刻本（1550 年）为翻译底本
译本在英美医学文化系统中的地位	基本不具备中医学价值，仅提供医史材料	边缘地位：作为“中医学最高权威”，以其中的中医学知识吸引读者	从边缘地位向中心地位迈进了一大步：被视为古代中医学及早期中国文明研究的有价值的重要参考书

6. 结论

本文首先介绍了多元系统理论及相应的描写性翻译批评方法，然后运用这一全新的方法对跨越近 80 年、产生 9 种译本的《素问》英译事业进行了描写性研究，包括不同时期译本的全面历时性描述以及对翻译历程脉络的勾勒。此项研究有力地证明了以下两点。

第一，用多元系统论的描写性翻译批评方法能够有效地解释一些由历史语境影响和决定的翻译现象，尤其适用于多年以前产生的翻译作品或是同一原作在不同历史条件下产生的不同译本进行研究。这一翻译批评的新方法可以弥补规定性翻译批评方法的局限性。

第二，《素问》英译事业的描写性研究表明：①中医学在国内及英美国家的兴衰消长对特定历史时期中医英译的规范产生重大影响，由此导致译者翻译意图、方法与倾向的不断变化；②作为译作，《素问》英译本在英语医学文化多元系统中的地位和功能随着社会、历史条件的变化而变化，《素问》的译介和研究正逐步走向高潮；③中医翻译批评研究，特别是中医经典的翻译批评研究，应涵盖规定性翻译批评方法与描写性翻译批评方法，以发展为完整的中医经典翻译批评系统，推动中医英译事业的发展。

参考文献

[1] 谢天振. 翻译研究新视野. 青岛：青岛出版社，2003：233－249.

[2] 王吉民，傅维康. 中国医史外文文献索引（1682—1965）. 上海：上海中医学院医史博物馆，1966：165.

[3] Veith I. The Yellow Emperor's classic of internal medicine. Berkeley，Los Angeles and London：University of California Press，1972：XIV－XV，110，127，100，115－125.

[4] Huang W. Nei Ching，the Chinese canon of medicine. Chin Med J，1950：68：1，2.

[5] 王吉民. 西译中医典籍重考. 中华医学杂志，1936，22（12）：1229－1234.

[6]《中国翻译》编辑部. 中译英技巧文集. 北京：中国对外翻译出版公司，1992：215.

[7] Ni，M. The Yellow Emperor' s classic of medicine. Boston，Massachusetts：Shambhala，1995：XIV.

[8] 周春才，韩亚洲.《黄帝内经》——养生图典. 北京：海豚出版社，1997.

[9] Wu NL，Wu AQ. Yellow Emperor's canon internal medicine. Beijing：China Science and Technology Press，1997.

[10] Zhu M. The medical classic of the Yellow Emperor. Beijing：Foreign Languages Press，2001.

[11] Unschuld PU. HUANG DI NEI JING SU WEN：nature，knowledge，imagery in an ancient Chinese medical text. Berkeley，LosAngeles and London：University of California Press，2003：IX.

[12] 马伯英，高晞，洪中立. 中外医学文化交流史——中外医学跨文化传通. 上海：文汇出版社，1993：602，605，611.

[13] 利玛窦撰. 利玛窦中国札记. 何高济，王遵仲，等译. 北京：中华书局，1983：34.

[14] 王吉民，傅维康. 中国医学外文著述书目（1656—1962）. 上海：上海中医学院医史博物馆，1963：19，65.

[15] 萧惠英. 王吉民、伍连德与《中国医史》. 中华医史杂志，2003，33（2）：92.

[16] 吴伯平. 美国中医药纵横谈. 国外医学·中医中药分册. 2003，25（1）：9－12，17.

[17] Nigel W. English-Chinese Chinese-English dictionary of Chinese medicine. 长沙：湖南科学技术出版社，1996：35，3，25.

[18] 程士德. 内经讲义. 上海：上海科学技术出版社，1984.

[19] 吉文辉，王大妹. 中医古籍版本学. 上海：上海科学技术出版社，2000：165－167.

[原文分为两篇，分别原载自《中国中西医结合杂志》，2004，24（10）：947－950；和《中国中西医结合杂志》，2005，25（2）：176－180.]

论《黄帝内经·素问》篇名的英译

——兼评两个英译本的英译篇名

兰凤利

《黄帝内经素问》（以下简称《素问》）是中医基本理论的渊薮，也是我国优秀文化遗产的重要组成部分。从现存《素问》的内容来看，这部著作决非出自一时一人之笔，而是在一个相当长的时期内各医家经验的总结汇编[1]，也就是一本论文集，而每篇论文的题目便是中医从业者所耳熟能详的篇名了。从某种意义上说，文题是作者给读者发出的“请柬”。就译者而言，如何替2000多年前的原作者发出这份“请柬”，邀请英语读者来欣赏这部传世之作呢？本文拟对国外出版的《素问》的两个主要英译本[2]的英译篇名进行评析，以探讨这一中医经典之作篇名的英译原则、标准及方法。

1. 两个英译本的英译篇名评析

1.1 Ilza Veith之英译篇名评析

Ilza Veith女士是一位医史学家，也是第一位将《素问》译成英文并公开出版的学者。Ilza Veith以西方的医史学家为读者对象，翻译了《素问》的第1—34章。《内科学档案》（*Archives of Internal Medicine*）称，“作者Ilza Veith创作了一部迷人的，但又具有学术性的著作”[2]。归结起来，她的英译篇名有如下特点。

1.1.1 直译为主，注重形合

直译法是指在不违背英语文化传统的前提下，在英译文中完全保留汉语词语的指称意义，求得内容与形式相符的方法。一般而言，直译所产生的译文均具有较好的回译性。我们可通过回译检验译文的准确性[3]，保持原文固有的特色。如：

1.1.1.1 生气通天论 题解：本篇论述人的生命活动与自然界息息相通的道理，故名篇。英译：Treatise on the Communication of the Force of Life with Heaven[2]。［注：除非标明参考文献，题解均参录：山东中医学院、河北医学院．黄帝内经素问校释（上、下册）．北京：人民卫生出版社，1991］

1.1.1.2 五脏生成篇 题解：本篇论述五脏与外环境及体内各组织的联系，体现了“人以天地之气生，四时之法成”的道理，故名篇。英译：Treatise on the Five Viscera in Relation to Their Part in Perfecting Life[2]。

1.1.1.3 三部九候论 题解：本篇主要论述三部九候的诊脉方法，并通过诊察三部九候脉象的变化，以判断疾病变化和预决死生，故名篇。英译：Treatise on the Three Regions and the Nine Subdivisions[2]。

以上篇名的英译不仅顾及形合，还兼顾意合，不失为佳译。但仅顾形合而误译篇名者，则为数更多。

1.1.1.4　异法方宜论　题解：本篇指出由于地域不同，所患疾病不同，因此治病方法亦不同，而是各有其所宜，故名篇。英译：The Different Methods of Treatment and the Appropriate Prescription[2]。改译：Suiting Methods of Treatment to Local Conditions。

1.1.1.5　诊要经终论　题解：本篇以论述诊病要道及十二经脉之终为重点，故名篇。英译：Treatise on the Important Examination of the Invariable Rules of Death[2]。改译：Essentials of Diagnostics and Collapse of Channels。

1.1.1.6　逆调论　题解：本篇主要论述由于阴阳、营卫等功能失调而引起的疾病，故名篇。英译：Treatise on Rebellion and Harmony[2]。改译：Disharmonies。

1.1.2　增译为辅，力求形意皆合

Ilza Veith 为了使译文与原文在内容、形式和精神等方面对等起来，翻译时，在原文的基础上添加了必要的单词或词组。如有下划线者为增译：

1.1.2.1　四气调神大论　题解：本篇主要论述人体应顺从四时气候的变化来调摄精神活动，使之适应自然界生长收藏的规律，从而达到养生防病的目的，故名篇。英译：Great Treatise on the Harmony of the Atmosphere of the Four Seasons with the（Human） Spirit[2]。

1.1.2.2　汤液醪醴论　题解：本篇首论古代制作汤液醪醴的意义，故名篇。英译：Treatise on the Treatment with Hot Water，Liquid Medicine，the Lees，of wine，and Sweet Wine[2]。

从 Ilza Veith 英译的篇名来看，Ilza Veith 一直在努力再现原文的形式与风格。Ilza Veith 的译文也确实得到了《科学》（*Science*）、《美国医学会会刊》（*The Journal of the American Medical Association*，*JAMA*）、《加州医学》（*California Medicine*）等权威杂志的高度评价。然而，仅就篇名的英译来看，限于译者的中文功底，仍存在不少因理解不当而造成的误译，如将“阴阳别论”“五脏别论”“经脉别论”的“别”译释为“separately”或“distinguish”，“灵兰秘典论”的“灵兰”译为“Ingenious and Subtlety”，“玉机真藏论”的“玉机”译为“Precious Mechanisms”，等。

1.2　Maoshing Ni 之英译篇名评析

Maoshing Ni 是一位美籍华裔中医师，他以中医学专业的学生以及对中医感兴趣的外行人为读者对象，将《素问》全部译成英文，并为此加入了大量的评论和解释。也正如译者所说，此译本是“A new translation of the Neijing Suwen with commentary”，可看成是《素问》的英文版“白话解”。他所译的篇名相当简练，归纳起来，有如下特点。

1.2.1 大量意译，注重意合

意译法是指译者在受到译语社会文化差异的局限时，不得不舍弃原文的字面意义，以求译文与原文的内容相符以及主要语言功能相似的方法[3]。如：

1.2.1.1 宝命全形论 题解：本篇指出人以天地之气生，四时之法成，欲保全形体，须宝惜天命，故名篇。英译：The Preservation of Health。

1.2.1.2 五常政大论 题解：本篇重点论述五运六气主时所引起的气象、物候变化及发病情况。因首先论及五运正常的政令，故名篇。英译：Rules of Phase Energetics。

说明："five phases"是国外很流行的"五行"的对应译语。

1.2.1.3 灵兰秘典论 题解：灵台兰室相传为黄帝藏书之所，是以本篇所述至关重要，作者意欲强调其为值得秘藏的典籍，故名篇。英译：The Sacred Teachings。

1.2.1.4 汤液醪醴论 题解：见1.2.2。英译：The Art of Medicine。

1.2.2 兼用直译，保持原文特色

1.2.2.1 金匾真言论 题解：作者以本篇所论至关重要，而喻之为可藏于金匾流传万世的真言，故名篇。英译：The Truth from the Golden Chamber。

1.2.2.2 刺齐论 题解：本篇论述以皮、脉、肉、筋、骨的不同分部作为针刺深浅不一的分剂，故名篇。"齐"与"剂"同，英译：Needling Depth in Acupuncture。

1.2.3 音译意译结合，译释某些论病篇名

音译意译结合法是指在英译中既保留原文的发音，又能体现原文的指称意义，以谐音又谐意的方式达到功能相似。Maoshing Ni 采用的是在拼音后加上一个表意的词，如：

1.2.3.1 痹论 英译：The Bi Syndrome。

1.2.3.2 痿论 英译：Wei Conditions。

1.2.4 省词翻译，力求简练

省词译法就是把原文中需要而译文中不需要的单词、词组等在翻译过程中加以省略[5]。如：

1.2.4.1 平人气象论 题解：本篇着重讨论平人的脉气与脉象，并以平人的脉象与病人的脉象相互对比，分析病情，故名篇。英译：Pulse Analysis。

1.2.4.2 离合真邪论 题解：本篇重点论述真气与邪气的离合同疾病的关系，故名篇。英译：Pathogens。

1.2.5 增词翻译，力求意明

对增译部分以下划线进行标注。

1.2.5.1 阴阳应象大论 题解：本篇将阴阳学说的理论体现于自然界具体事物及其发展变化的现象之中，并加以阐述，故名篇。英译：The Manifestation of Yin and Yang from the Macrocosm to the Microcosm。

1.2.5.2　咳论　题解：本篇重点讨论了咳嗽的病因、病机、症状和治疗原则，故名篇。英译：Etiology，Diagnosis，and Treatment of Cough。

1.2.6　依内容重新译写篇名

1.2.6.1　玉机真藏论　题解：本篇因论述真藏之气在诊断方面的价值好似用天文仪器玉机窥测天象那样重要，故名篇。英译：Seasonal Variations and Abnormalities in Pulses。

说明：本篇主要说明四时太过与不及的病脉，以及真脏脉的病象，并阐述了疾病传变规律，最后讨论了五虚和五实的病状和预后[6]。

1.2.6.2　三部九侯论　题解：见 1.1.3。英译：Determining Life and Death。

说明：本篇讨论了三部九侯的诊脉及各种脉象的病证、刺法和死期[6]。

1.2.7　使用副标题

此外，译者还会偶尔添加副标题。如厥论，英译：Jue Conditions：the Separation of Yin and Yang。

可见，Maoshing Ni 的英译篇名既简练又切题，且选词通俗易懂，是一本难得的"普及版"优秀译著。

2.《素问》篇名英译的原则、标准及方法

2.1　理解是翻译的基础

著名学者 George Steiner 在他 1975 年出版的翻译理论方面的鸿篇巨作《通天塔——语言与翻译面面观》（*After Babel——Aspects of Language and Translation*）的第 1 章就专论"Understandings Translation"，即"理解就是翻译"，也就是说，翻译取决于理解的程度[7]。Ilza Veith 的误译主要是望文生义，即对原文理解不当造成的。即使是作为中医师的 Maoshing Ni 也因理解不当而误译了一些篇名。如"厥论"，译者添加副标题将其译成"Jue Conditios：the Separation of Yin and Yang"，这本身是个好办法，但是此副标题却使《素问》所论及的本不互相矛盾的医理前后矛盾（按：《生气通天论》曰："阴阳离决，精气乃绝"；又《调经论》曰："血之与气并走于上，则为大厥，厥则暴死，气复反则生，不反则死"）。又如"缪刺论"专论"缪刺"，《素问识》云："左病刺右，右病刺左，交错其处，故曰缪刺"。那么，译者何以将副标题译成"Acupuncturing the Superficial Luo"？

笔者认为，要理解和翻译《素问》这样的中医古籍，就必须同时掌握中医学知识，具备扎实的古汉语（医古文）基础，并精通外语，具备一定的语言学和翻译学素养，了解西医的理论与实践，还要熟悉中国古典哲学。

2.2 信守原文的内容意旨，灵活运用各种翻译方法和技巧，吸引心目中预定的读者

王佐良教授说："吸引心目中预定的读者——这是任何译者所不能忽视的大事"[8]。英国维多利亚时代的优秀学者 Matthew Amold（1822—1888 年）就曾提出"翻译为谁"的问题——译文是仅仅忠实于原作，还是应更多地把译文读者放在心里[7]？Ilza Veith、Maoshing Ni 分别以西方的医史学家、中医学专业的学生及对中医感兴趣的外行人为读者对象，因此，他们的英译篇名也就各有千秋。

在把握原文的内容意旨之后，如何依不同的读者对象来翻译《素问》这样一部独具中国医学文化特色的经典篇名呢？刘士聪教授在谈到翻译文学作品里所包含的中国特有的文化因素时，提到应运用注释、或增或舍。在译文中作出解释、努力再现原文的形式与风格等方法来加以处理。这些方法均可借鉴。以下就不同的读者对象，就《素问》篇名的英译分别加以说明。

2.2.1 以中医学教学、科研、临床工作人员为读者对象

针对这群读者，译者应努力再现原文的内容、形式与风格，所译的译本应是一个学术性的、严肃的译本。David Hawks 在他的《红楼梦》英译本"序言"里谈到这个问题时说："我自始至终遵守一个不变的原则：就是把所有的一切——甚至双关语——都译出来……我敢假定小说中的一枝一叶都有其作用，必须用各种方式加以交代。我不能自命在这方面完全成功，可是如果我可以将这部中国小说所给予我的满足之感传达读者以万一，那我就不虚此生了。"[9] 实际上他讲了两个原则，即"把所有的一切都译出来"以及"用各种方式加以交代"，以传达"满足之感"。为此，笔者建议：

2.2.1.1 直译为主，强调回译性　鉴于《素问》是一部经典之作，国内中医从业者都熟谙各篇篇名，因此，强调回译性有利于国内外同行进行学术交流。当然，为了明意、简练，在直译的同时，也可适当地增词或省词。

2.2.1.2 运用注释，解释篇名的命名含义或对篇名中的病名做必要的解释

在直译的同时，以注释解释篇名的命名含义，让读者知其所以"名"。涉及病名的，如"痹论"，在据该篇所限定的意义译好之后，还应对中医的"痹"以注释的形式加以解释。

2.2.1.3 适当使用副标题　如"灵兰秘典论"主要讨论了人身十二脏腑的生理功能。翻译时，在直译篇名之后，再使用副标题点明本篇的内容，可译为：Secret Records from Royal Library：Functions of Yin and Yang Organs。

2.2.2 以中医学专业低年级学生及对中医感兴趣的外行人为读者对象

针对这群读者，译者应对全书各篇的内容及篇名的命名含义有透彻的理解，尽量不用或少用注释，注重意合，抓住各篇的核心内容，突出主题，以吸引读者的注意力。必要时，可据该篇内容重新译写篇名。Maoshing Ni 的《素问》英译

篇名尽管也有一些不当之处，但瑕不掩瑜，其翻译方法仍值得学习和借鉴。

2.3 英译篇名风格一致，切合原文的语体语域

当《素问》中文篇名的风格一致时，英文篇名的风格也应相应一致。如吴氏父子[10]将“刺热”“刺疟”“刺腰痛”三篇分别译为“Acupuncture for Treating the Febrile Diseases of the Viscera”“On Treating Malaria with Acupuncture”“The Pricking Therapy for Lumbago of Various Channels”，可见，英文的用词、形式与风格均互不相同。建议分别译为“Acupuncture Treatment of Febrile Diseases”“Acupuncture Treatment of Malaria-like Illnesses”“Acupuncture Treatment of Lumbar Pain”，以使译文的形式与风格同原文一致。

不管是学术性还是普及性译本，《素问》都是国内外公认的中医经典之作，因此，其英译也应符合国内外中医英译的发展趋势，不宜另造译语。也就是说，术语应在国内外流行的两种主要术语体系中选择，并应注意同一译著中同一术语的英译应前后一致。Maoshing Ni 的英译篇名中便存在很多同一术语的英译前后不一致情况，如“经脉”，时而译为“meridian”，时而译为“channel”；“络”，时而译为“collateral”，时而又音译为“Luo”； “热病”，时而译为“febrile disease”，时而译为“Wen Bing”，等等，应力戒。

2.4 遵从译语的语言习惯，符合英文文章标题

要求译者要在忠实原意的前提下把篇名译得符合英文读者的习惯，就应参照英文标题的特点：省略冠词，且篇名中的“……论（大论）”也可不必译出，从而将篇名译得简练、切题、醒目。

参考文献

[1] 程士德．内经讲义．上海：上海科学技术出版社，1984：2.

[2] Veith I. The Yellow Emperor's Classic of Internal Medicine. Berkeley and Los Angeles：University of California Press，1972：Back Cover，102，105，140，147，151，155，186，251.

[3] Ni MSH. The Yellow Emperor's Classic of Medicine，Massachusetts：Shambhala，1995：Ⅶ-Ⅸ.

[4] 陈宏薇．汉英翻译基础．上海：上海外语教育出版社，2002：88，94，101.

[5] 冯庆华．实用翻译教程．上海：上海外语教育出版社，2002：469，61.

[6] 郭霭春．《黄帝内经素问》校注语译．天津：天津科学技术出版社，1999：115，128.

[7] 申雨平．西方翻译理论精选．北京：外语教学与研究出版社，2002：364，168.

[8] 王佐良．思考与试笔．北京：外语教学与研究出版社，1989：42.

[9] 中国翻译编辑部．中译英技巧文集．北京：中国对外翻译出版公司，1992：102-114.

[10] 吴连胜，吴奇．黄帝内经（汉英对照）．北京：中国科学技术出版社，1997：Ⅰ-7.

［原载《中国中西医结合杂志》，2004，24（3）：265-268.］

《黄帝内经·素问》书名英译探讨

兰凤利

《黄帝内经》分为《素问》与《灵枢》，为我国现存最早的较为系统和完整的医学典籍。《黄帝内经》集中反映了我国古代的医学成就，创立了中医学的理论体系，奠定了中医学发展的基础，2000 多年来一直指导着中医学的发展。直到今天，《黄帝内经》仍列“四大经典”之首，为学习中医者的必读之书，也是世界各国研究我国古代文明史、医学史的重要著作。因其中保存了中医学丰富的理论知识和实践经验，已引起世界许多国家的重视，其部分或全部内容已相继被译成日、英、德、法文出版。据 1992 年 8 月 2 日法新社消息，法国尼斯市的一名医生塞内尔·德波尔特已将《素问》译成法文，并将书名定为《病状与根源》。因《素问》为中医学的奠基之作，从而使中医对西方人来说不再具有神秘色彩。日本京都大学人文科学研究所早就翻译出版了《皇帝内经·素问》的日译本[1]［注：该书“黄帝”误作“皇帝”。笔者推测，这可能是据 Yellow Emperor 回译的结果。另见该书第 680 页：中国科学研究院讲师罗希文曾翻译了带注释的《伤寒杂病论》《金匾安略》（“安”应作“要”）、《黄帝内经》第一卷的英译本，向国内外发行，颇受欢迎］。

1．《黄帝内经》的英译

长期以来，这一经典的英译名称极不统一。目前，书名为《黄帝内经》的主要有以下几种译文（括号内为译者）：

The Yellow Emperor's Classic of Internal Medicine（Ilza Veith）[2]

Inner Classic of the Yellow Emperor（Ted J. Keptchuk）[3]

The Yellow Emperor's Inner Canon（Nigel Wiseman）[4]

The Yellow Emperor's Classic of Internal Medicine（Giovanni Maciocia）[5]

The Yellow Emperor's Classic of Medicine（Maoshing Ni）[6]

Emperor's Canon of Medicine（欧明）[7]

Yellow Emperor's Canon Internal Medicine（吴连胜、吴奇）[8]

The Medical Classic of the Yellow Emperor（Zhu Ming）[9]

我们知道，“黄帝”并非一个“黄色的皇帝”（Yellow Emperor），而“内经”也并非是“内科学”（Internal Medicine）的经典。

关于“黄帝”，战国秦汉时期许多旧史学家都把他说成是古代的一个帝王。例如《辞海》说“黄帝”为：“传说中中原各族的共同祖先。姬姓，号轩辕氏、有熊氏。少典之子。”实际上，黄帝并非一个人名，它原是我国原始社会末期的一个氏族。这个氏族原先居住在我国西北方，据《中国通史简编》记载：“据传说，黄帝曾居住在涿鹿（河北宣化鸡鸣山）地方的山湾里，过着往来不定、迁徙无常的游牧生活。后来打败了九黎族和炎帝族，逐渐在中部地区定居下来。”到了春秋时期，这个氏族又被称为“华族”，这就是中华民族的始祖，也就是汉以后所谓“汉族”的祖先。正因为黄帝氏族是华族的始祖，所以历代人们都以自己是黄帝子孙为荣，而且为了追本溯源，也常把一切文物制度推源到黄帝，托名为黄帝的创造。正如《淮南子》所说：“世俗之人，多尊古而贱今，故为道者，必托之于神农，黄帝而后能入说”[10]。

从上述译文可以看出，Yellow Emperor 几乎成了“黄帝”约定俗成的译语。关于“黄帝”的英译，《中国翻译》也曾不止一次探讨过。在 1989 年第一期汉译英练习中就有这样一句话：作为炎黄子孙还可以去拜谒离西安不远的黄帝陵。译文是：If you are of Chinese descent，you may tribute to the tomb of Huangdi (Yellow Emperor)，first Chinese emperor。后来，张震久先生提出异议，认为从社会发展史的观点看，“黄帝”译为 Yellow Emperor 或 first Chinese emperor 似不妥，因为“皇帝”（emperor）为君主制国家的国家元首名称之一，而中国的“皇帝”是自秦王嬴政始。他将“炎黄子孙”译为：the descendants of Yan Di and Huang Di（All the Chinese people are supposed to be descendents of Huang Di and Yan Di，two chiefs of famous ancient tribes in the Huanghe River valley）[11]。笔者基本同意张震久先生的观点，但对括号内的注释持保留态度。鉴于以上对“黄帝”的阐释以及对“炎黄子孙”的公认理解，建议将“黄帝”音译为 Huang Di (the earliest ancestor of Chinese)。

在古典医学著作中，以“经”为书名的除《黄帝内经》外，尚有《难经》《本草经》《针灸甲乙经》《中藏经》等。对“经”字的含义，陆德明的解释为“常也，法也，径也”。指出“经”就是常道、规范的意思。医书名“经”，也无非是说明本书是医学的规范，也就是医者们必须学习和遵循的意思。译者一般采用 classic 或 canon 来对译“经”。《朗文当代高级英语辞典》[12]将 classic 释义为：a book，play，or other work of art that is regarded as being a very fine example of its type and having lasting importance，即经典作品，杰作，名著。将 canon 释义为：an established law of the Christian church，即（基督教）教规；a generally accepted standard of behavior or thought，即（伦理或思想行为上的）规范，准则，标准；an official list of writings that are recognized as being truly the work of a certain writer or as being part of a larger collection of writings。而《黄帝内经》是一部医学经典，“黄帝”又系伪托之辞，因此，笔者认为以 classic 对译“经”为妥。

“内”是与“外”相对而言的。例如《汉书·艺文志》所载书目，医经七家中就有《黄帝内经》《黄帝外经》《扁鹊内经》《扁鹊外经》《白氏内经》《白氏外经》等，说明书名分内外，并无深意。正如《医籍考》所说：“犹《易》内外卦及《春秋》内外传，《庄子》内外篇，《韩非子》内外储说，以次第名焉者，不必有深意。”但也有人认为医经分内外，是理论与临床，或理论的纯、驳而分的。例如《四库提要辨证》就认为纯者为内经，驳者为外经。近代《中医学概论》则谓《黄帝内经》是讲述医学基本知识的，《黄帝外经》是讲述医疗技术的。由于《黄帝外经》久已亡佚，因而据其内容的说法，也就无从查考，因此，“内”不宜译释为“internal medicine”（内科学）。

鉴于此，在保持回译性的前提下，笔者建议将《黄帝内经》译为 Huang-Di's Inner Classic。

2.《素问》的英译

《素问》是《黄帝内经》的重要组成部分，详尽地论述了有关人体生理、病理、诊断、治疗等医学领域中的各方面内容，突出了阴阳五行的哲学思想，强调了人与自然密切相关和人体内部高度统一的整体观念。《素问》不但是中医基本理论的渊薮，也是我国优秀的文化遗产的重要组成部分。目前，书名《素问》主要有以下几种译文（括号内为译者）：

Questions and Answers（Ilza Veith）[2]

Simple Questions（Leon Wieger，Ted J. Kaptchuk，Giovanni Maciocia）[2,3,5]

Interpretation of Problems（Homer H. Dubs）[2]

Elementary Questions（Nigel Wiseman）[4]

Questions of Organic and Fundamental Nature（Maoshing Ni）[6]

Familiar Conversation（欧明）[7]

Plain Questions（欧明，吴连胜，吴奇）[7,8]

从以上译文可以看出，“问”多译作 questions、conversation 或 problems；而“素”则多译作 simple、elementary、familiar 或 plain。严格意义上说，Questions of Organic and Fundamental Nature 不是翻译，而是译者个人对书名的解释。那么，“素问”到底为何义？国内学者对《素问》的名义，历来有不同的看法。段逸山教授将其归纳为以下 8 种：

（1）黄帝向岐伯询问性情之源、五行之本。素者，本也。问者，黄帝问岐伯也。方陈性情之源、五行之本，故曰《素问》。（《素问》通行本卷第一新校正引全元起语）

（2）黄帝询问太素。“按《乾凿度》（即《周易·乾凿度》）云：‘夫有形者生于无形，故有太易、有太初、有太始、有太素。太易者，未见气也；太初者，气之始也；太始者，形之始也；太素者，质之始也。’气形质具，而疴瘵由是萌生，故黄帝问此，太素质之始也。《素问》之名义或由此。”（《素问》通行本卷第一北宋林亿等新校正）

（3）黄帝问素女。天降素女，以治人疾，黄帝问之，而作《素问》。（北宋张君房《云岌七签·真仙通鉴》）

（4）用白绢书写黄帝之问。昔人谓《素问》以素书黄帝之问，犹言素书也。（南宋赵希牟《郡斋读书后志》）

（5）平素问答之书。平日讲求，谓之《素问》（明代吴良《素问注》）。

《素问》者，黄帝与岐伯、鬼臾区、伯高、少师、少俞、雷公六臣平素问答之书（明代马莳《内经素问注证发微》）。明代张介宾《类经》、王九达《黄帝内经素问灵枢合类》等均持此观点。

（6）黄帝向岐伯询问《黄帝太素》。《素问》之名，人难卒晓。予按《汉志》阴阳家有《黄帝太素》，此必取其“素”字，又以与岐伯问，故曰《素问》也。（清代姚际恒《古今伪书考》）

（7）黄帝向岐伯询问治病之法。素者，法也……黄帝问治病之法于岐伯，故其书曰《素问》。素问者，法问也，犹后世扬雄著书谓之《法问》矣。（清代胡澎《黄帝内经素问校义》）

（8）质问。考《管子》云：“素也者，五色之质也。”而《礼记》“仲尼燕居”注、《吕览》“上德”注、《韩诗章句》（《文选·舞赋》注引）等，直训为“素，质也”，而“质”字假为质问之质。故《广雅》云：“质，问也。”《礼·曲礼》“质君之前”注：“质犹对也。”然则素问乃质问之谓，犹言黄岐对问之书也（按皇甫谧称此经“论病精辨”，又《八十一难经》，“难”字亦为问难之义，是古人以问答为书名之一证也）。（日本喜多村直宽《素问札记》）

对以上说法，段逸山教授从语文及合理性的角度进行评判分析，认为《素问》的名义是“平素问答”，这“不仅符合古人确定书名崇尚质朴的风格，更与《素问》内容与体裁的实际相吻合”[13]。笔者颇以为是。据此，我们应将《素问》译为 General Questions and Answers。而段逸山教授的这一研究成果竟与 Ilza Veith 女士的理解惊人地相似［注：据现有资料，Ilza Veith 女士是研究《素问》并将之译成英文并公开出版的第一位西方学者，这也是她在美国约翰·霍普金斯大学医学史研究所（Institute of the History of Medicine of the John Hopkins University）攻读博士的学位论文］，因此，笔者建议将《素问》译为 General Questions and Answers from Huang Di's Inner Classic。

参考文献

［1］马祖毅，任荣珍汉籍外译史．武汉：湖北教育出版社，1997：675.

［2］Veith I. The Yellow Emperor's classic of internal medicine. Berkeley and Los Angeles：University of California Press，1972：8.
［3］Kaptchuk TJ. Chinese medicine：the web that has no weaver. London：Rider，2000：465.
［4］Wiseman N，Ellis A. Fundamentals of Chinese Medicine. Massachusetts：Paradigm Publications，1996：499.
［5］Maciocia G. The foundations of Chinese medicine. New York：Churchill Livingstone，1989：487.
［6］Ni MSH. The Yellow Emperors classic of medicine. Massachusetts：Shambhala，1995：12.
［7］欧明．汉英中医辞典．广州：广东科技出版社；香港：三联书店香港分店，1986：654.
［8］Nelson LW，Andrew QW. Yellow Emperor' s canon internal medicine. 北京：中国科学技术出版社，2002.
［9］Zhu M. The medical classic of the Yellow Emperor. 北京：外文出版社，2001.
［10］程士德．内经讲义．上海：上海科学技术出版社，1984：2.
［11］《中国翻译》编辑部．中译英技巧文集．北京：中国对外翻译出版公司，1992：277－278
［12］艾迪生·维斯理·朗文出版公司辞典部．朗文当代高级英语辞典．北京：商务印书馆，1998：199，258.
［13］段逸山．《素问》全元起双研究与辑复．上海：上海科学技术出版社，2001：1－5.

［原载《中国中西医结合杂志》，2004，24（2）：175－177.］

关于《黄帝内经》书名英译的商榷

刘 伟

《汉英中医辞典》（广东科技出版社和三联书店香港分店，1986年联合出版）、《汉英医学大辞典》（人民卫生出版社，1987年）是近10年来中医药汉译英翻译工作者的案头必备工具书，在促进中医药学走向世界、中医学界与世界医学界进行学术交流方面起到了不可或缺的作用。但是，犹如一块美玉也有瑕疵一样，这两本词典中也不可避免地存有不足之处。本文试就有关《黄帝内经》书名的英译问题，提出与这两本词典的英译书名的不同翻译意见，并就此书名的翻译问题与从事中医药汉译英翻译工作的同行们进行商榷。

1. 在《汉英中医辞典》中，《黄帝内经》的书名被英译为“Emperor's Canon of Medicine”。笔者认为，此一英译的《黄帝内经》的书名似有不妥。

在英语语言中，“emperor”一词的含义为“皇帝”。皇帝是一个“职位”，不同姓名的人都可以担当此职位。如：我国历史上的李世民、弘历等，法国历史上的拿破仑以及马其顿历史上的亚力山大等，都曾位居皇帝职位。黄帝确实是中国历史上传说的一位皇帝（编者按：对于“黄帝”的看法目前存在争议）。但是，笔者认为，我们可以说黄帝是一位皇帝，可是我们不能说皇帝是黄帝；而该英译书名“Emperor's Canon of Medicine”中，把“黄帝”译为了“emperor”（皇帝）。如果我们把该英译的书名译回为汉语，只能译为《黄帝内经》，而不能译为《黄帝内经》；而“Emperor's Canon of Medicine”（《黄帝内经》）的英译书名也极易使人产生误解，以为该书是论述古代宫庭帝王的内科学的书，而不是反映中国古代的医学成就、创立了中医学理论体系的《黄帝内经》一书。把《黄帝内经》的书名译为“Emperor's Canon of Medicine”显然不妥。

2. 在《汉英医学大辞典》中，《黄帝内经》的书名被译为“The Yellow Emperor's Internal Classic；The Yellow Emperor's Canon of Internal Medicine”。从定义上讲，《黄帝内经》的此种英译书名比《汉英中医辞典》中的英译书名要明确得多。但是，不妥之处也是明显的。

该英译书名中，在“emperor”前面增加了一个英语定冠词“the”和一个修饰词“yellow”。其目的无非是想把该“Emperor”（皇帝）指定为“黄帝”。但是，在英语语言中，“yellow”一词的含义为“黄色的、黄皮肤的，黄色、黄种人”等。如果我们把该英译书名“The Yellow Emperor's Canon of Internal Medicine”译回汉语，则该书名成了《黄色（黄皮肤）黄帝内经》或是《黄种人黄帝内经》。从历史上看，黄皮肤、黄种人的皇帝有很多，读者不知该书所指的是哪一位“黄皮肤、黄种人”皇帝。该英译书名把“黄帝”译为“The Yellow Emperor”，其意思与《黄帝内经》书名中所指的“黄帝”相差甚远，读者甚至不知所云。此种译法显然也是不妥的。

我们再从历史学的角度来看这个书名的翻译。黄帝是我国人民传说中的历史人物，为“少典之子，姓公孙，名曰轩辕”[《史记》，（汉）司马迁]。那么，“公孙轩辕”怎么改称为“黄帝”了呢？据《史记》中记载，“有土德之瑞，土色黄，故称黄帝，犹神农火德王而称炎帝然也”[《史记索隐》，（唐）司马贞]；“生日角龙颜，有景云之瑞，以土德王，故曰黄帝”[《史记·正义》（唐）张守节]；“有土德之瑞，故号黄帝”[《史记》，（汉）司马迁]。据此，我们得知“黄帝”一名称是由于轩辕的金、木、水、火、土五行中，土行旺盛而被称为“黄帝”的，因此，我们知道黄帝是一个具体的人，名称为“黄帝”，是中国历史上远古时期的一个皇帝。用现代话讲，黄帝当时的“职位”是皇帝。

我们知道，虽然书名称为《黄帝内经》，但只是假托，作者实与传说中的历史人物黄帝并无关系。但是，既然汉语的《黄帝内经》一书假托黄帝之名成书，而该书从古流传至今，一直指引着中医学的发展，并在世界范围内产生了影响，那么，在英译该书的书名时，我们自然而然地也要按照原作的精神，仍然要假托黄帝之名来译。不能把“黄帝”英译为“emperor”（皇帝），或英译为“the yellow emperor”（黄色的、黄皮肤、黄种人皇帝），而应按其汉语名字“黄帝”英译为“Huang Di”。

综上所述，《黄帝内经》书名的英译似应译为“Huang Di's Canon of Internal Medicine”为宜。

[原载《中国中西医结合杂志》，2000，20（7）：553.]

当代翻译理论在《黄帝内经》英译研究中的应用

冯文林　伍海涛

中医学理论的奠基之作——《黄帝内经》，由《素问》和《灵枢》两部分组成，受到历代医家的推崇。近一个世纪以来，《黄帝内经》中的《素问》已经被译为多种语言传播到世界很多地区。据资料显示，目前已有多达 9 个甚至 11 个《素问》的不同英译本[1-12]，对于《黄帝内经》英译的研究也越发受到国内外学者的重视。本文从西方和国内不同的翻译理论在《黄帝内经》英译研究中的应用为契机来探讨《黄帝内经》英译的现状。

1. 西方翻译理论在《黄帝内经》英译研究中的应用

1.1　尤金・奈达

尤金・A・奈达（Eugene A. Nida，1914—2011），著名的美国语言学家、翻译家及翻译理论家。在当代西方翻译理论中，奈达的翻译理论在我国介绍得最早、最多，影响最大[13]。他的理论在《黄帝内经》翻译研究中已经凸显其重要性。奈达把“通讯论和信息论用于翻译研究，认为翻译就是交际”[14]，即“翻译是跨语言、跨文化的交际活动”[13]。奈达指出，合格的翻译者在翻译过程中必须考虑语言交际的一切有关因素，必须从作者、内容、读者、背景、作品表达手段等各方面对原作进行全面分析，然后将其转换成类似交际作用的译品，以便使读者看懂[13]。刘九茹[15]在评析吴连胜、吴奇父子的英译本[9]基础上，提出了《黄帝内经》英译的两条原则，其中以信息传译为主的原则就是运用了奈达的交际学理论。刘九茹[15]认为，《黄帝内经》等中医翻译之首要的是信息的内容，为了让译文读者理解所传达的信息，译者只有从译文接受者的角度出发，将中医典籍中包含的基本理论和精华译成英语并把信息的意思表达清楚，才能实现译本的信息传递和交流的功能，促进中医药学的国际交流，从而达到有效交际的目的。奈达还提出了“动态对等要求对译文进行相应调整以满足不同接受者的要求”[13]。张登峰等[16]选取英译《黄帝内经》的 3 个译本［即医药高校教材《英语》（中医分册）[6]、李照国的英汉对照《黄帝内经》[12]以及《内、难全集》（为《黄帝内经》和《难经》的合译本[2]］中两段常见的当代今译与英译形式，分析比较了这些译本的同工异曲之处和细微差异。张登峰等依据奈达理论，即同一源语信息可能有不同形式的译文以适应不同层次读者群的需要，提出了《黄帝内经》不同译本不仅是出于读者的需要，也符合时代发展的要求。

1.2 彼得·纽马克

彼得·纽马克（Peter Newmark，1916—2011），英国著名的翻译理论家和翻译教育家。中国译界最早译介了纽马克翻译理论最重要的两种翻译方法，即语义翻译（semantic translation）和交际翻译（communicative translation）。纽马克根据不同的内容和文体，将文本分为表达功能（expressive function）、信息功能（informative function）和呼唤功能（vocative function）[13]。以表达功能为主的文本如文学作品，其核心是表情达意，所以译者应主要采用语义翻译为主的方法；以信息功能为主的文本如非文学作品，其核心是语言之外的现实世界，所以译者应采用交际翻译法[13]。纽马克虽然指出不同的文本类型采用不同的翻译方法，但语义翻译和交际翻译是一个整体，两者在翻译中常交替使用，或侧重不同或合二为一[13]。段晋丽[17]分析了《素问》的两个英译本《*The Yellow Emperor's Classic of Internal Medicine*》（Ilza Veith 译，1972）[5]和《*The Yellow Emperor's Classic of Medicine*》（Maoshing Ni 译，1995）[7]，按照信息论的观点，医学翻译的本质是通过语种变换把源语所承担的信息转换成目标语承载的信息；医学翻译的目的是介绍国内外的先进医学经验和技术，使不同国家和民族的人们得以进行医学文化交流，因此，要求准确传达原文语义，既要力求做到"信息等价"（information equivalency），又要有较强的信息传递性（information transitivity），所以段晋丽根据纽马克的翻译理论，认为由于科技语篇在功能上的特殊性，中医古籍中的隐喻一般不必译出。译者在翻译的过程中，既要力求避免误译，又要结合科技语篇的特点，选择适当的翻译策略，尽量避免出现译文对于原文信息的不"信"、不"达"现象，避免造成"虽译犹不译"的结果。

1.3 乔治·斯坦纳

乔治·斯坦纳（George Steiner，1929—）是当代著名学者、文学评论家、散文家、哲学家、小说家、翻译理论家和教育家，精通英、法、德三种语言。斯坦纳的代表作《通天塔之后：语言与翻译面面观》被翻译学界广泛评价为"一部里程碑式的著作"[14]，20 多年来再版多次，也被视为西方现代翻译研究领域一部具有一定特色和较高理论价值的重要文献[13]。斯坦纳从阐释学角度提出了翻译的步骤，即信赖（trust）、侵入（aggression）、吸收（incorporation）和补偿（restitution）[13]。王治梅等[18]以阐释学为视角，运用斯坦纳阐释翻译理论的四个翻译步骤，分析了《黄帝内经》两个译本（李照国译本[12]和 Veith 译本[5]）中省略辞格的典型英译实例，总结了译者翻译的策略与规律，认为阐释翻译理论的四个翻译步骤阐述了翻译的全过程，每一步都是不可或缺的。李照国和 Veith 的译文都做到了前三步，但是对于第四步"补偿"；两者都局限于各种自身和客观因素而不能完全准确地作出补偿：不论是作为本族语的译者和作为目标语的译者在翻译过程中应对语言、文化、风格等方面做出适当的补偿，不能完全"译古如古”，也不能完全脱离源语的语言体系。

1.4　汉斯·弗米尔

汉斯·弗米尔（Hans J. Vermeer，1930—2010）是德国翻译功能学派（也被称为目的学派）的创始人，其提出的目的论（skopos theory）是功能派翻译理论的重要理论[13]。王继慧[19]从文化资本理论的角度，运用翻译功能目的论原理，要求译文应该达成翻译活动的特定目的，着重关注《黄帝内经》书名的含义、书名英译的文化目的和具体的翻译策略及方法，对现有的各种译文进行分析和比较。王继慧通过研究发现，为了达到良好的中国传统优秀文化对外传播效果，《黄帝内经》书名的英译应凸显中国文化特色和准确传达其医学科学价值，在多个不同译名中，王继慧认为张庆荣教授对《黄帝内经》书名的英译 Huangdi Neijing（Huangdi's Inner Classic of Medicine）[20]是目前最佳译名。王继慧倡导尽快推行该译名在译界和国际文化交流中的标准化工作，通过世界文化消费者的接受和肯定，中国优秀文化资本在世界范围将实现更为顺畅的运行，该文化资本的潜在价值也将全面提升。

1.5　莫娜·贝克

莫娜·贝克（Mona Baker），当代英国翻译理论家。贝克开辟了以语料库方法展开的翻译研究的先河，这是一种全新的翻译研究的途径[14]。雷燕等[21]认为现有的《黄帝内经》英译研究基本是思辨性总结，利用语料库的方法做一些实证性研究可弥补目前研究现状的不足。《黄帝内经》的英译研究可以借鉴语料库的方法，收集《黄帝内经》中文及多个译本的电子文本，建成一个小型平行语料库，并对语料做各种带有研究目的的标注，利用检索工具对标注语料做方便快捷的收寻和分析。这种实证性研究可发现以往因条件所限未能发现或未注意的语言事实和特征，找到某些可循的规律，突破现有的思辨性研究，指导《黄帝内经》及其他中医古籍的翻译。李苹等[22]在分析了中医英语语料库研究现状的基础上，指出了《黄帝内经》汉英语料库建设的意义和必要性，也对《黄帝内经》汉英语料库建库提出了设想。

1.6　埃文-佐哈尔

伊塔玛·埃文-佐哈尔（Itama Even-Zohar），以色列学者。埃文-佐哈尔通过观察翻译对社会的影响，于 20 世纪 70 年代初提出了多元系统理论（polysystem theory），对翻译理论产生了很大的影响，其被视为“翻译研究学派”的先驱之一[13]。兰凤利[2,23]介绍了多元系统理论及相应的描写性翻译批评方法论，并运用多元系统理论的方法对跨越近 80 年产生的 9 种译本的《素问》英译事业进行了描写性研究。兰凤利将《素问》的英译历程分为三个历史时期，根据不同时期译本的特征，力图考证特定历史背景中译者的意图，不同历史时期《素问》英译本在英美文化（医学文化）多元系统中不同的地位及功能，以及特定历史条件之下中医古籍英译的规范与倾向，由此证明了用多元系统论的描写性翻译批评方法能有效地解释一些由历史语境影响和决定的翻译现象，尤其适用于对多年以前产生的翻译作品或是同一原作在不同历史条件下产生的不同译本进行研究，这一翻译批评的新方法可以弥补规定性翻译批评方法的局限性。同时，兰凤利还指出，《素问》英译本在英语医学文化多元系统中的地位和功能随着社会、历史条件的变化而变化，《素问》的译介和研究正逐步走向高潮。

1.7 道格拉斯·罗宾逊

道格拉斯·罗宾逊（Douglas Robinson，1954—），美国著名翻译家。他的主要译学著作之一是1991年出版的《轮到了译者》，书中提出了“翻译应当以译者为中心”[14]的理论。罗宾逊强调“翻译应当从人出发”，翻译的过程中“译者的中心能动性作用”[14]。兰凤利[24]分析了1925—2003年近80年间出现的9种《素问》英译本，在探讨了“谁在翻译《素问》”之后，认为译者的学术背景和知识结构对《素问》的英译过程影响最大，译者主体性也最为明显，译者主体性对译文的影响也就最大，这也是目前翻译界在译者主体性方面探讨最多的问题；翻译中的“创造性叛逆”现象往往是研究译者的译入语医学文化意识和读者意识的突破口，这些意识受到译者的文化身份、文化取向以及译者身处的外部大环境的影响，从而体现在他（她）的翻译策略、翻译目的、具体的翻译方式等方面；《素问》的翻译是典籍翻译，也是科技翻译，故译者需要依据能影响甚至决定译者主体性良性发挥的各种因素而进行翻译。兰凤利还提出了《素问》的译者所应具备的修养，即具备一定的中医古籍版本学、训诂学、校勘学知识；具备中医学学术背景和较强的古汉语阅读能力；具备扎实的译入语语言功底和翻译素养；具备译入语医学文化意识以及读者意识等[24]。雷燕等[25]认为译者主体性指译者在翻译活动中表现的主观能动性，它贯穿于翻译的始终；译者主体性具有自主性、能动性、目的性、创造性等特点，译者应充分发挥挖掘自身潜能，有效进行翻译操作；但同时译者主体性又是“忠实”标准下的主体性，忠实是译者翻译的底线。雷燕[25]以《素问》4个英译本的某些译文为例，认为《内经》的翻译是一项艰难而浩大的工程，4名译者均为此做出了不懈努力：其中朱明[10]、李照国[12]有较完备的中医知识，故译本较少误译，但由于译入语（英语）不是母语，译文句式稍显简单，表达效果欠佳；Maoshing Ni[7]和Iliza Veith[5]以译入语为母语，译文倾向使用长句、复句，表达流畅、地道，但由于中医师Maoshing Ni的译本旨在传播中医，面向普通读者，故译文中加入较多个人理解，难免有些偏颇，Iliza Veith对古汉语并不十分精通，故造成不少误译。由此证明了译者的知识结构、双语能力及翻译前确立的翻译目的、方法等主体性因素对译文质量产生较大的影响。

1.8 罗伯特·布格兰德和沃尔夫兰·威尔斯

罗伯特·布格兰德（Robert de Beaugrande，1946—2008），美国翻译理论

家。布格兰德于 1978 年发表了以语篇语言学思想为指导的翻译理论，他始终以语篇语言学视角来阐释语言与翻译的问题，确立了他在英美翻译研究领域中语篇语言学派带头人的重要地位。他指出："翻译单位不是单个的词或句子，而是整个语篇"[14]。沃尔夫兰·威尔斯（Wolfram Wilss，1925—）是德国"萨尔派"（是以联邦德国萨尔大学为基础的一个流派）的主要代表。他也认为翻译应以语篇作为基本单位，翻译是把源语篇变成最适当的对等的目标语篇[14]。李振[26]认为翻译研究与实践中离不开语篇分析理论，语篇在翻译实践中的完整性与一体性，就是要把握中西语言语篇构成的差异，注重语篇的衔接、连贯以及情景语境与文化语境因素的作用，形成符合译文读者的语篇形式，所以医古文翻译同样要体现语篇意识；李振以医古文经典——《黄帝内经》英译为例进行翻译语篇分析，探讨了医古文翻译中的语篇意识，认为当前医古文英译中语篇意识不强仍是影响其译文读者接受程度的一大问题，在医古文连贯及语境方面的分析尚有很大的研究空间。

2. 国内翻译理论在《黄帝内经》英译研究中的应用

2.1　胡庚申

胡庚申（1949—），国内著名的跨文化/国际交流语用研究专家和翻译理论家。胡庚申以达尔文"适应/选择"说为理论支撑，创立了"翻译适应选择论"的基本理念，该理论的构建将为中国译坛，特别是为翻译理论研究拓宽了新的研究视角。李英照等[27]选取了《素问》的李照国[12]、Maoshing Ni[7]、吴连胜和吴奇父子[9]的译本，运用胡庚申的"翻译适应选择论"，通过对《素问》同一原文语句的对应翻译加以比较分析，发现译者们面对不同翻译生态环境时具有各自不同的适应与选择过程，这是造成不同译者对原文中的同一词汇的译词不同的根本原因；同一译者在同一章节中相关词汇的翻译方法并非随意确定，而是译者们能动地适应选择的结果。李英照[27]以《黄帝内经》中包含"痹"的病名的英译为契机，分析了译者的知识结构、翻译发起人的意图以及目标读者定位，认为了解译者的适应选择过程可以帮助自己在同类图书中做出选择，并且在图书的阅读过程中更好地理解和利用译文，从而最大限度地实现译者意欲达到的翻译目的。比如，选择忠实谨慎的李照国本[12]的读者可以了解原汁原味的中医经典；选择通俗易懂的 Maoshing Ni 本[7]的读者大多是外行或者刚入门的中医学习者；吴氏父子本[9]尽管在选词的精确性方面尚有待商榷，但从译词的信息密度和与之相关的阅读效率来看可以帮助读者快捷地从临床应用的角度来挖掘《黄帝内经》。

2.2　李照国

李照国（1961—），国内知名的中医英语翻译、教学和研究者。李照国的著作和论文很多，对中医英语翻译特别是《黄帝内经》的英译贡献很大，其《黄帝内经》英译本为世人所推崇。李照国认为《黄帝内经》由于年代久远，语言晦涩，理论深奥，再加上各家注解不一，将其译为今文已颇为不易，译为英语便更是难上加难[28]。所以李照国翻译《黄帝内经》时遵循两个基本原则[28]：一是“与时俱退，立足实际”，李照国认为虽然古今思维方式、语言结构和思想观念的变化，“与时俱退”的理念有时也很难落实，但在思想观念和认识方式上可以回归到《黄帝内经》产生的那个时代，以避免以今释古，所以李照国在翻译《黄帝内经》中某些含有浓厚的中国国情的核心概念时均予以音译，再用括号将现行译法作为文内注解附于有关音译概念之后，以帮助读者理解。另在译文之后附加详细注解，以帮助读者完整准确地理解相关概念的实际内涵。二是“译古如古，文不加饰”。李照国尽可能在译文中保持原文的结构形式和表达方式，尽量不增词语。但由于古文文简趣深，翻译时若不增加字词，有时很难表达清楚，所以凡因表达需要而增加的词语，李照国均将其置于中括号之内，以便使读者理解从而防止衍文的出现。

3. 小结

研究中国医药古籍英译，特别是《黄帝内经》，具有社会文化传播的重要意义，也具有典籍英译的理论与方法论研究空间。西方翻译理论在《黄帝内经》翻译研究中的运用体现了《黄帝内经》翻译研究走国际化交流的轨道，这种理念对于学术界交流和教学都是有益的。《黄帝内经》翻译研究需要融合现代交叉学科（语义学、认知语言学、语用学、西方诠释学、接受美学、阐释学、翻译学等）的理论认识，将经验层面的认识经过提炼、加工、改造、分类、概括、综合而成为中国医药古籍的翻译理论思想与方法论相统一的比较系统的理论框架。《黄帝内经》翻译研究既需要有宏观理论（目的、原则、策略、准则）的阐释，又需要有微观理论［技术理论（技巧与方法）］的可印证性、可操作性的照应性说明，这样有利于有效地指导中医药典籍的翻译实践。然而，《黄帝内经》内容复杂，所涉范畴极广，仅拟定一两个简单的原则与方法难以解决所有的问题。国内有些《黄帝内经》翻译研究者仅从经验原则表述，所论笼统含糊，难以在遇到具体问题时指导具体实践；有些仅对《黄帝内经》翻译的个案比较说明，没有将其视为一“类”现象进行研究，没有进一步对此类现象中的问题本质认识作出阐发，只有特殊性认识，没有普遍原理概括性认识。我们应该认识到《黄帝内经》等中医药典籍英译并非是为“原则”而翻译，应是为特定目的—需求而翻译，特别是重译本的翻译更需要理论指导。

参考文献

[1] 张斌，杜福荣．《黄帝内经》比喻辞格英译研究回眸．时珍国医国药，2011，22（12）：

3001 - 3003.
[2] 兰凤利．《黄帝内经素问》英译事业的描写性研究（1）．中国中西医结合杂志，2004，24（10）：947 - 950.
[3] 王吉民，傅维康．中国医史外文文献索引（1682—1965）．上海：上海中医学院医史博物馆，1966：165.
[4] Wen H. Nei Ching，the Chinese canon of medicine. Chin Med J，1950，68（1，2）：1 - 33.
[5] Ilza V. The Yellow Emperor's classic of internal medicine. Berkeley：University of California Press，1972：101 - 177.
[6] 上海第二医学院主编．英语・中医分册．北京：人民卫生出版社，1980：6，9，10 - 11.
[7] Ni MS. The Yellow Emperor's classic of medicine. Massachusetts：Shambhala，1995：160 -162.
[8] 周春才，韩亚洲编绘．《黄帝内经》——养生图典（汉英）．北京：海豚出版社，1997：133 - 135.
[9] 吴连胜，吴奇，译．黄帝内经（汉英对照）．北京：中国科学技术出版社，1997：208 -212.
[10] Zhu M. The medical classic of the Yellow Emperor. Beijing：Foreign Languages Press，2001：5 - 10，110 - 116，230 - 236.
[11] Unschuld PU. Huangdi Neijing Suwen：nature，knowledge，imagery in an ancient Chinese medical text. Berkeley：University of California Press，2003：Ⅸ-Ⅻ.
[12] 李照国，译．Yellow Emperor's canon of medicine：plain conversation. 西安：世界图书出版公司，2005：2 - 240，1234.
[13] 李文革．西方翻译理论流派研究．北京：中国社会科学出版社，2004：91 - 106，112 - 131，139，184 - 185，255 - 263.
[14] 谭载喜．西方翻译简史．2 版．北京：商务印书馆，2004：216，223 - 225，231 - 240，240 - 241，246 - 248，252 - 254.
[15] 刘九茹．《黄帝内经》英译两原则．河南职工医学院学报，2008，20（6）：609 - 611.
[16] 张登峰，孙红梅，史文君．《黄帝内经》翻译比较．陕西中医学院学报，2011，34（1）：92 - 94.
[17] 段晋丽．《〈黄帝内经・素问〉翻译实例分析》之商榷．菏泽医学专科学校学报，2008，20（1）：93 - 96.
[18] 王治梅，张斌．从阐释翻译论看《黄帝内经》省略辞格的英译．中西医结合学报，2010，8（11）：1097 - 1100.
[19] 王继慧．中医药典籍《黄帝内经》书名英译探讨．辽宁中医药大学学报，2011，13（9）：161 - 165.
[20] 张庆荣主译．中医基础理论（中英文对照）．2 版．北京：人民卫生出版社，2007.
[21] 雷燕，施蕴中．《黄帝内经》英译研究．辽宁中医药大学学报，2008，10（4）：172 -173.
[22] 李苹，施蕴中．语料库语言学和《黄帝内经》汉英语料库．中国科技信息，2009，(3)：

259，261.

[23] 兰凤利.《黄帝内经素问》英译事业的描写性研究（2）. 中国中西医结合杂志，2005，25（2）：176－180.

[24] 兰凤利.论译者主体性对《黄帝内经素问》英译的影响.中华医史杂志，2005，35（2）：74－78.

[25] 雷燕，施蕴中.译者主体性对《黄帝内经素问》译文的影响.江西中医学院学报，2007，19（6）：84－86.

[26] 李振.从《黄帝内经》英译看医古文翻译的语篇意识.云南中医学院学报，2009，32（2）：7－10.

[27] 李英照，施蕴中.《内经·痹沦篇》中含“痹”病名的英译——“翻译适应选择论”观照下的翻译解读.中国科技信息，2009，(1)：221－223.

[28] 李照国.《黄帝内经》英译得失谈.中国科技翻译，2009，22（4）：3－7.

[原载《中国中西医结合杂志》，2014，34（1）：101－105.]

"Huangdi" 还是 "Huang Di"?

——关于"黄帝"名字英译的商榷

刘　伟

近几年出版的汉英辞典上关于"黄帝"名字的英译形式不一致，使中医英译工作者在进行中医文献的英译工作时无所适从，造成中医术语英译工作的混乱现象。笔者试就"黄帝"名字英译的英文形式与同行商榷。

1. "黄帝"是人名

"黄帝"一名在中医药学中占有极其重要的位置。目前国内现存最早的奠定中医药学理论的经典著作《黄帝内经》就是假托"黄帝"之名成书的。该书以黄帝提问、岐伯作答的二人对话形式来阐述中医学理论。例如，"黄帝问曰：少阴何以主肾？肾何以主水？岐伯对曰：肾者至阴也，至阴者盛水也，肺者太阴也，少阴者冬脉也，故其本在肾，其末在肺，皆积水也。"《黄帝内经・素问》[1]。另《史记》记载：生日角龙颜，有景云之瑞，以土德王，故曰黄帝。"[2]由此可以确认，"黄帝"是一个人的名字。

2. "黄帝"名字目前的英译形式及其分析

关于"黄帝"的英译，目前有以下几种方式：①"Yellow Emperor"[3]。②"Huangdi"，"Yellow Emperor"。[4]上述"黄帝"名字的英译形式分析如下：①、②中的"黄帝"英译名"Yellow Emperor"中，"emperor"一词在英语中的意思是"皇帝"，并非"黄帝"。把"yellow"加在"emperor"的前面，作为"emperor"的修饰语，懂英语的中国人可能会猜其是指"黄帝"，但是，不懂中国历史、医史的外国人也只能理解为"某位黄种人皇帝"或"某位黄色的皇帝"，无法理解为"黄帝"，因为"yellow"一词在英语语言中的意思是"黄色的、黄皮肤的、黄色人种的"，没有表示中国人姓名的"黄"字的意思。②中的"黄帝"英译名"Huangdi"是按照音译法以汉语的读音把"黄帝"翻译为英文的。尽管该英译名字读音与汉语"黄帝"的读音相同，但是在英译中医理论和中医文献中应用却行不通。我们已知"岐黄"这一中医术语成为了"中医"的代名词，如果采用了"黄帝"英译名字"Huangdi"的形式，则"岐黄"只能英译为"Qi Huangdi"，显然是行不通的。

3. 中医术语“黄帝”的英译形式

1982年经联合国批准用汉语拼音拼写中国的人名和地名，并在全世界推广使用。我们把“黄帝”这一人名英译时，应遵照联合国批准的译法，采用中国人名汉语拼音的形式这一国际通用规则，译为“Huang Di”，这样，不但中国人明白“Huang Di”所指的是“黄帝”，使用英语为母语的对中医学感兴趣的外国人也立即明白“Huang Di”所指的是“黄帝”。中医“岐黄”这一术语就可以英译为“Qi Huang”。

综上所述，笔者提出：从中医学的角度来考虑，“黄帝”的名字英译为“Huang Di”较为妥当。

参考文献

[1] 黄帝内经素问. 北京：人民卫生出版社，1981：326.
[2]（汉）司马迁 . 史记 . 北京：中华书局，1982：2 .
[3] 金魁和 . 汉英医学大辞典 . 北京：人民卫生出版社，2004：1796.
[4] 吴景荣，程镇球 . 新时代汉英大辞典 . 北京：商务印书馆，2001：672.

[原载《中国中西医结合杂志》，2007，27（11）：1015.]

第二节　中药方剂英译实践

中药方剂名的英译技巧与原则

张　昀

把中药方剂名进行英译，目的是让我国独特的中药方剂学走出国门，使外国人能准确了解所指的中药方剂，为世界人民的健康事业做出应有的贡献，同时也为中西医结合进行学术交流做出贡献。正因为如此，中药方剂名的准确英译显得极为重要。中药方剂的命名具有其内在的理据。一般来说，中药方剂大多采用以药命名、药物的效能命名、药名加功效和药的味数四种方法进行命名。从语法结构看，方剂名称绝大多数为偏正词组，分别以名词为中心词表示主要药材、剂型，以表示药物功效的短语构成修饰结构。以常用方剂“明目地黄丸”为例，主药“地黄丸”构成中心词，功效“明目”为修饰结构。方剂的命名模式和构词方法使方剂名称的英译有规可循、有据可依。本文试图揭示中药方剂名英译的一些技巧和原则。

1　英译技巧

1.1　确立中心词

中药方剂中有许多是以药品主要药材加剂型命名，英译时以该药学名即药材的拉丁文为标准译成相应的中心词。值得注意的是，这些药材往往被加工成各种不同剂型：膏、片、胶囊、丸、糖浆、冲剂、汤、饮、散、丹、栓以及复方类。它们与主要药材一起构成中心词来体现方剂的性状。例如：益母草膏，semifluid extract of motherwort；穿心莲，andrographis tablet；天麻胶囊，gastrodia capsule；木香槟榔丸，pill of aucklandiae and arecae；止咳枇杷糖浆，cough syrup of loquat leat；感冒退热冲剂，cold-fever-treating infusion；两地汤，decoction of rehmanniae and lyciiradicis；生脉饮，pulse-activating decoction；通幽汤，decoction for dysphagia；泻白散，powder for expelling lung-heat；小活络丹，small bolus for activating channels and collaterals；妇宁栓，suppository for relieving woman disease；复方丹参注射液，compound injection of red sage root 等。此外，还有一些方剂是以药的味数作中心词的，例如：四物汤，decoction of four drugs；六味地黄丸，bolus of six drugs including rehmannia。

1.2 转化偏正词

在确定中心词后，接着选择表示药物效能的短语作修饰结构，从而把汉语的偏正词组转化为英语的名词短语。

1.2.1 以-ing分词作前置修饰语 中药方剂中表示药物主要功效和作用的部分可以用相应的-ing分词来翻译，在方剂名中作前置修饰语。例如：牛黄解毒片，detoxicating tablet of cow-bezoar；伸筋丹胶囊，relaxing muscles and tendons capsule。也可以在-ing分词前加名词，用连字符连接，构成复合词作前置修饰语。例如：麝香镇痛膏，pain-alleviating adhesive plaster of musk；胃康灵胶囊，stomach-recovering capsule；理气舒心片，Qi-regulating and heart-soothing tablet；舒肝丸，liver-soothing bolus；生脉饮，pulse-activating decoction。

1.2.2 形容词作前置修饰语 例如：止咳枇杷糖浆，cough syrup of loquat leaf；元胡止痛胶囊，analgesic capsule of corydalis tuber。

1.2.3 介词短语作后置修饰语 在中药方剂名的英译中，还可以用for表示药物功效，构成后置修饰语修饰中心词。如：羚羊感冒片，tablet of antelope's horn for common cold；当归补血汤，decoction of angelicae sinensis for enriching blood；枳实导滞丸，pill of aurantii immaturus for relieving stagnation。

1.2.4 -ing分词作后置修饰语 有些方剂名称含有药的味数和主要药材两部分，是以味数作中心词，主要药材作修饰语。这类方剂的英译可使用-ing分词作后置修饰语。例如：六味地黄丸，bolus of six drugs including rehmannia；九味羌活汤，decoction of nine ingredients containing notopterygii。

2. 英译原则

中药方剂的命名除以药命名、药物效能命名及药病结合命名等直接理据外，还涉及中国历史、地理、宗教、哲学等文化因素，再加上中医是中国所特有的传统医学，因此，中药方剂的翻译不仅要考虑中医所具有的特性，还要跨越英汉语言和文化上的障碍。想要让英美人确实理解并接受中药方剂，翻译时必须遵循一些相关的原则。

2.1 避虚就实原则

有些方剂为了修辞或避讳的需要采用别名或异名，其独特的文化含义是西方人无法解读的。在这种情况下，就应当注重语义的翻译。通常的做法是避虚就实，将实质性的药名理据进行英译，损失其中的一些文化含义。例如，泰山磐石散实际上是安胎的中药，其药名中的泰山、磐石表示稳固的意思，要照实翻译的话，西方人无法理解或引起误解，因此，最好根据药物的功效实译为“powder for calming fetus”。又如三鞭补酒、通幽汤，要对等翻译的话，解释上要花一番工夫，而且也不符合译名的规范，因此，应当分别实译为“tonic tincture of three-animal penes”和“decoction for dysphagia”。类似的例子还有：保济丸，health pill；通关丸，pill for relieving trismus and resuscitation；雏凤精，oral liquid of chicken fetus；香砂六君子丸，pill of costus and amomum with six noble ingredients；二仙膏，semifluid extract of ginseng and antler glue。

2.2 舍繁就简原则

在对中药方剂的功效进行描述性、解释性翻译时应当力求简洁，因为这不是辞典释义，用词不能太长。如果与原方剂名相比，译语冗长繁杂，则交际功能就差，翻译后很难被外国人记住和接受，因此，应该力求简明扼要[1]。例如，“止咳枇杷糖浆”可译成 cough syrup of loquat leaf，省去 alleviating（止）。又如“香砂养胃丸”可译成 stomache pill of aucklandia and amomum fruit，省去 nourishing（养）。

2.3 音译原则

音译是保持中药方剂特色的一种重要方法。中药方剂名里有许多“气”“阴”“阳”等多义词，这类词概念独特，含义丰富，具有特殊文化因素。事实上，这些词的音译形式已被国际中医界广泛接受，并经常运用在临床实践中，因此，当方剂名中含有这类词时可用音译原则，例如：固阴煎，decoction for keeping Yin；补中益气丸，bolus of rein forcing middle-Jiao and replenishing Qi；理气舒心片，Qi-regulating and heart soothing tablet。有些中药方剂含有的语汇具有浓厚的中国文化含义，是传统中医所特有的，没有对应的英语词汇，如果直译容易引起误解，在这种情况下，也可用音译的原则。如在有些词典里，“乌鸡白凤丸”被直译为 black cock and white phoenix decoction。但在英文中，cock 一词与性有关，是禁忌语，而乌鸡白凤丸是一种治疗妇科病的药。西方女士在看到这样的药名时一定不会购买。如果译成 Wuji Baifeng pill，既可避免误解和文化休克，又可以保持译名的回译性，即如果读者想了解进一步的信息，可以根据汉语拼音查出其中文原文[2]。

类似的音译例子还有：一贯煎，Yiguan decoction；再造散，Zaizao powder；失笑丸，Shixiao pill；舟军丸，Zhouju pill；驻军丸，Zhujun pill；虎潜丸，Huqian bolus；一捻金，Yinianjin powder for infants[3]。当然我们应当尽量少用、慎用音译，毕竟对外国人来说汉语拼音是外来词，理解上有困难。

中药方剂名的英译是一个不断实践和探索的过程。随着人们对传统中药方剂学的进一步深入研究，中西医结合与交流趋势的增强以及英汉语言和文化的相互影响，中药方剂的命名将发生变化，由此会给中药方剂名称的英译带来诸多不确定因素。但只要我们恪守一些基本原则，就能够不断提高译名的质量。

参考文献

[1] 李照国．中医英语翻译技巧．北京：人民卫生出版社，1997：393－402.
[2] 李永安．音译在中医名词翻译中的应用．中国中西医结合杂志，2001，21（10）：792－793.
[3] 李宗友．最新英汉药名词典．北京：中医古籍出版社，1994：825－835.

［原载《中国中西医结合杂志》，2004，24（7）：664－665.］

谈中药药性理论有关术语的英译

袁洪仁

中药药性理论的内容，包括四气、五味、升降浮沉和归经等。它是古代医家在长期的医疗实践中对药物作用的认识，其中四气、五味因来自于自然界的气化，故以“司岁备物”（《素问·至真要大论》）之运气理论做指导。中药药性理论有关术语的英译应忠实于此事实，现分述如下。

1. 四气的英译

四气是指寒、热、温、凉四种不同的药性，是古代医家在长期的医疗实践中总结出来的：能治热性病的药物多属寒凉性质，能治寒性病的药物多属温热性质。寒与凉、热与温仅是程度上的区别。故“四气”译作“four drug-Qi”，意为“四种药气”“四种药性”。后缀“-Qi”既表达了作为中药四种药性的四气称呼，又表达了药性与自然界气化、药物临床功效（中医脏象学说中 Qi 有“功能”之意）的相关性。相应地，四气所包括的寒、热、温、凉四性分别译作“cold-Qi”“hot-Qi”“warm-Qi”“cool-Qi”。以“cool-Qi”为例，意为“寒性”“气化之性寒”“功效之性寒”，余类推。至于平性，是指药性平和，微有偏温偏凉之异，仍在四性之中，可译作“mild-Qi”。平性偏温或偏凉，分别译作“mild warm-Qi”“mild cool-Qi”。因“mild”有“轻的、温和的、非极端的”之意。

2. 五味的英译

五味指辛、甘、酸、苦、咸五种不同的药味。五味与药物作用密切联系，人们又常据药物功效反过来推断药味，与口尝不符。事实上，五味实质上是天地四季五气气化产生的，即风化、热化、湿化、寒化、燥化的结果。故“五味”译作“five taste-Qi”，意为“五种气化之味” “五种功效之味”。这种译法，前缀“tase-”表达了药味原本是直接口尝感觉出的味道，后缀“-Qi”则不仅表达了药味是对药物功能的认识（脏象学说中 Qi 有“功能”之意），而且表达了药味来自于自然界的气化。相应地，五味所包括的辛、甘、酸、苦、咸分别译作“acrid-Qi”“sweet-Qi”“sour-Qi”“bitter-Qi”“salty-Qi”。以“acrid-Qi”为例，意思就是指“气化之味辛”“功效之味辛”，余类推。至于淡味和涩味，其作用分别近于甘味、酸味，仍在五味之中，故分别译为“tasteless-Qi”“astringent-Qi”。

3. 升、降、浮、沉和归经的英译

升、降、浮、沉是药物在治疗作用中的趋向，升浮药主向上、向外，沉降药主向下、向内，故升、降、浮、沉分别译作 upward-Qi、downward-Qi、outward-Qi、inward-Qi。以“upward-Qi”为例，意思为“升性”“上升之效”，余类推。相应地，升浮药和沉降药分别译作 up-outward-Qi drug、down-inward-Qi drug。至于归经，是指药物归向以五脏为核心的经络联通的身体各组织部分，译作“emstem of neurovaso-Qiduct”，意为“所入经脉”[1]。与此相关的引经药，指某些具有引导其他药物到达病变部位之作用的药物，故译作“guide-drug”，意为“向导药”。

参考文献

[1] 袁洪仁．谈经络学说术语的英译．中国中西医结合杂志，2001，21（3）：198.

[原载《中国中西医结合杂志》，2003，23（12）：917]

中药名词英译标准化的探讨

范为宇　杨秋铭　谢　琪　胡艳敏

随着中医药对外交流不断增加，中医药英译工作近年来广泛展开，大大促进了中医药走向世界的进程。但是，由于缺乏标准规范，中医药英译工作中存在着名词不统一的问题，从而在一定程度上影响了对中医药学的对外交流。本文力图通过较为客观的统计方法，对规范中药复方名词的英译标准化做出探索和尝试。

1. 研究方法

我们认为，以目前文献中使用词频率最高的英译法为首选译法，应当是较客观的英译标准化方法，因此，本研究对世界上最大的医学文献数据库 MEDLINE 里中医药学名词术语的各种英译法进行了词频统计。

1.1　研究样本

研究样本以《中华人民共和国药典》（1995 年版）[1]、全国高等中医院校统编教材《中药学》[2]、《中国中医药学主题词表》[3]为依据，选取了其中 600 个中药复方名词（含中药药物作用名词 36 个，中药名词 350 个，方剂名词 70 个，中成药名词 68 个，剂型名词 20 个，炮制加工名词 20 个，中药理论名词 36 个）作为研究样本。

1.2　译法来源

译法来源为 20 余种工具书。选择了近年来比较流行或权威的 22 本工具书作为中药名词英译法的来源。

1.3　词频来源

美国国立医学图书馆 MEDLINE 数据库是目前世界上收录范围最广、收录文献最多、最权威的医学文献数据库。该数据库是用英文编制的，因此，将其作为中药复方名词英译法的词频来源是具有相当的说服力的。

1.4　研究方法

我们利用 Microsoft Access 数据库软件建立了中药复方名词英译名数据库，其中设有中药复方名词、工具书、英译名、MEDLINE 出现频率等字段。将每一名词在不同工具书中的不同译法及其在 MEDLINE 中出现的次数分别输入数据库，进行各种英译法词频量统计排序，并根据统计排序结果了解各种英译法被接受的程度，从而确定各名词术语的首选英译法。

2. 结果

2.1 译法数据库

通过本研究，建成了一个中药复方名词译法数据库。数据库采用 Microsoft Access 软件，收集了 600 种中药复方名词在 20 余种工具书中的不同译法，及其在 MEDLINE 数据库中的词频量，共有 18 525 条记录。

2.2 从词频统计看中药复方名词英译的规律

通过词频量分析可以看出，目前中药复方名词的英译具有以下规律。

2.2.1 中药植物药名词的英译

以英文译名最为常用，其次为拉丁学名，再次为汉语拼音音译。例如大黄的译法见表 1。

表 1 “大黄”的各种英译法在 MEDLINE 中出现的词频统计

来源工具书	译名	出现次数
《英汉对照中医本科系列教材——中药学分册》[4]	Rhubarb	236
《汉英医学大辞典》[5]	Rhubarb	236
《简明汉英日中医药词典》[6]	Rhubarb	236
《中华人民共和国药典》[1]	Rhubarb	236
《汉英中医药分类辞典》[7]	Rhubarb	236
《汉英双解中医大辞典》[8]	Rhubarb	236
《英汉实用中医药大全》[9]	Rhubarb	236
《英汉汉英中医词典》[10]	Rhubarb	236
Practical TCM & Pharmacolog (*Herbal Formulas*)[11]	Rhubarb	236
An Introduction to Chinese Materia Medica[12]	Rhubarb	236
Practical TCM & Pharmacolog (*Medicinal Herbs*)[11]	Rhubarb	236
《新世纪汉英科技大词典》[13]	Rhubarb	236
《英汉对照实用中医文库》[14]	Rhubarb	236

续表

来源工具书	译名	出现次数
《新世纪汉英科技大词典》[13]	Rheum	139
《慈禧光绪医方选议》[15]	Radix et Rhizoma Rhei	18
《汉英医学大辞典》[5]	Radix et Rhizoma Rhei	18
《简明汉英日中医药词典》[6]	Radix et Rhizoma Rhei	18
《汉英中医辞典》[16]	Radix et Rhizoma Rhei	18
《中华人民共和国药典》[1]	Radix et Rhizoma Rhei	18
《汉英常用中药手册》[17]	Radix et Rhizoma Rhei	18
《汉英中医药分类辞典》[7]	Radix et Rhizoma Rhei	18
《新世纪汉英科技大词典》[13]	Radix et Rhizoma Rhei	18
Advanced Textbook on TCM an Pharmacology Vol. 2[18]	Radix et Rhizoma rhei	18
《中国中医药学主题词表》[3]	Rheum Officinale	15
《新世纪汉英科技大词典》[13]	Chinese Rhubarb	12
《简明汉英日中医药词典》[6]	Dahuang	10
《新世纪汉英科技大词典》[13]	Rhizoma Rhei	0
《新世纪汉英科技大词典》[13]	Chinese Reasel Root	0
Chinese Herbs and Compatibility[19]	Rhubarb Root and Rhizome	0

2.2.2　中药动物药名词的英译

对中药动物名词的翻译，同样以英文译名最为常用，其次为拉丁学名，再次为汉语拼音音译，例如“蟾酥”的译法见表 2。

表 2 “蟾酥”的各种英译法在 MEDLINE 中出现的词频统计

来源工具书	译名	出现次数
《汉英中医药分类辞典》[7]	Toad Venom	41
《汉英英汉中医大辞典》[20]	Toad Venom	41
《英汉实用中医药大全》[9]	Toad Venom	41
《英汉汉英中医词典》[10]	Toad Venom	41
An Introduction to Chinese Materia Medica[12]	Toad Venom	41
《汉英中医药分类辞典》[7]	Toad Venom	41
《汉英英汉中医大辞典》[20]	Bufotoxin	8
Advanced Textbook on TCM and Pharmacology Vol. 2[18]	Venenum Bufoni	5
《中国中医药学主题词表》[3]	Venenum Bufonis	5
《汉英医学大辞典》[5]	Venenum Bufonis	5
《慈禧光绪医方选议》[15]	Venenum Bufonis	5
《英汉汉英中医词典》[10]	Bufonis Venenum	5
An Introduction to Chinese Materia Medica[12]	Venenum Bufoni	5
《汉英中医药分类辞典》[7]	Venenum Bufoni	5
《汉英中医辞典》[16]	Venenum Bufoni	5
《英汉实用中医药大全》[9]	Venenum Bufoni	5
《汉英中医药分类辞典》[7]	Venenum Bufoni	5
《中华人民共和国药典》[1]	Venenum Bufoni	5
《汉英常用中药手册》[17]	Venenum Bufoni	5
《中华人民共和国药典》[1]	Chansu	3
《汉英英汉中医大辞典》[20]	Toad-cake	3
《汉英英汉中医大辞典》[20]	Cake of Toad Skin	0
《汉英英汉中医大辞典》[20]	Dried Venom of Toads	0
《慈禧光绪医方选议》[15]	Chan Chu	0

2.2.3　中药矿物药名词的英译

中药矿物药名的英译，仍然是以英文译名最为常用，其次为拉丁学名，再次为汉语拼音音译，例如“自然铜”的译法见表3。

表3　“自然铜”的各种英译法在MEDLINE中出现的词频统计

来源工具书	译名	出现次数
《英汉实用中医药大全》[9]	Pyrite	111
《汉英中医药分类辞典》[7]	Pyrite	111
An Introduction to Chinese Materia Medica[12]	Pyrite	111
《新世纪汉英科技大词典》[13]	Pyrite	111
《汉英医学大辞典》[5]	Pyrite	111
《汉英英汉中医大辞典》[20]	Pyrite	111
《简明汉英日中医药词典》[6]	Pyrite	111
《汉英双解中医大辞典》[8]	Pyrite	111
《英汉汉英中医词典》[10]	Pyrite	111
《中华人民共和国药典》[1]	Pyrite	111
《简明汉英日中医药词典》[6]	Pyritum	3
《汉英中医辞典》[16]	Pyritum	3
《汉英常用中药手册》[17]	Pyritum	3
《新世纪汉英科技大词典》[13]	Pyritum	3
《中国中医药学主题词表》[3]	PYRITUM	3
《汉英医学大辞典》[5]	Pyritum	3
《中华人民共和国药典》[1]	Pyritum	3
《慈禧光绪医方选议》[15]	Pyritum	3
《汉英中医药分类辞典》[7]	Pyritum	3
《英汉汉英中医词典》[10]	Pyritum	3
Advanced Textbook on TCM and Pharmacology Vol. 2[18]	Pyritum	3
An Introduction to Chinese Materia Medica[12]	Pyritum	3
《英汉实用中医药大全》[9]	Pyritum	3
《中华人民共和国药典》[1]	Zirantong	1
An Introduction to Chinese Materia Medica[12]	Zirantong	1
《汉英英汉中医大辞典》[20]	Zirantong	1
《中国中医药学主题词表》[3]	Zirantong	0
《新世纪汉英科技大词典》[13]	Native Copper	0

2.2.4 方剂名词的英译

以单一汉字分别用汉语拼音音译最为常用，其次为两个以上汉字的拼音组合音译加剂型英译词，再次为意译。如“小柴胡汤”的译法见表4。

表4 “小柴胡汤”的各种英译法在MEDLINE中出现的词频统计

来源工具书	译名	出现次数
Chinese Herbs and Compatibility[19]	Xiao Chai Hu Tang	34
《英汉对照实用中医文库》[14]	Xiao Chaihu Tang	3
《汉英医学大辞典》[5]	Xiao Chaihu Tang	3
《简明汉英日中医药词典》[6]	Xiao Chaihu Tang	3
《汉英中医药分类辞典》[7]	Xiao Chaihu Tang	3
《新世纪汉英科技大词典》[13]	Xiao Chaihu Tang	3
Practical TCM & Pharmacology (Herbal Formulas)[11]	Xiao Chaihu Tang	3
《中国中医药学主题词表》[3]	Xiaochaihu Decoction	2
《汉英医学大辞典》[5]	Minor Decoction of Bupleurum	1
《简明汉英日中医药词典》[6]	Minor Decoction of Bupleurum	1
An Introduction to Chinese Ma-teria Medica[12]	Xiaochaihu Tang	1
An Introduction to Chinese Ma-teria Medica[12]	Minor Decoction of Bupleurum	1
《英汉对照实用中医文库》[14]	Minor Decoction of Bupleurum	1
《汉英双解中医大辞典》[8]	Minor Decoction of Bupleurum	1
《新世纪汉英科技大词典》[13]	Minor Decoction of Bupleurum	1
Advanced Textbook on TCM and Pharmacology Vol. 2[18]	Decoction of Bupleuri for Regulating Shao Yang	1
《英汉对照中医本科系列教材被方剂学分册》[4]	Minor Bupleurum Decoction	0
《汉英中医辞典》[16]	Decoction of Bupleurum for Regulating Shao Yang	0
《英汉汉英中医词典》[10]	Minor Bupleurum Decoction	0
《汉英中医药分类辞典》[7]	Minor (Mild) Bupleurum Decoction	0
Practical TCM & Pharmacology (Herbal Formulas)[11]	Decoction of Little Bupleurum Combination	0

2.2.5　中药剂型名词的英译

多译为相对应的英文词。

2.2.6　其他相关名词的英译

由于中成药、中药的药物作用、炮制加工煎服法及中药理论及学科类名词在MEDLINE中出现的频次极少，故未能找出其译法的规律。

3. 讨论

通过对22种工具书中600个中药名词英译法在MEDLINE的出现频率统计研究，可以从中找出目前中药名词英文翻译的一些规律。根据这些规律，我们建议，为了实现中药名词的英译标准化，应当作如下规定。

（1）对于中药材名词的译法，应以英文译名为标准，在学术性较强的中药专业文献中，可加注拉丁译名，以区别不同种属。尽量少用汉语拼音音译，必要时，可在英译或拉丁译名后附汉语拼音译名。

（2）对于方剂名或中成药名，以中文逐字汉语拼音音译为标准，或可加剂型英译词。

（3）对于剂型名词，以相应的英文词为标准译法。

（4）对于其他类型的中药复方名词，译法标准应视具体词汇而定，但原则应为简洁、符合英语习惯且不失中医特色。

参考文献

[1] 郭济贤．中华人民共和国药典．北京：化学工业出版社，1997.

[2] 凌一揆．中药学．上海：上海科学技术出版社，1984.

[3] 吴兰成．中国中医药学主题词表．北京：中医古籍出版社，1996.

[4] 北京中医药大学．英汉对照中医本科系列教材——中药学分册．北京：学苑出版社，1998.

[5] 汉英、汉法、汉德、汉日、汉俄医学大辞典编纂委员会．汉英医学大辞典．北京：人民卫生出版社，1987.

[6] 史载祥．简明汉英日中医药词典．北京：人民卫生出版社，1998.

[7] 谢竹藩．汉英中医药分类辞典．北京：新世纪出版社，1994.

[8] 原一祥．汉英双解中医大辞典．北京：人民卫生出版社，1997.

[9] 徐象才．英汉实用中医药大全．北京：高等教育出版社，1994.

[10] 魏迺杰．英汉汉英中医词典．长沙：湖南科学技术出版社，1996.

[11] 耿俊英．Practical TCM & pharmacology（herbal formulas）．北京：新世界出版社，1991.

[12] 刘昌孝．An introduction to Chinese materia medica. 北京：北京医科大学、中国协和医科大学联合出版社，1993.

[13] 柳闻．新世纪汉英科技大词典．北京：电子工业出版社，1997.

[14] 张恩勤．英汉对照实用中医文库．上海：上海中医药大学出版社，1990.
[15] 陈可冀．慈禧光绪医方选议．北京：外文出版社，1996.
[16] 欧明．汉英中医辞典．广州：广东科技出版社，香港：三联书店香港分店，1986.
[17] 欧明．汉英常用中药手册．广州：广东科技出版社，香港：三联书店有限公司，1992.
[18] 国家中医药管理局．Advanced textbook on TCM and pharmacology Vol. 2. 北京：新世界出版社，1995.
[19] Chen P. Chinese herbs and compatibility. 北京：科学出版社，1997.
[20] 郑风钦．汉英英汉中医大辞典．天津：天津大学出版社，1994.

[原载《中国中西医结合杂志》，2003，23（2）：150-152.]

中药商品名称的美学特征与英语名称的翻译

罗　磊

中医药学有着悠久的历史和丰富的内容。过去的中药商品仅限于丸、散、膏、露等成药，现代随着中药煎剂包装机械的出现，中药煎剂也具备了商品的条件。作为将商品推向国际市场并占领国际市场的重要工具，中药产品的名称除了能够反映商品属性之外，还具有自身独特的美学特征。当前，一方面是越来越多的国内中药产品要打入国际市场，另一方面是我国中药产品在国外市场的销售举步维艰，如何给国内中药商品取一个恰当的英语商品名称，怎样正确地翻译中药产品商标品牌名称，就显得现实意义更加重大。关于中药商标品牌名称的英译，国内英语界已从英汉语言及文化对比的角度作了诸多阐述。本文将结合中药商品名称的美学特征，从美学角度探讨英语中成药商标品牌名称的翻译问题。

众所周知，一个国家的商品在他国市场上成功与否的诸因素中，是否拥有广大的消费者是一个不容忽视的因素。而最大限度地拥有消费者，一方面与商品的效用、质量、颜色、设计、图案等有关，另一方面也与商品名称是否通俗易懂，是否符合他国广大消费者的审美需求有关[1]。在我国，Coca-cola（可口可乐）、Goldlion（金利来）、Boeing（波音）、Cannon（佳能）、Microsoft（微软）的品名现在已成为中国消费者熟悉的著名品牌。这些商品名称首先具有通俗美。所谓通俗美，是指商品名称要通俗易懂，容易为广大消费者所理解，同时符合普通群众的审美需求和审美能力，并为他们所接受和欣赏。同样的道理，在将中药翻译成英文时，应该以通俗美为基本出发点，使译名符合外国人的审美取向。只有这样，才能拉近产品和消费者的距离，增强产品的亲和力，从而激起消费者购买的欲望。目前，中药商品名称的翻译方法有音译、意译和音义译结合三种方法，但不管是哪一种，都应以具有通俗美为出发点。应该在简洁朴实、一目了然、易懂易记、引人入胜方面予以注意。下面我们根据以上原则，结合中药商品所固有的美学特征，把中药商品的英语翻译方法分成三类进行介绍。

1. 根据药物功效、主治病症取名

例如：保和丸，Digestion-promoting Pill；泻白散，Lung-heat Expelling Powder；肾气丸，Pill for Invigorating Kidney Energy；消风散，Wind-dispersing Powder；抗白喉合剂，Anti-diphtheria Mixture；温脾汤，Spleen-warming Decoction；败毒散，Antiphlogistic Powder；温经汤，Meridian-warming Decoction；宫外孕方，

Extrauterine Pregnancy Decoction；疝气方，Hernia Decoction；三痹汤，Triple Arthralgia Decoction；涤痰丸，Phlegm-eliminating Pellet；和胃片，Tablet for Regulating the Stomach；护肝养肾片，Tablet for Nourishing the Liver and Kidney；撮风膏，Paste for Relieving Wind-syndrome；宣青发表膏，Ointment for Letting out the Toxic Material；抗白喉流浸膏，Anti-Diphtheria Liquid Extract；补中益气煎膏，Decocted Paste for Strengthening Middle Warmer and Benefiting Vital Energy；收口膏药，Adhesive Plaster；定喘汤，Decoction for Relieving Asthma；补阳还五汤，Decoction for Invigorating Yang；咳喘糖浆，Syrup for Relieving Asthma & Cough 等。

根据商标学原理，商品名称应有记忆功能，具有简朴美。只有简洁朴实，才能明快，才能一目了然，才能易读、易懂、易记。以上这类中药商品的名称只包含有药物功效和剂型两个内容，满足了上述要求，并符合商标的主要功能。

2. 根据药料取名

例如：木香槟榔丸，Aucklandiae and Areca Pill；藿香正气散，Herba Agastachis Powder for Restoring Healthy Energy；鳖甲煎丸，Carapac Trionycis Bolus；苍耳子散，Xantbii Powder；人参汤，Ginseng Decoction；大柴胡汤，Large Bupleuri Decoction；乌梅饮，Mume Decoction；芍药汤，Paeonia Decoction；地黄饮子，Rehmanniae Decoction；黄芩汤，Radix Scutellariae Decoction；牡蛎散，Concha Ostreae Powder；苏合香丸，Resina Liquidambaris Orientals Bolus；桂枝汤，Ramulus Cinnamomi Decoction；附子汤，Aconiti Praeparata Decoction；大黄牡丹汤，Rhei and Moutan Radicis Decoction；大黄附子汤，Rhei and Aconiti Decoction；桑菊饮，Mori and Chrysanthemi Decoction；五仁丸，Five-semen Pill；柏子养心丹，Semen Biotae Pill for Nourishing the Heart；五仁露，Five Seeds Syrup 等。以上有以君药取名的，有以君药臣药共同取名的。

根据药材取名进行翻译，可使外国消费者了解中医成药的主要药物是什么，也利于外国消费者记忆药品的品牌，符合商标的简洁、明快的要求。

3. 根据中药商品名的奇特美取名

例如：碧玉散，Jasper Powder；玉女煎，Jade Maid Decoction；回春丹，Resliscitation Pill；鸡苏散，Rooster-weking Powder；鸡鸣散，Rooster-crowing Powder；桃花汤，Peach Blossom Decoction；紫雪丹，Purple Snow Pellet；白虎汤，White Tiger Decoction；青龙汤，Blue Dragon Decoction 等。

商品名称还应具有引人入胜的功能，使消费者产生购买商品的欲望。一般而言，使消费者对商品名称产生兴趣，进而对产品感兴趣的方法很多，而使商品名称具有奇特美不失为一种好方法。所谓奇特美就是指商品名称采用异乎寻常的表现手法，真实而又传神地反映商品的属性和效用。商品名称合乎事理的奇特，不仅可以收到出奇制胜的效果，使消费者对商品产生强烈的兴趣，而且其本身的美可以给消费者以强烈的美的感受。商品名称用的是普通词汇，品名与产品属性毫无瓜葛，这本身就给消费者以奇特的感受。对国外产品的汉语翻译就有不少成功的例子，如 canon 意为“大炮”，但是（佳能）却是复印机和打印机的品名。另外，一些药物由于字母组合异乎寻常，这些品名新颖独特，给人留下深刻印象。上面的译名中有以中文的比喻法译名译过来的，如碧玉散（Jasper Powder）、王女煎（Jade Maid Decoction），都有朦胧的诗意美；有以服药时间命名译名译过来的，如鸡苏散（Rooster-weking Powder）、鸡鸣散（Rooster-crowing Powder），强调了服药时间，易理解，易记忆；有以颜色命名的，如：桃花汤（Peach Blossom Decoction）、紫雪丹（Purple Snow Pellet），这些译法引人入胜，让人遐想，美不可言；有以动物命名的，如白虎汤（White Tiger Decoction）、青龙汤（Blue Dragon Decoction）。这两个品名对国外消费者是新奇的，也易于记忆。

将“白虎汤”“青龙汤”分别译成 Baihu Decoction 和 Qinglong Decoction[2] 是欠妥的，这就像世界著名品牌服饰 Crocodile，可以按源语的语义译成“鳄鱼”，而不必一定要采用音译一样。中国消费者听到“鳄鱼”，也并没有因为鳄鱼是可怕的动物而产生恐惧和厌恶。相反，译为 White Tiger Decoction 和 Blue Dragon Decoction，所产生的新奇、易于记忆的特点，也可以留给消费者鲜明的记忆。中药商品名称的翻译和人名等的翻译一样都可采用音译、意译、半音半意译或几种译法同时使用的方法。在音译、意译、半音半意译或几种译法同时可以使用的情况下，应该首先考虑意译，因为意译能够更充分地体现中药商品的内涵和文化气氛。但音译只适宜用于确实难以用其他译法表达其概念的术语，应尽量控制其数量[3]。如果我们过多地采用音译，就会使国外消费者产生难以理解诸多中药商品的感觉，影响记忆，就像我们常看到的诸多国外以汉语音译的商品名称易于混淆、难以理解一样，不能引起他人兴趣。比喻性词语也常出现在中药商品名称中，利用事物之间的相似特征，通过具体形象来比喻某种事物。运用比喻性词语是为了使语言生动、逼真，富有感染力。这是中医语言一种重要的修辞手段。汉语和英语都有丰富的比喻性词语，但因使用汉、英两种语言的人民有着不同的民族历史和风俗习惯，对比喻性词语的使用也有所不同。在英译中药商品名称注意利用比喻特征的同时，也必须注意汉英语言比喻特征的差别，力求能正确地表达原文思想内容，同时又能保持原文语言的修辞效果。另外，中药商品已有通行译法的，就要照用，不要与众不同，独出心裁。中药商品名称的翻译要按照“名从主人”与“约定俗成”的公认原则。新的中药商品名称的确立必须以认真的态度对待和创制。

总之，中药商品名称的翻译，可充分利用中药商品原本的意境和原本商品名称的美学特征，展示其通俗美、简朴美、奇特美，使国外消费者产生丰富而美好的联想，从而也有利于将中药推向世界。

参考文献

[1] 胡开宝．商品名称的美学特征与英译．中国翻译，2000，5：51-53.
[2] 李照国．中医英语翻译技巧．北京：人民卫生出版社，1997：401.
[3] 谢竹藩．关于中医名词术语英译的讨论．中国中西医结合杂志，2000，20（9）：706-708.

[原载《中国中西医结合杂志》，2003，23（3）：225-226.]

论中药七情的英文翻译

许凌之　施蕴中

中药配伍是中药临床应用的重要形式，它是中药向方剂过渡的一个桥梁。中药配伍之后，再确定恰当的剂量和剂型，即成为方剂。中药配伍是中医的一大特色。“七情”作为传统中药配伍理论的核心内容，在介绍传统中药配伍理论时必然要提及。现行《中药学》教材也仍将《神农本草经》中的中药“七情”作为中药配伍的主要理论和内容要求学生学习和掌握。鉴于“七情”的重要性，本文拟讨论中药“七情”的英文翻译现状、存在问题，并就如何翻译的问题提出个人见解。

1. 中药“七情”英文翻译现状

中药“七情”一说首见于《神农本草经》。经云：“药有单行者，有相须者，有相使者，有相畏者，有相恶者，有相反者，有相杀者。凡此七情，合和视之。当用相须相使者良，勿用相恶相反者。若有毒宜制，可用相畏相杀者；不尔，勿合用也。”笔者从《中药学》[1]《汉英英汉中医大词典》[2]、*Interactions Between Chinese Herbal Medicinal Products and Orthodox Drugs*[3]三本较有代表性的中医药著作中搜集了中药“七情”翻译的资料。因《汉英英汉中医大词典》有多种翻译形式，为了便于比较，笔者根据翻译信息密度原则[4]，略去解释性翻译。比较结果发现，中药“七情”的英文翻译多种多样（表 1）。之所以选择这三本著作，是因为这三本书代表了三类不同的情形：《中药学》为 2001 年出版，出版日期较近，且作为国内为数不多的中药学英译版教材，在国内外有一定影响，代表了当前比较流行的翻译方法。《汉英英汉中医大词典》成书年代较早（1994），该词典涵盖了其出版前多数的传统表达形式。*Interactions Between Chinese Herbal Medicinal Products and Orthodox Drugs* 一书是国外学者关于中药和西药相互作用的论著，书中提出了一些不同于国内的表达形式，反映了国外学者的理解和翻译。

表1　三本书中中药"七情"译法一览表

《中药学》	《汉英英汉中医大词典》	*Interactions Between Chinese Herbal Medicinal Products and Orthodox Drugs*
七情 seven prescriptions	seven emotions	the compatibility of herbs
单行 going alone	①using a single drug ②going alone	single application
相须 mutual reinforcement	mutual reinforcement	①synergism ②mutual reinforcement
相使 mutual assistant	mutual assistance	①mutual assistance ②mutual enhancement
相杀 mutual detoxication	mutual detoxication	mutual detoxification
相畏 mutual restraint	①incompatibility between two drugs ②mutual restraint	mutual inhibition
相恶 mutual inhibition	mutual inhibition	mutual antagonism
相反 antagonism	① antagonism between two drugs ② antagonism, incompatibility between two drugs	incompatibility

2. 中药"七情"一词的英文翻译

翻译"七情"一词关键在于区分"中药七情"和"情感七情"。《汉英英汉中医大词典》中"七情"仅有 seven emotions 一种译法。中医有"喜、怒、忧、思、悲、恐、惊"之"七情"。中药"七情"一词，作为中药学独特的专业术语，说的是中药七种配伍关系，翻译时如果局限于"情"（emotion），则会丧失原文的本意。compatibility 一词在西医药学中是"配伍"的意思。《泰伯百科医学词典》（*Taber's Cyclopedic Medical Dictionary*）对 compatibility 一词的解释是："state of suitability to be mixed or taken together without unfavorable results, as drugs"[5]，因此，可以借用此词，把中药"七情"译为 seven features of compatibility[4] 或者 the compatibility of herbs[3]。

3. 中药“七情”各词的英文翻译

翻译“七情”各词的关键在于区分单、双向关系。除单行外，“七情”其余配伍方式均以“相”字开头。“相”很自然的英文联想是“mutual”，因此，人们常将“相”译成 mutual，如“相使”译为 mutual assistance。先看“相”和 mutual 的含义。在《古汉语常用字字典》[6]中“相”（xiang，阴平）的解释有两个：①互相。②表示动作偏指一方，如好言相劝。在《牛津高阶英汉双解词典》[7]中 mutual 的解释有：①（of a feeling or an action）felt or done by each towards the other，指感想或行为相互的、彼此的，如 mutual affection、mutual suspicion 等。②［作定语］（of people）having the same specified relationship to each other（指人）有相同关系的。③〔作定语〕shared by two or more people（人与人之间）共同的、共有的、共享的。目前所知，“相”身兼两职，既可表示单向关系，也可表示双向关系。在中药“七情”中的“相”，有时表达单向（A 药仅作用于 B 药，或 B 药仅作用于 A 药）关系，有时表示双向（A、B 两药相互作用)。然而，mutual 却没有此功能，仅表示双向关系，因此，在选词时，并非“相”就和“mutual”一一对应。

3.1 翻译中药“七情”各词时 mutual 的使用

我们所查到的资料，除《中医英语翻译技巧》外，其他书[8-10]的译法基本与《汉英英汉中医大词典》一致（表 2）。《汉英英汉中医大词典》的作者已经注意到，对“相反”不用 mutual。《中医英语翻译技巧》一书的作者进一步认识到，对“相杀”“相恶”不用 mutual，但翻译其他各词时，是否都要用 mutual?

表 2 两本书翻译中药“七情”各词时 mutual 的使用

	《汉英英汉中医大词典》	《中医英语翻译技巧》
相须	mutual reinforcement	mutual promotion
相使	mutual assistant	mutual enhancement
相杀	mutual detoxication	detoxication
相畏	mutual restraint	mutual antagonism
相恶	mutual inhibition	inhibition
相反	incompatibility	incompatibility

3.2 “相须”和“相使”的英文翻译

相须和相使皆属于有利配伍。《神农本草经》云：“相须相使者良。”相须指性能相类似的药物配合应用，可增强原药物疗效。如石膏和知母配合能明显增强石膏、知母的清热泻火的疗效。相使指性能、功效方面有某些共性，或性能、功效虽不相同，但治疗目的一致的药物配伍应用，但以一药为主，另一药为辅，两药合用，提高主药的疗效。如补气利水的黄芪与利水健脾的茯苓配伍时，茯苓能提高黄芪补气利水的治疗效果[11]。要翻译好这两个词，关键在于区分相须和相使的同时，突出相使的单向主辅关系。

“相须”以往常译为 mutual promotion 和 mutual reinforcement，笔者认为把“相须”译为 potentiation 较为合适。在陆再英等编写的《英汉医学词汇》[12]（第 2 版）中解释道：promotion：促进作用、催化作用；reinforcement：增强、增力、加固；potentiation：增强、强化。此三词虽然有着近似的解释，但 promotion 和 reinforcement 是常用词，potentiation 则专指两药合用时的协同作用，在西医中广泛应用。《临床药理学》（*Clinical Pharmacology*）[13]一书对 potentiation 的解释是：“（to make more powerful）occurs when one drug increases the action of another。”《丘吉尔医学词典》（*Churchill's Medical Dictionary*）一书的解释是：A phenomenon in which the effect produced when two agents act together is greater than the sum of their effects when they act separately”[14]。《斯特德曼医学词典》（*Stedman's Medical Dictionary*）一书的解释是：“Interaction between two or more drugs or agents resulting in a pharmacologic response greater than the sum of individual responses to each drug or agent”[15]。借用西药的常用词，可以便于理解，建议用 potentiation 翻译“相须”。

“相使”，从字义分析，“使”，伶也（《说文》），从也（《尔雅》），役也（《广韵》）。此处当取役使、佐使，含襄助、辅佐之意[16]。根据主辅关系，assistance 是一个不错的选择。相使是单向的主从关系，“A 药、B 药为之使”，即 A 药为主，B 药为仆，B 药辅助 A 药发生作用。如人参、甘草为之使，加强人参补气之功；黄芪、茯苓为之使，可增强黄芪补气利水之功；附子、桑枝为之使，可增强附子散寒止痛、治上肢痹证之功，后者均为前者之使，绝不可能同时又出现“B 药、A 药为之使”的情况。正如陶弘景所说：“诸芝使署预，署预复使紫芝，计无应如此。”如果把“相使”译为“mutual assistance”，读者会认为“A 药、B 药为之使”的同时“B 药、A 药为之使”也成立，这是不符合原意的，因此，“相使”不应使用 mutual，只用 assistance 就足够了。

3.3 “相杀”和“相畏”的英文翻译

相杀，即一种药物能减轻或消除另一种药物的毒性或副作用。“杀”，戮也（《说文》），克也（《尔雅》），转义为减省（《广雅》）。故“A 药杀 B 药的毒”，即 A 药能减耗 B 药的毒力。如生姜能减轻或消除生天南星的毒性或副作用，所以说生姜杀生南星。相畏即一种药物的毒性反应或副作用能被另一种药物减轻或消除。“畏”，惧也（《广雅》），如生南星的毒性能被生姜减轻或消除，所以说生南星畏生姜。通常认为相杀与相畏是同一配伍关系的主动、被动两种提法。既说“生姜杀生半夏”，也说“生半夏畏生姜”。但有人提出，在实际临床使用中，相畏与相杀是有区别的，并非同一配伍的两种提法。当运用某种毒性药物的常用功效治疗疾病时，必须用相杀的配伍，以减轻或消除其毒性或副作用。当运用某种毒性药物的毒性或副作用治疗疾病时，应尽量避免相畏配伍，以保留其毒性或副作用，因此，相杀是毒性药物运用的常用配伍方式，相畏是毒性药物运用时的配伍禁忌[17]。

综上所述，“相杀”才是真正的 detoxification，“相畏”则可译为 toxicity restraint，这样既体现了相杀、相畏的侧重点，又不至于与“相恶”混淆。

3.4　“相恶”和“相反”的英文翻译

相恶，即两药合用时，一种药物能使另一种药物原有功效减弱，甚至丧失。“恶”，本义为过失，即不善（《说文》），引申为憎恶（《广韵》）。A 药恶 B 药，A 药不欲与 B 药相共也[18]。如人参恶莱菔子中，人参为补气药之首，大补元气，但是莱菔子的消积导滞作用能使人参补气作用削弱。同时，“相恶”是单向的，A 药恶 B 药，绝没有同时 B 药恶 A 药的情况出现。如陶弘景说：“牛黄恶龙骨，而龙骨得牛黄更良，此有以相制伏故也”，因此，笔者认为相恶不用 mutual，而建议用 inhibit。inhibit 的解释为：hinder，restrain，or prevent（an action or process），例如，cold inhibits plant growth[18]。人参恶莱菔子可译为 Lai Fuzi（semen raphani）inhibits Renshen’s（radix ginseng）effect，因此，“相恶”选用 inhibition 是合理的。相反即两种药物合用时能产生或增强毒性反应或副作用，如“十八反”“十九畏”中的若干药物。以往常用 incompatibility[2]（配伍禁忌[12]）作为“相反”的译文，但笔者认为并不合适。相恶和相反，一个减效，一个增毒，均属配伍禁忌。incompatibility 的词义覆盖了这两个词，因此，用其翻译“相反”不合适。“相反”一词的另一种常见译法是 antagonism。antagonism 一词来源于西医，指 mutual opposition or contrary action，即拮抗作用，包含以下两种情况[13]：①the action of one drug opposes the action of another（一种药物与另一种药物的作用相对抗）；②They compete reversibly for the same drug receptor（两者对同样的药物受体发生相反的作用），与中医所指并不相同。而且其相应的动词是“antagonize”，表示“对……起反作用、中和、抵消、对抗”[19]，也没有“产生或增强毒性反应或副作用”的意思，因此，不能采用。建议“相反”译为 negative-effect inducing。

参考文献

[1] 刘公望．中药学．北京：华夏出版社，2001：10－11.

[2] 郑凤钦．汉英英汉中医大辞典．天津：天津大学出版社，1994：305－306.
[3] Chank，CL. Interactions between Chinese herbal medicinal products and orthodox drugs. Singapore：Harwood Academic Publishers，2000：33.
[4] 李照国．中医英语翻译技巧．北京：人民卫生出版社，2001：133，76.
[5] Taber's cyclopedic medical dictionary. Philadelphia：F. A. Davis Company，1981：320.
[6]《古汉语常用字字典》编写组．古汉语常用字字典．北京：商务印书馆，1998：312.
[7] 霍恩比．牛津高阶英汉双解词典．4 版．李北达译．香港：牛津大学出版社（中国）有限公司，1997：973.
[8] 汉英、汉法、汉德、汉日、汉俄医学大词典编纂委员会．汉英医学大词典．北京：人民卫生出版社，1987：1781.
[9] 原一祥，任继学，黄龙，等．汉英双解中医大辞典．北京：人民卫生出版社，1996：676－677.
[10] 李照国．简明汉英中医词典．上海：上海科学技术出版社，2002：363－364.
[11] 雷载权．中药学．上海：上海科学技术出版社，1995：20.
[12] 陆再英，唐锦治，梁扩寰，等．英汉医学词汇．2 版．北京：人民卫生出版社，2000：1277，1350，1258.
[13] Laurence DR，Bennett PN，Brown MJ. Clinical pharmacology. 8 版．北京：科学出版社，1999：116－117.
[14] Koenigsberg，Ruth KR. Churchill's medical dictionary. New York：Churchill Livingstone Inc，1989：1502.
[15] Pugh MB. Stedman's medical dictionary. Baltimore：Lippincott Williams & Wilkins，2000：1434.
[16] 王家葵，张瑞贤．神农本草经研究．北京：北京科学技术出版社，2001：92－97.
[17] 李新旺，任钧国．中药七情探析．中医研究，2000，13（5）：11，21.
[18] 皮尔素．新牛津英语词典．上海：上海外语教育出版社，2001：939.
[19] 陈维益．英汉医学辞典．2 版．上海：上海科学技术出版社，1997：105.

[原载《中国中西医结合杂志》，2004，24（11）：1043－1046.]

中成药说明书“功能与主治”的文体特点与翻译

李俊梅

中成药说明书的“功能与主治”是其精华，是患者的用药指南，是医师和药剂师指导患者用药的依据。中成药说明书的“功能与主治”属于严谨的科技文体，“科技论文的翻译，辞藻在其次，文字要力求简单易懂，但内容知识一定正确无误地译出来”[1]。马谷城在谈到科技翻译时说“正确、通顺、易懂”三者是一个不可分割的整体[2]。我国生产的许多中成药疗效非常好，但其说明书的英文翻译误译较多。误译主要出现在中成药说明书中的“功能与主治”中。“功能与主治”的翻译主要涉及中医术语的翻译，应采取“对等翻译”或“等效翻译”。由于受中成药说明书文体的限制，在方寸之间为患者传递更多、更准确的信息尤为重要。

1. 中成药说明书“功能与主治”的特点

中成药说明书“功能与主治”涉及中医学知识和中医术语。中医术语是一种哲学语言、文学语言及日常生活用语的混合产物。中医术语貌似平常，实则内涵深邃，且一词往往具有多义性。中医术语是中医学中基本的、重要的成分，它们体现了中医语言的文体特征，其特点是直截了当、言简意赅，属于严谨的科技文体。

2. 中成药说明书“功能与主治”的翻译

中成药说明书“功能与主治”是说明中成药的药效范围，其翻译方法取决于中医术语和西医英文术语相对概念的差异情况。其翻译主要涉及中医术语的翻译。中医术语的翻译应遵循以下原则：中西医学术语差异不太大的采取对等翻译，差异较大的采取等效翻译，中西医学术语毫无相近之处者，采取音译。中成药说明书“功能与主治”常译为 Function and indication，Action and indication，Function and action，Function and usage。常用的句型为 It is indicated for...，It is indicated that... 等。

2.1 对等翻译（equivalence in translation)

中成药说明书“功能与主治”中只有一小部分的中医术语与西医术语有对应术语，或者中西医术语之间差异不太大，可采取对等翻译的方法。也就是说，对于中西医学概念的内涵和外延完全一致，术语严格对应者，可直接引用相对应的西医术语[3]。

例 1：中成药喉疾灵的功能与主治为：清热解毒，散肿止痛。用于腮腺炎、扁桃腺炎、急性咽炎……采取对等翻译的方法，可直接翻译为：Action and indication：antipyretic and antidote，detumescence and acesodyne. It is indicated for parotitis，tonsillitis，acute pharyngitis...。

例 2：中成药“ -月见草”的主治为：... 降脂、减肥、抗衰老。可译为：Indication：.... lipolysis，antiobesic and antiaging。

例 3：鸡谷草丸的功能为：清热解毒，消炎止痛。译为：Efficiency：antipyretic，antidote，antiphlogitic and pain-killing。

由于中西文化的差异，只有一部分中成药主治中的中医术语可采取对等翻译，如：心烦意乱 restless，失眠多梦 insomnia and dreaminess，心悸怔忡 palpitation，谵语发狂 delirium and mania，半身不遂 hemiplegia，大便秘结 constipation，体倦乏力 fatigue，不思饮食 losing appetite，月经不调 irregular menstruation，血漏血崩 metrorrhagia，视物模糊 poor vision，胃脘疼痛 ache in the stomach，头痛咽干 headache and pharyngoxerosis 等。

2.2　等效翻译（equivalence value in translation）

大部分的中成药“功能与主治”中的中医术语在西医学术语中找不到相应的术语，或者中西医术语内涵差异较大，采用等效翻译，特别是中医的四字术语，如采用直译不能准确表达原术语的整体含义，可采取解释性翻译，将中成药“功能与主治”中的中医术语译为名词短语、动词短语和动名词短语。

2.2.1　译为名词短语

如：气郁不舒 uncomfortable feeling due to the stasis of vital energy，肝郁不舒 uncomfortable feeling caused by liver congestion，贫血身虚 weakness due to anemia，肺瘀血咳 cough due to blood stasis in the lung，脾虚水泛 edema due to hypofunction of spleen，头晕自汗 dizziness and night sweat，气短心悸 shortness of breath and palpitation，表里俱实 exterior and inferior heat，外寒内热 exogenous cold-evil and interior heat-evil，恶寒壮热 chillness and high fever，眩晕耳鸣 dizziness and tinnitus，气血不足 insufficiency of the vital energy and blood，气血两虚 deficiency of vital energy and blood，肝肾阴亏 Yin-deficiency of the liver and kidney。

例 4：蜜炼川贝枇杷膏的功能与主治为：……用于伤风感冒，痰多痰稠，气喘不适，咽喉干痒及声音沙哑。译为：Actions and indications：... For relief ofcough due to cold，copious cough phlegm，discomfort throat，aphonia and hoarse。

2.2.2　译为动词短语

如：消积化滞 promote digestion to relieve dyspepsia，补气养血 invigorate the vital energy to nourish the blood，行气止痛 regulate vital energy circulation to relieve pain，胃脘满闷 feeling depressed and full in the gastric cavity，祛瘀调经 regulate menstruation by removing blood stasis。

例 5：三金片的功能主治为：……利湿通淋，补虚益肾。译为：Action and indication：... dispel dampness to relieve stranguria，tonify the human body and benefit the kidney。

例 6：活血通脉胶囊的功能与主治为：活血化瘀，通脉止痛。译为：Action and indication：promote blood circulation to remove stasis，dredge the meridium passage to alleviate pain。

例 7：乳康片的功能与主治为：疏肝解郁、软坚散结、消积化痰……。译为：Actions and indications：soothe the liver and regulate the circulation of Qi，resolve hard lumps，promote digestion to remove phlegm...

2.2.3 译为动名词短语

例 8：天麻丸的功能与主治为：祛风湿、舒筋通络、活血止痛，用于肢体拘挛、手足麻木、腰腿痛。译为：Actions and indications：It has the effects onrheumatism，relieving rigidity muscles and activating the channels，invigorating blood circulation to relieve pain. It is indicated for stiff limbs，numb extremities，lumbocrural pain。

例 9：冠参片的作用与用途为：本品有活血化瘀、通利络脉、养血安神等功用。译为：Function and usage：It is indicated for promoting blood circulation by removing blood stasis，dredging the meridium passage，nourshing the blood and tranquilizing the mind。

例 10：蜜炼川贝枇杷膏的功能与主治为：清热润肺，止咳平喘，理气化痰。译为：Actions and indications：clearing away heat and moisturizing lungs，stopping cough and asthma，regulating Qi and removing sputum。

3. 音译

随着东西文化的交流和相互影响，一些医药英语新词已逐渐成为人们日常生活和工作中家喻户晓的词汇。这些新词以英语的本来面目出现，不需要翻译成汉语。有些中医术语也是这样。拿中医学的“气”来讲，有功能之气，也有物质之气；有先天之气，也有后天之气；还有元气、宗气、营气、卫气、正气、肾气、中气等。翻译时可直接用拼音“Qi”来代替。其他常见的音译还有：阴阳 Yin-Yang，五行 Wuxing，推拿 Tuina，气功 Qigong，三焦 Sanjiao，足三里 Zusanli，太阴 Taiyin，少阳 Shaoyang，命门 Mingmen。要使中医学某些特有的概念在英译中保持特有的内涵，音译恐怕是唯一可行之法[4]。

例 11：地奥心血康的功能与主治为：活血化瘀，行气止痛。译为：Action and indication：Promote blood circulation by removing blood stasis，promote the Qi circulation to relieve pain。

例 12：脑血栓片的功能与主治为：活血化瘀，醒脑通络，潜阳熄风。译为：Action and indication：The medicine is able to promote blood circulation by removing blood stasis，refresh the brain and remove the obstruction in the channels，suppress the hyperfunction of liver-Yang to eliminate wind evil。

要想译好中成药说明书中的“功能与主治”，译者首先要弄懂中医术语的内涵，也就是理解原文。在理解原文的基础上，用规范语言来表达原义。译者要认真推敲每个词的用法，切记望文生义，绝不能硬译、死译。

参考文献

[1] 张树柏．谈科技论文的翻译．北京：外语教学与研究出版社，1984：331－334.

[2] 马谷城．漫谈科技英语翻译——“信、达、雅”小议．北京：外语教学与研究出版社，1984：345－347.

[3] 李俊梅．词汇空缺与中医术语的翻译．中国中西医结合杂志，2007，27（3）：272－273.

[4] 李照国，朱忠宝．中医英语翻译技巧．北京：人民卫生出版社，2001：58－60.

[原载《中国中西医结合杂志》，2009，29（4）：357－358.]

中医方剂名称英译的归化与异化

蒋基昌

随着中外文化交流的增加，当前的翻译理论对译文文化因素的要求日益提高。归化和异化翻译作为与语言及文化密切相关的翻译策略逐渐受到人们的重视，对它们的争论也不曾终止。译者一方面要忠实于原文，另一方面又要使译文流畅，符合译文读者的思维习惯。异化与归化两种方法均有其自身的价值，应相辅相成，共同使翻译起到跨越不同文化的桥梁作用。笔者从中医方剂名称翻译的具体情况出发，阐述归化及异化翻译各自的优势与劣势，以及这两种翻译策略对中医方剂名称的理解与学习造成的影响。

1. 中医方剂的命名

中医方剂的名称是几千年来众多医家治疗疾病、综合运用中药的文化反映。由于历史、学派、地域、宗教等方面的原因，方剂的命名方法各种各样，名称也五花八门，有些还具有浓厚的宗教和民族文化特色。通常来说，方剂的命名方式有：①以主要药物命名，如银翘散；②以中心功用命名，如回阳救急汤；③以治疗效用命名，如失笑散、泰山磐石散；④以适应证命名，如五淋散；⑤以脏腑配合五行特征命名，如白虎汤、大青龙汤；⑥以数字和数量命名，如四妙勇安汤；⑦以历史典故命名，如诸葛行军散；⑧以特殊性命名，等[1]。

2. 中医方剂名称的翻译

国内外使用的英文版中医教材中，方剂名称的翻译都是以汉语拼音加上英语翻译。在翻译这类中医专有名词时，译者会碰到诸多问题，例如，如何正确理解方剂名称的科学属性和文化内涵，如何选择正确的对应词语，如何做到译文既忠实可信又能被西方读者理解接受等。在翻译以主要药物命名、中心功用命名和适应证命名的方剂名称时，相对来说比较简单，直接把剂型和药物名或疗效或适应证翻译出来即可。容易产生文化冲突的英译往往来自于以其他几种方法命名的方剂名称。目前，对此类方剂名称的翻译主要有归化和异化两种方法。

2.1 归化翻译

中医方剂名称的归化翻译可把方剂的作用和功效直接表达出来，外国读者一看便懂，更不会有文化的冲突和误解。以白虎汤为例，“白虎，西方金神也。应秋而归于肺。热甚于内者，以寒下之；热甚于外者，以凉解之；其有中外俱热，内不得泄，外不得发者，非此汤则不能解之也。夏热秋凉，暑暍之气，得秋而止，秋之令曰处暑，是汤以白虎命之，谓能止热也”[2]，因此，有人提出白虎汤应该译为 Decoction for Eliminating Heat[3]。若翻译成“White Tiger Decoction”[4]，会让人误解为此方是治疗白虎的疾病，或者是取白虎的某个器官入药。由金魁和主编《汉英医学大辞典》中的中医方剂名称在翻译基本上采用归化翻译，如失笑散译为 Wonderful Powder for Relieving Blood Stagnation；保和丸译为 Pill for Promoting Digestion；泰山磐石散译为 Miscarriage Preventing Powder；疏凿饮子译为 Decoction for Diuresis 等[5]。从上述例子可以看出，归化法翻译后的译本易于使中医文化被西方本土文化读者接受，获得读者的身份认同。简单、易懂的“归化法”译本可以帮助西方读者了解中医，为孕育中医的中国传统文化和英语国家的固有文化相容提供肥沃的文化土壤。

2.2 异化翻译

与归化翻译不同，异化翻译强调源语言的主导作用，译文应保留源语言的语言特点，尊重源语言文化的身份和地位，或试图故意保留其异域性。如，失笑散能活血祛瘀、散结止痛，患者服用后，于不知不觉中诸证悉除，不禁欣然失笑，故名“失笑散”。采用异化翻译，把失笑散译成 Sudden Smile Powder[6] 和 Breaking into a Smile Powder[4] 能充分表达该方的命名意图。又如，四妙勇安汤仅有四味，功效绝妙，且量大力专，勇猛迅速，使邪祛病除，身体健康，平安无虞，故称四妙勇安汤。英译有 Mysterious Four Resting Hero Decoction[6]，Decoction of Four Wonderful Drugs for Quick Restoration of Health[5] 等。本方的异化翻译值得商榷。“四妙”是指四种巧妙配伍的中药，用“mysterious”来翻译欠妥。姑且把第一种英译回译成中文，为“神秘的四个休息英雄汤”，与原方的含义风马牛不相及。第二种英译与原方的含义非常接近，但把“安”翻译成“康复”，似乎过于宽泛。针对本方的主治，“安”有两种含义：一者本方主治足趾溃疡，十指连心，疼痛异常，患者不停地大声呻吟；再者本方主治病证属热入血分，火毒内蕴，患者夜间烦躁，亦不得入睡。服用本方后，热清痛止，血分得安，患者即可安静而入睡。而且把“中药”译成“drugs”值得商榷。“drugs”指西药、毒品，而用“herbs”则比较恰当。“妙”字用“wonderful”来翻译，本身没有错，但如果用“well matched”来翻译也许更能反映原方巧妙的配伍。古人云：治身如治国，用药如用兵。从原方特点出发，笔者探索性地把“勇”译为“potent”，把“安”译为“stopping groaning”，将“四妙勇安汤”翻译成 Decoction of Four Well Matched Potent Herbs for Stopping Groaning，也许更能完整地体现原方的命名意图。这种异化的翻译方法保留了源语言的语言特征和药剂名称内涵的文化意义，同时又符合目标语的表达习惯。

综上所述，异化法译本较归化法译本更能体现中医英译的简洁性原则、民族性原则和回译性原则，有着不可取代的优势。异化法译本能保持中医用语简明扼要的特点，能反映一个国家和民族的文化特色，是一种文化区别于另一种文化的象征，能较为准确地再现源语言所含信息，减少翻译过程对信息的损益程度，有利于提高翻译质量，限制滥译。

3. 归化与异化翻译的优劣

在翻译中医方剂名称时，归化法与异化法各有千秋。归化翻译能够从目标语言的视角进行阐述，结合目标语的文化特征及语言习性，特别适用于初学者及对中医不甚了解者，有利于中医的快速传播和推广。但由于归化法忽视了源语言的文化特征及方剂所包含的历史渊源或特殊含义，读者无法知道方剂命名的真正科学内涵和文化属性。从某种意义上说，中医方剂名称的归化翻译是对源语言和文化的背叛，是对读者的欺骗。如“失笑散”译为 Wonderful Powder for Relieving Blood Stagnation，其字面意义为活血化瘀的好药，与“失笑散”的命名内涵相差甚远；而且中医活血化瘀的方剂有数十甚至数百。长此以往，将不利于外国学习者对中医中药的深入了解，甚至可能造成他们学习中的障碍。异化翻译注重将方剂名称异域化，尽量保留源语言中方剂名称的特点和文化气息，虽不如归化翻译那样简单易懂，但却更接近方剂命名的本意，更能体现出方剂名称的精髓。如，疏凿饮子为治水肿之峻剂，适用于外而一身尽肿，内而口渴、便秘之上下表里俱病之候。方中既有宣降肺气、疏散表邪之药，又有温运脾阳、渗湿利水之药，使上下疏通，表里透达，内外照应，标本同治。其消散上下内外之水势，犹如夏禹治水，疏江凿河，开其闭塞，从而使水道通畅，江河顺流，不致横溢泛滥成灾矣，故称“疏凿饮子”。“Decoction for Diuresis”这种归化翻译仅说明了该方的作用，无法体现该方药效峻猛，犹如夏禹治水、疏江凿河的特点。源语言的“疏”和“凿”分别有疏通和开凿的意思，比喻该方剂功效之强大，见效之迅速。笔者试图将其翻译成 Dredging and Canalizing Decoction，还原了源语言的特点及意义，不仅对于了解中医方剂的读者来说易于接受，更能反映出该方剂名称的原本含义。

4. 结语

归化和异化是翻译界长期争论的一个问题。主张归化处理者，旨在保证读者对译文接受的顺畅程度不因异质语言文化因素而受影响；坚持异化处理者，目的恰恰在于求异，希望能通过引入异质文化因素而丰富本国文化，促进世界文化在真正意义上的互补交流[7]。世界各种文化具有普遍性，但又有特殊性；翻译不仅仅是两种文字之间的文字转换活动，更是两种语言背后的文化交流活动。中医是几千年来中华民族的文化结晶，她是一门独立完整的科学，我们必须保持其语言特色和风格，并进一步发扬光大，而无权使她变得支离破碎，或使其变成一个大杂烩。中医英译者必须不断地完善自己，始终站在本民族文化的最大利益上，以民族文化为核心，展开较深层次的研究，提高中医英译质量[8]。在方剂名称的翻译中，应该以异化翻译为主，同时结合归化翻译，让学习者能够更好地理解方剂的命名缘由及其语言文字与文化特点，深入掌握中医方剂的文化特征、历史渊源及语言特征，从而触及中医药的本质，同时亦能将中华民族传承千年的传统文化发扬光大，让中医中药这块瑰宝在国际舞台大放异彩。

参考文献

[1] 张养生，张卫华．方剂命名目的性与原则性的探索．中国中医基础医学杂志，2006，12(9)：652-654.

[2] 成无撰．伤寒明理论．上海：上海科学技术出版社，1959：63.

[3] 康广盛，周洪伟．浅谈中医英译中方剂名称的翻译．中国中西医结合杂志，2008，28(6)：555-556.

[4] Maciocia G. The foundations of Chinese medicine. London：Churchill Livingstone Publishers Limited，2005：1149，1162.

[5] 金魁和．汉英医学大辞典．北京：人民卫生出版社，2004：1737，1877，1889，1893，1894.

[6] 魏迺杰．英汉汉英中医辞典．长沙：湖南科学技术出版社，1996：631，749.

[7] 吴建．中英口译中的文化输出．上海翻译，2008，96(3)：41.

[8] 欧阳勤，卢晓青，郑坚英．文化对中医英文翻译的影响．福建中医学院学报，2007，17(2)：53-56.

[原载《中国中西医结合杂志》，2012，32(8)：1144-1145.]

"Zhibai Dihuang" 还是 "Zhibo Dihuang"?

——也谈中医方剂名英译

刘九茹

方剂名英译是中医术语英译的一个重要组成部分。根据 2004 年全国科技名词术语审定委员会和中医名词术语审定委员会主持召开的"中医名词术语审定会议"确立的简洁、统一、易于回译等中医术语翻译原则，目前方剂名英译实践中多采用音译加意译的翻译方法，如麻黄汤：Ma Huang Tang（Ephedra Decoction），乌梅丸：Wu Mei Wan（Mume Pill）等。

然而，笔者研究发现，方剂名英译中译名不统一的现象时有发生，其中最常见的是由汉语多音字带来的译名不统一，严重影响了方剂名英译的规范化、科学性和统一性。以中医经典名方知柏地黄丸的英译为例。笔者通过 CNKI 检索发现，知柏地黄丸（汤）中的"知柏地黄"四字目前至少存在以下不同的译法：

（1）Zhibodihuang：HPLC 法测定知柏地黄丸浓缩丸中马钱苷的含量：Determining the contents of Loganin in Zhibodihuang Concentrated Pill by HPLC[2]。

（2）Zhi Bo Di Huang：知柏地黄丸浸液对大鼠嗜铬细胞内钙的作用：The effects of extract of Zhi Bo Di Huang Wan on the Ca^{2+} of rat chromaffin cell[3]。

（3）Zhibai Dihuang：双波长薄层扫描法测定知柏地黄丸中盐酸小檗碱的含量：Determination of berberine hydrochloride in Zhibai Dihuang Wan with scanning method of two-wave lengths thin layer chromatography[4]。

（4）Zhi-Bai-Di-Huang：知柏地黄汤对解脲脲原体感染大鼠精子活力的影响：Experimental study of Zhi-Bai-Di-Huang Decoction in treating ureaplasma urealyticum and enhancing spermatozoa motility[5]。

（5）ZhiboDihuang：知柏地黄汤联合二甲双胍治疗 2 型糖尿病 52 例临床观察：Clinical observation on the treatment of 52 cases of DM Ⅱ with ZhiboDihuang Decoction and metformin[6]。

由以上例子可以看出，对知柏地黄丸中的多音字"柏"字的不同认识是导致该方剂名英译不统一现象出现的主要原因。根据《现代汉语词典》，"柏"字有三个读音：① 柏，bǎi，柏树，乔木，木材质地坚硬，用来做建筑材料。② 柏，bó，柏林，德国城市名。③柏，bò，黄柏，同黄檗，乔木，木材坚硬，茎可制黄色染料，树皮可入药，也作黄柏。知柏地黄丸由六味地黄丸加知母、黄柏（黄檗）两味中药配伍而成。由此看来，知柏地黄丸中的"柏"字应读作 bò，译成英语就是 bo（Bo）。

多音字是汉字中常见的现象。所谓多音字就是一个字有两个或两个以上的读音。不同的读音表义不同，用法不同，词性也往往不同。汉字多音现象由来已久，现代汉字中多音字数量很大。在国家语言文字工作委员会、国家教育委员会颁布的《现代汉语常用字表》中，常用字 2500 字，其中多音字 411 字，占全部常用字的 16.4%；次常用字 1000 字，其中多音字 110 字，占全部次常用字的 11%左右。汉字多音常常造成人们出现误读现象，因此，应当引起人们的重视。由于汉字读音有区别词性和词义的作用，翻译中的拼音错误无疑会影响到方剂名翻译的准确性和科学性，如将 Baizi Yangxin Wan（柏子养心丸）译成 Bozi Yangxin Wan 等。

古汉语中也有多音字，这种现象称为异读。异读词是指一个词有几个不同的读音，而这几个不同的读音表达的完全是同一个意思。例如把“波浪（bō làng）”说成“pō làng”，把“机械（jī xiè）”说成“jī jiè”，把“比较（bǐ jiào）”说成“bǐ jiǎo”。异读词给普通话学习增加了负担，所以从 1956 年开始，国家就组织人员对普通话异读词的读音进行审定，给大量异读词确立了规范读音，排除了其他读音。并于 1963 年和 1985 年公布了《普通话异读词审音表》初稿和修订稿，因此，现在异读词的读音应该以 1985 年公布的审音表为准。此后的辞书（如《现代汉语词典》，1996 年版）已按该表注音。

语言国情学认为，凡是含有国情的概念均应音译，以利于保持其基本内涵。中医翻译是科技翻译，科学用语力求客观、严密、准确、简洁。汉语多音字的存在是客观现实，我们在方剂名音译过程中要特别注意汉语多音字的问题，勤查词典，将中医方剂名准确完整地传播到世界各地。

参考文献

[1] 中国社会科学院语言研究所词典编辑室．现代汉语词典．北京：商务印书馆，2004：14，48，50.

[2] 徐桂香，杨婕，陈钟文．HPLC 法测定知柏地黄丸浓缩丸中马钱苷的含量．河南中医学院学报，2007，22（4）：30－31.

[3] 叶琴，陈良怡，张春光，等．知柏地黄丸浸液对大鼠嗜铬细胞内钙的作用．华中理工大学学报，2000，28（6）：108－110.

[4] 张明昶，李健，张小勇．双波长薄层扫描法测定知柏地黄丸中盐酸小檗碱的含量．贵阳医学院学报，2002，27（6）：511－513.

[5] 郑毅春，刘朝圣．知柏地黄汤对解脲脲原体感染大鼠精子活力的影响．辽宁中医药大学学报，2007，19（3）：205－207.

[6] 罗学林，赵郴．知柏地黄汤联合二甲双胍治疗 2 型糖尿病 52 例临床观察．中医药导报，2005，11（6）：15－18.

[原载《中国中西医结合杂志》，2010，30（11）：1221－1226.]

方剂学“君、臣、佐、使”英译的探讨

蒋基昌

君、臣、佐、使是中医方剂学的重要组方原则。目前对这些中医术语的英译国内外有各种不同的译法。笔者就国内外的常见译法，与 2007 年 10 月 16 日颁布的《世界卫生组织西太区传统医学国际标准名词术语》中的译法进行比较分析，辨别优劣，旨在进一步规范统一这些中医术语的英译。

1. “君、臣、佐、使”的常见译法

常见英译有“monarch、minister、assistant、guide”[1]，“sovereign（chief）、minister（associate）、adjuvant（assistant）、courier（guide）”[2]，“sovereign、minister、assistant、envoy”[3]，“principal、assistant、adjuvant 、guiding”[4]，“emperor、minister、assistant、courier”[5]等。《世界卫生组织西太区传统医学国际标准名词术语》把“君、臣、佐、使”分别翻译成 sovereign、minister、assistant、courier[6]。

2. “君、臣、佐、使”的英译分析

2.1 “君”的英译

常见的有 monarch、sovereign、emperor、principal、chief。principal 和 chief 意思非常接近，都有“重要的、主要的”的含义。《韦伯斯特大辞典》对 monarch、sovereign、emperor 的解释为[7]：monarch 是指“国王或一个拥有极高地位或权力的人；sovereign 是指在一定范围内拥有至高权力的人或公认的领袖”；emperor 是指“国王或一个帝国的至高统治者”。方剂学中的君药是指针对病因或主证起主要治疗作用的药物，是方剂组成中最重要的药物。以上的英译都能表达“君药”的含义，但 principal 当名词用时是“负责人、校长、主犯”等意思，与“君”的词义相差甚远。从忠实的角度来看，“君”翻译成“sovereign”最为贴切准确。

2.2 “臣”的英译

“臣”的英译比较一致，大多数译为 minister，以辅助 sovereign。associate 当名词用时意为“同伴、朋友”。assistant 意为“助手、帮手”，级别较低。associate和 assistant 都不如 minister 准确贴切。

2.3 “佐”的英译

佐药有 3 种含义：①佐助药，即配合君药、臣药以加强治疗作用，或治疗兼病与兼证的药物；②佐制药，即起到制约君药、臣药的峻烈之性或减轻消除君药、臣药毒性的药物；③反佐药，即病重邪甚，可能拒药时，配用与君药性味相反而又能在治疗中起相成作用的药物。“佐”的英译有 assistant 和 adjuvant。adjuvant 是西医术语，指免疫佐剂，用它来翻译容易引起误解和混乱。assistant 基本上能表达佐药的三种含义，而且在级别上比 sovereign 和 minister 要低，用它来翻译“佐”最为恰当。complement 当名词用时意思是“补足物、定额人数和装备”，无法表达“佐”的含义，更不能体现君、臣、佐、使的等级内涵。

2.4 “使”的英译

使药有两种含义：①引经药，即引导方中诸药达到病所的药物；②调和药，即调和方中诸药性味的药物。“使”的英译有 guide、courier、envoy。guide 当名词用为“导游”的意思，无法充分承担带有特殊任务的“使药”的文化内涵。《韦伯斯特大辞典》对 courier、envoy 的解释为：courier 是指“信使或军队中的传令兵”；envoys 是指“外交事务中的全权特使或特别代表。”[7] 从《韦伯斯特大辞典》的解释来看，用 courier 来翻译比较恰当。

3. 讨论

“君、臣、佐、使”是将古代社会治国的行政和人际关系移植于方剂学中，从而来说明方中诸药的配伍关系。《世界卫生组织西太区传统医学国际标准名词术语》把“君、臣、佐、使”分别翻译成 sovereign、minister、assistant 和 courier 是非常贴切的翻译，既能准确表达“君、臣、佐、使”的科学属性，又能传递中医的文化哲学内涵。中医术语的英译应该采用 WHO 颁布的标准翻译，而不应闭门造车，以免引起更多的误解和混乱。尽管这些标准译法有值得商讨的地方，但作为一名中医翻译工作者应带头去遵守国际组织所制定的标准，也只有这样才能正确翻译中医术语，更好更快地促进中医的对外传播与发展。

参考文献

[1] 金魁和．汉英医学大辞典．北京：人民卫生出版社，2004：1812.
[2] 谢竹藩．新编汉英中医药分类辞典．北京：外文出版社，2002：376.
[3] 魏迺杰．英汉汉英中医辞典．长沙：湖南科学技术出版社，1996：532.
[4] 杨育周，储利荣．方剂学．北京：人民卫生出版社，2001：109.
[5] Qiu J. Traditional medicine：a culture in the balance. Nature，2007，448：126.
[6] WHO Western Pacific Region. WHO international standard terminologies on traditional medi-

cine in the Western Pacific Region，2007：264.

[7] Webster M. Webster's ninth new collegiate dictionary. Massachusetts：Merriam Webster Inc，1987：299，417，408，765，1128.

[原载《中国中西医结合杂志》，2010，30 (10)：1105.]

浅谈中医英译中方剂名称的翻译

康广盛　周洪伟

目前中医药术语英译的研究与实践都有了长足的进展，但仍未形成统一的规范。笔者认为，中医方剂名称英译一般均可采用以英语直译为主、意译为补充的方法，有特殊含义的方剂名称英译时可采用拼音音译与意译相结合的方法。

1. 采用以英语直译为主、意译为补充的方法

尽管中医方剂名称命名方法多种多样，但一般均可采用以英语直译为主、意译为补充的方法。

1.1　以方中药味数目为主命名的方剂

以方中所含药味数目命名的代表方剂十灰散，可译为 Powder Made of Ashes of Ten Herbs；四物汤，可译为 Four Herbs Decoction；四君子汤，可译为 Decoction Made of Four Noble Herbs。

1.2　以方中药物为主命名的方剂

以方中君药命名的代表方剂桂枝汤，可译为 Ramulus Cinnamoni Decoction；以方中臣药命名的代表方剂炙甘草汤可译为 Honey-Roasted Radix Glycyrrhizae Praeparatae Decoction；以方中使药命名的代表方剂十枣汤，可译为 Ten Fructus Ziziphi Jujubae Decoction；以方中所含诸药名命名的代表方剂大黄甘草汤，可译为 Radix et Rhizoma Rhei and Radix Glycyrrhizea Uralensis Decoction。

1.3　以方剂功效或主治命名的方剂

以方剂功效命名的代表方剂止嗽散，可译为 Powder for Relieving Cough；越鞠丸，可译为 Pill for Relieving Stagnation。以方剂主治命名的代表方剂四逆散，可译为 Powder for Treating Cold Limbs。

1.4　以方中君药加功效命名的方剂

代表方剂黄连解毒汤，可译为 Rhizoma Coptidis Decoction for Relieving Toxin。

1.5　以方中药味数目加君药命名的方剂

代表方剂九味羌活汤，可译为 Decoction of Nine Herbs Containing Rhizoma seu Radix Notopterygii。

1.6　以方中药味数目加功效命名的方剂

代表方剂三子养亲汤，可译为 Decoction of Three Kinds of Seeds for the Aged。

1.7　以方中药味用量比例关系命名的方剂

代表方剂六一散，可译为 Six-to-One Powder。

需要指出的是，在中医方剂名称英译的具体实践中，存在着对方剂中所含中药名称的两种翻译方法，一种为中药名称的拉丁语翻译，另一种为中药名称的英语翻译。由于拉丁语翻译中药名称较为规范，能够有效避免中药误译与误用，故笔者认为应采用拉丁语译法。

2. 具有特殊含义的中医方剂名称采用拼音音译与意译相结合的方法

中医方剂名称中有些是具有特殊含义的，单纯采用英语直译容易造成明显的错译，此时则应采用拼音音译与意译相结合的方法为好。举例如下。

2.1　白虎汤

当前有许多译者直接将其译为 White Tiger Decoction，这种翻译不能将白虎汤的本意表达出来，而且会给读者造成极大困惑，笔者认为是不足取的。成无己[1]指出："白虎，西方金神也。应秋而归肺。热甚于内者，以寒下之；热甚于外者，以凉解之；其有中外俱热，内不得解，外不得发者，非此汤则不能解之也。夏热秋凉，暑暍之气，得秋而止，秋之令曰处暑，是汤以白虎命之，谓能止热也。"由此笔者认为，白虎汤可译为 Bai Hu Tang（Decoction for Eliminating Heat）。

2.2　右归丸

也有译者直接将其译为 Backing to the Right Bolus，这种译法也同样不能将右归丸的中医内涵表达出来。《难经・三十九难》指出："肾两者，非皆肾也，其左为肾，右为命门。"[2]陈士铎认为，"命门者，先天之火也"[3]。右归丸"温补肾阳，填精益髓"，主治"肾阳不足，命门火衰证"[4]。由此笔者认为，"右归丸"可译为 You Gui Wan（Bolus for Reinforcing Kidney-Yang）。

中医学是以中国传统文化为背景所形成的一门独特的医学理论体系，所以要准确地将中医学翻译为英语，不仅要有扎实的英语基础及较渊博的现代医学知识，还必须精通中医学理论。以上笔者对中医英译中方剂名称翻译的探讨，希望能对中医药术语英译的统一化和规范化略尽绵薄之力。

参考文献

[1] 成无己撰．伤寒明理论．上海：上海科学技术出版社，1959：63.
[2] 南京中医学院校释．难经校释．北京：人民卫生出版社，1979：94－95.
[3] 陈士铎．石室秘录．北京：中国中医药出版社，1991：277.
[4] 段富津．方剂学．上海：上海科学技术出版社，1995：142－143.

[原载《中国中西医结合杂志》，2008，28（6）：555－556.]

试论方剂学“君、臣、佐、使”的英译

陈　金　张庆荣

“君、臣、佐、使”是中医方剂学用来分析和说明方剂结构和功能的重要说理工具，是将产生于古代社会人际从属关系的概念移植于方剂学中，从而借人际从属关系来说明一首方剂之中诸药的相互关系，通常被称作“组方原则”，也有称之为“组方结构”者。自从成无已在《伤寒明理论·药方论》中将之具体地应用于方论之中以后，“君、臣、佐、使”就成为分析方剂的重要内容之一。尽管“君、臣、佐、使”在中医方剂学研究中有如此悠久的应用历史，但其含义却经历了较为纷繁的变化。同时，正是由于其含义比较复杂，所以对于“君、臣、佐、使”的英译，各家又多有不同之处。

在此本文试图通过对“君、臣、佐、使”含义的源流变化加以归纳和整理，并分析说明现在公认的“君、臣、佐、使”含义，从而进一步分析“君、臣、佐、使”的英译方法并找出较为合理的英译形式。

1. 君药

1.1　源流

根据历代较为一致的观点，取《素问·至真要大论》：“主病之谓君”之义，而非《神农本草经》：“上药一百二十种为君”。

1.2　含义

君药，有“一方之中群药之尊首”的含义。“君，尊也”（《说文》）、“君也者，掌令者也”（《春秋繁露》）、“君者，治辨之主也”（《荀子·礼论》）、“克长克君”（《诗·大雅·皇矣》）。在《广雅疏证》中有：“君，群也……君者，善群也……”，表明君为“群”的组织者。在一首方剂中，君药应当是治疗疾病的最重要的药物，对疾病的治疗发挥着主要和主导作用，是必不可少的，为方中诸药之长。

1.3　英译

翻译君药时常用的单词有：principal、monarch、sovereign、chief。其中principal作为名词，有“a head，ruler，or superior”的含义。作为形容词含有“重要的、首要的、主要的”意思，如在《简明牛津英语词典》（*The Concise Oxford English Dictionary*，第9版）中其释义有：“①first in rank or importance；chief；②main，leading”等。monarch主要是对君主制国家元首的正式称呼，更多的

是象征极权。sovereign 的含义与 monarch 相近，指国家元首而言。而 sovereign remedy 是万能药、灵丹妙药的陈旧用法。《简明牛津英语词典》中的这一义项的解释为：excellent；effective。容易引起对方剂学中所指君药的错误理解。chief 一词从词源上来讲来自于拉丁语 caput，有“head”的意思，一般指部落首领、组织的领导人等，作形容词时有“最重要的、主要的、首席的、最高级别的”含义。综上，“君药”一词应以 principal 一词对应为优。

2. 臣药

2.1 源流

“臣”取《素问》“佐君之谓臣”这一含义，而《本经》中“中药一百二十种为“臣”的含义为后世所不用，故不予分析。其中“佐”字的含义为以下助上，故在《素问》中臣药有“较为主动地辅助君药”的含义。

2.2 含义

臣药，为辅佐君药而设。臣药必须服从、增强并扩大君药的治疗作用。“臣，事君者也。象屈服之形。”(《说文》)、“仕于公曰臣”(《礼记·礼运》)、“事君不贰是谓臣”(《国语·晋语》)。

2.3 英译

对臣药的翻译经常使用 assistant、minister、adjuvant、associate。

assistant 一词在《简明牛津英语词典》中的解释为：“a person who assists, esp. as a subordinate in a particular job or roll”，较为接近方剂学中臣药的定义。另外，assistant 有动词形式 assist，翻译时行文较为方便。

minister 指的是“a head of a government department”，在作动词使用时，有给“某人以帮助”的意思。

adjuvant 的含义为“an adjuvant (helpful, auxiliary) person or thing”。这一含义与臣药含义是较为接近的，但却不能反映臣药在级别上要低于君药这一情况。此外，在医学方面有免疫佐剂的含义：“a substance which enhances the body's immune response to an antigen”，故易引起对臣药的误解。

associate 的含义为“a business partner or colleague”或者“a friend or companion”，即伙伴、同事、朋友，与臣药的含义不符。

故对臣药的英译应以 assistant 为宜。

3. 佐药

3.1 源流

前述臣药内容中，已有“佐”的字样，其含义为辅助，而金·成无己在《伤寒明理论·药方论》中使用“佐”时为受臣药宣摄之意。此外，《素问·至真要大论》中有这样一句话："奇之不去则偶之，是谓重方。偶之不去则反佐以取之。所谓寒热温凉反从其病也"，王冰以"声气相合"注之，为后世"反佐"一说之肇始。此外，明·何瑭《医学管见·论君、臣、佐、使第十六》曰："热药之过甚而有害也，须少用寒凉药以监制之，使热药不至为害，此所谓佐也"的观点与后世医家佐制的提法十分相近。此外，《医原》一书中又出现了"正佐""反佐"这样两相对应的提法。综上，成氏之佐为正佐、佐助，王氏之佐为反佐，何氏之佐为佐制，而反佐、佐制二义又构成广义的反佐。

3.2　含义

佐药，以下助上为佐，以其位低而能助君臣药得名。"太宰之职，常建邦之六典，以佐王治邦国"（《周礼·天官》）。

在现代中医方剂学中，常将佐药分为佐助、佐制、反佐三种，又有以佐助为正佐，佐制、反佐二者为反佐的观点。正佐或佐助体现了佐药的本义，是指与君臣药药性相同而力不及之而言。反佐（佐制、反佐）为后世派生出的意义，指与君臣药药性相反而稍稍用之，以制毒纠偏或引君臣药与病相合，从而有利于君臣药治疗疾病作用的合理发挥的药物。佐制，是指对君臣过偏之药性或其毒性的制约或消除作用。反佐，强调药性与君臣药相反而与病邪性质相同或相似，按"同气相求"之理，可以引君臣药与病邪相合，从而有助于祛除病邪。

3.3　英译

佐药常用 assistant、adjuvant 两词，但 assistant 一词已用于臣药，故不再适宜单独用于翻译佐药，可以考虑以 secondary assistant 的方式表述。而 adjuvant，正如前述，作为一个已经存在的西医学词汇，再用于中医方剂学中亦难免引起误会。

若从用词简洁及一致的角度考虑，secondary assistant 的表述方式略嫌繁琐，故佐药用 complement 一词更为适宜。作名词时，可以解释为：something that completes，作动词其含义为 complete。词源为拉丁词 complementum，含义为 fill up，即填满的意思。在方剂学中使用此词，寓有"将一方药物补充完满，对方中主要药物的补充"之意。

对佐助药的翻译可以用 due complement，这一形式也可用于对正佐药的英译。

对佐制药的翻译可以为：diminution complement。

diminution 作为名词有"变小、减少"的意思，在《简明牛津英语词典》中解释为："the act or an instance of diminishing"。其词源为拉丁语 diminut，意为"break up small"。两词相合，有"减少"和"消除"的含义。故佐制药可以以"diminution complement"的方式表达。

在翻译反佐时，常用的词有 corrigent、contrary、paradox 等。

corrigent 一词的含义为矫味剂、矫正剂，减轻药物过强作用或改善药味的物质。似乎容易与“使药的调和作用”这一含义相混淆。

contrary adjuvant 也是对佐药的一种表达方法，但表达为 contrary assistant 更为合适一些。从前后一致的角度来讲，“反佐”可译为 contrary complement。另外，也有人将“反佐”译为 contrary treatment，这种译法将反佐与反治两个不同级别的概念相混淆，是不可取的。此英译形式也可以用作与正佐相对应的广义的反佐的英译。另外，与 contrary 一词意义较为接近的 opposite、reverse 等词也可以用在反佐的翻译中。

paradox 一词意为“矛盾”，或“似是而非、似非而是”，与“反佐”的含义相去甚远，故不宜使用。

所以，翻译“佐药”宜用 complement 一词，应以 due complement 表示“正佐”（佐助），diminution complement 表示“佐制”，contrary complement 表示“反佐”。

4. 使药

4.1　源流

《素问》：“应臣之谓使”，即使药是受臣药支配、差遣之药。《本经》曰：“下药一百二十五种为佐使”，这一观点与方剂学的观点所不符。何瑭曰：“引经及引治病之药于病所者使也”，其义似从中药学“引经报使”一说变化而来。后世又混合“引经”与“药引”两种说法，遂产生“使药调和诸药”的观念。

4.2　含义

现代方剂学中使药的第一层含义为专入一经，直达病所，与病相遇，即所谓引经报使。杜佑《通典·职官典》曰：“设官以经之，置使以纬之。按察、采访等使以理州县。节度、团练等使以督府军事。租庸、转运、盐铁、青苗、营田等使以毓财货。其馀细务因事置使者，不可悉数。其转运以下诸使，无适所治，废置不常，故不别列于篇。”——可见，“使”多专为一事所设，具有专一性和临时性。使药的另一含义为“沟通，调和方中诸药之关系，使方中诸药药力、药性及功效虽不同而能协和，有上下协调”之意。故简言之，使药的含义在于引药到达病所和协调诸药（也有据此认为矫味的药物为使药者）之意，是为方中其他药物服务的药物。当然，本经及某些后世医家也有以被众药驱使之药为使药者，在此不予讨论。

4.3　英译

使药常用 guide、courier、messenger、mediating 等形容词或名词，若词性为形容词，往往加在 drug、herb 等代表药物或中药的单词前面构成相关词组。

guide 一词可以作名词使用。作名词时其含义为：①a person who leads or

shows the way, or directions the movements of a person or group; ②a person who conducts visitors or tourists on tours, etc.; ③a professional mountain climber in charge of a group 等。guide 与引经报使的含义非常契合，可以直接用作为“使药是引经药”这一层含义的英语形式。

courier 指“信使、专业导游”而言，与引经报使含义略有差别，但也可以使用。

messenger 的含义为：①a person who carries a message; ②a person employed to carry messages，即送信者、信使、通信员，故不适合做使药的英语对应词。与 messenger 类似的词还有 dispatcher，其动词 dispatch 含义为发送（send off to a destination or for a purpose），另外还有“结束、消灭”的含义。dispatcher 一词本身还可以解释为“发报机”。故 messenger 和 dispatcher 两词不适合用作“使药”的英语对应词。

此外，还有 conductant 一词，其名词及动词形式为 conduct，与 lead 或 guide 词义相近，但似乎现有英文字典并无此词。

从调和药的角度翻译使药，常用的词为 mediating，其动词形式 mediate 的意思是 intervene (between parties in a dispute) to produce agreement or reconciliation，即“调停、调解、斡旋”的意思。可以作为“使药是调和药”的这一层意思的对应词。也可以使用 harmonizing 一词。即作为调和药性的使药，在其翻译时可以为 mediating guide 或 harmonizing guide。在需要行文简洁及强调调和作用时，也可以使用 mediator 一词来表达有调和作用的使药。

综上所述，中医方剂学中“君、臣、佐、使”可以相应地译为 principal、assistant、complement、guide，而“佐助”（或“正佐”）“佐制”“反佐”可以译为 due complement、diminution complement、contrary complement，使药的“引经药”这一含义应作为其本义，不予变化，仍用 guide 一词，而在需要特别强调其“调和诸药”这一含义时，译作 mediating guide，或简洁表述为 mediator。

[原载《中国中西医结合杂志》，2007，27（10）：946－948.]

中成药名的常见英译结构

周 珏　曲凡　南睿

中成药名的英译是中医英译的重要组成部分。笔者在实践中总结了 8 种中成药名常见的英译结构，现简述如下。

1. 病（症）名＋剂型

直译即可。如“肺痈汤”译为“Pulmonary Abscess Decoction”。

2. 功效＋剂型

可译为“剂型＋for＋功效”。如“疏经活血汤”译为 Decoction for Dredging Meridians and Promoting Blood Circulation；“补中益气汤”译为 Decoction for Strengthening Middle Warmer and Benefiting Vital Qi；“血府逐瘀丸”译为 Bolus for Eliminating Blood Stasis in Chest。

3. 药物＋剂型

可译为“剂型＋of＋药物”。如“牡蛎散”译为 Powder of Concha Ostreae；“防己黄芪汤”译为 Decoction of Stephaniae Tetrandrae and Astra gali seu Hedysari。

4. 药物＋功效＋剂型或功效＋药物＋剂型

可译为“剂型＋of＋药物＋for＋功效”。如“安宫牛黄丸”译为 Bolus of Calculus Bovis for Resurrection；“藿香正气散”译为 Powder of Agastachis for Restoring Healthy Qi。

5. 病（症）名＋功效＋剂型

可译为“剂型＋for＋病（症）名＋to＋功效”。如“乙肝扶正胶囊”译为 Capsule for Hepatitis B to Support Healthy Qi。

6. 病因（机）＋病（症）名＋剂型

可译为“剂型＋for＋病（症）名＋due to＋病因（机）”。如“三痹汤”译为 Decoction for Arthralgia due to Wind，Cold and Dampness。

7. 含有“特色词汇”的中成药名

需要结合中医药学知识将中成药名中的“特色词汇”的含义翻译出来。如“缩泉丸”，“缩”有减缩收敛之意；“泉”原指水泉，这里形容功能同水泉的膀胱。缩泉丸能使肾虚得补，精气益固，寒气温散，遗尿自止，好像泉水缩敛一般，故命名缩泉丸，译为 Bolus for Decreasing Urination。再如对“更衣丸”的翻译，“更衣”，古时称大、小便之婉辞，因此，将其译为 Bolus for Removing Constipation。

8. 需要音译的特例

有些中成药名的命名很特殊，在这种情况下，笔者建议音译为妥。如“二至丸”中的“二至”指夏至和冬至两个节气，是以药物的采集时间命名。“一贯煎”中的“一贯”体现创立者“一以贯之”注重肝肾阴虚辨证观点的医学思想。类似于这种内涵丰富、命名特殊的中成药名还无法将其简明准确地英译出来，音译实为无奈之举。总之，中成药名的英译应遵循科学性、简洁性、标准性和信息性的原则。

[原载《中国中西医结合杂志》，2007，27（7）：616.]

方剂名称英译

杨伊凡

中医药学有数千年的历史，据完备的方剂书籍刊载，已经有 5 万多个方剂，但临床常用的不过是数百个。就这些方剂的名称英译而言，均还没有比较统一的译法标准。有直译的，如“白虎汤”译为 White Tiger Decoction；有意译的，如“逍遥散”译为 Ease Powder，“龙胆泻肝汤”译为 Bolus of Geniana for Purging Liver Fire；有根据功效译的，如“左金丸”译为 Liver Fire Purging and Stomach Regulating Pill；有以药物的名称译的，如“香连丸”译为 Aucklandia-Coptis Pill；有混合意思译的，如“香砂六君子汤”译为 Decoction of Costus and Amomum with Six Noble Ingredients。这些译法看上去比较混乱，不利于学生学习和医师临床使用。笔者认为目前也没有一种固定的译法是最好的，比如说统一采取直译，或意译，或功效译，或药名译等，都无法达到最佳效果。中医药英译是一门新兴的学科，没有现成的词汇，大多都是创造的。对一些词汇的翻译，谁先使用，然后大家跟着用，时间长了，就习惯了，虽然回过头来看可能并不是最好的译法，但已经得到约定俗成，也就变成了大家共同的标准了。如小青龙汤译为 Xiao Qing Long Tang (Minor Blue Dragon Formula)，六味地黄丸译为 Liu Wei Di Huang Wan (Rehmannia Six Formula) 等。

关于方名使用中文拼音的问题，我们认为需要使用，并且建议大写，至少音节第一个字母大写，并且音阶之间要间隔。所以所有方剂都是由“拼音＋英文方名”两部分所组成。因为对于所有的中药我们都是用拼音作为教学和临床方式使用的。

方名采取这种翻译方式，清楚、易区分，避免单纯使用拼音或单纯使用英文或拉丁文容易混淆的缺点。如用于日常教学和临床，则可单用拼音名；如用在书面或写文章等较正规的场合，则采取两部分合成法。

至于中药处方名是否要采用拉丁文的问题，我们认为主要是不实用。澳大利亚联邦药物管理局使用的规范“中草药名”是 Name of Therapeutic Herbs，相当于有效植物药名，并不是拉丁文，也不同于植物名——Botanical Name。中药方剂的中文方名有的用汤、丸、散、丹等，因此，人们翻译时也是跟着使用不同的单词相对应，如“汤”——decoction，“丸”——pill，“散”——powder，等。笔者认为，由于所有中药方剂都是复方的方剂，是否可以以“方剂”——formula 来作统一规范。所以在教学和临床使用时，我们都一律使用这种表达，也很实用方便。

方剂毕竟是由有治疗作用的中药组成的，要做到方剂翻译既要表达中文方名的意思，又要保持医学词汇比较严肃的特色，我们认为拼音加主药（一般英文名）的译法可取。如“八珍汤”，如其按“八种珍贵的药物组成的方剂”来翻译，不如使用 Bazhen Tang（Ginseng and Danggui Eight Formula（英文名的意思是由人参和当归等 8 种药物组成的方剂）来得简洁而朴实，也达意。有些方剂名称因古代沿袭的原因，比较夸张，如“仙方活命饮”等，直译起来似乎不太严肃。

现将常用的中医十大名方的英译列举如下：逍遥散 Xiao Yao San（Bupleurum & Danggui formula），六味地黄丸——Liu Wei Di Huang Wan（Rehmannia Six formula），补中益气汤 Bu Zhong Yi Qi Tang（Ginseng & Astragalus formula），龙胆泻肝汤——Long Dan Xie Gan Tang（Gentiana formula）；小柴胡汤 Xiao Chai Hu Tang（Minor Bupleurum formula）；归脾丸——Gui Pi Wan（Ginseng & Longan formula）；黄连解毒汤——Huang Lian Jie Du Tang（Coptis & Scute formula）；银翘散——Yin Qiao San（Lonicera & Forsythia formula）；血府逐瘀汤——Xue Fu Zhu Yu Tang（Persica & Cnidium formula）；温胆汤——Wen Dan Tang（Bamboo & Hoelen formula）。

［原载《中国中西医结合杂志》，2005，25（8）：713.］

中医方剂名英译问题探讨

——格式及其内涵

申　光

方剂是中医学中的一个重要组成部分，其命名方式基本上可以归纳为：①以方剂的组成命名，如麻黄汤、桑菊饮等；②以方剂的主要功效作用命名，如生化汤、承气汤等；③以方剂主治病症命名，如鹭鸶咳丸等；④以方剂用法、制剂等特点命名，如十灰散、鸡鸣散等；⑤以立方者的思想内容命名，如白虎汤等。总之，方剂的命名不仅是为了区别，更重要的是它还表达了立方人的思想内涵，因此，在将其翻译成英语的时候一定要注意到其内涵。再者，中医方剂名属于药品名称，为了使其符合药名的国际通用标准规范统一，在翻译时应参照拉丁语药品命名法。

《汉英医学大词典》翻译方剂名的方法是音译加意译。笔者认为这种方法是对的，既能反映中医方剂名的特色，又有助于外国人理解。但是，在具体翻译中，却存在着两个方面的问题。一是译名在格式上不符合药名的国际通用标准——拉丁语药品命名法，如："丹参饮"译为 Red Sage Drink，"泰山磐石散"译为 Miscarriage Preventing Powder，等。二是有些方剂名的英语翻译忽视了名称的内涵，只是简单地将其直译出来，这样就会使外国人产生误解或文化休克。如"白虎汤"译成"White Tiger Decoction"，"二妙散"译成"Two Wonderful Drugs Powder (Pill)"，"大青龙汤"译成"Major Decoction of Green Dragon"，"小青龙汤"译成"Miner Decoction of Green Dragon"等。下面笔者就以这几个译名为例阐述一下自己的观点。

首先，在译名的格式上，笔者认为应该遵循拉丁语药品命名法的格式，这样既符合国际惯例，也能使方剂的英语译名在格式上规范统一。具体到方剂的译名上，笔者认为应该比照拉丁语药品命名法中的制剂类药品命名法的公式，即：剂型（名词主格）＋原料药（名词属格）。如 Pulvis Rhei Compositus（复方大黄散）。说明制剂的性质、用途等时，用介词短语，如 Aqua pro Injectione（注射用水）等。虽然英语的语法与拉丁语的语法有所不同，如英语的名词没有变格的概念等，但在格式上却是可以比照的，也就是说应该把剂型放在前面。如上例中的"丹参饮"应该比照 Pulvis Rhei Compositus（复方大黄散）的译法译成 Drink of Red Sage，"泰山磐石散"比照 Aqua pro Injectione（注射用水）的译法译成 Powder for Preventing Miscarriage。

其次，在翻译方剂名时，一定要注意其内涵，千万不要做望文生义的翻译。如上面提到的白虎汤、二妙散、小青龙汤的翻译。这几例翻译不仅存在着格式上的问题，而且还存在着意义上的问题。下面阐述个人的一点见解。

1. 白虎汤

根据《中国古方方名考》，白虎汤中的“白虎”并不是“白色老虎”的意思，而是四象之一。《三辅黄图》中说：“苍龙、白虎、朱雀、玄武，天之四灵，以镇四方。”四象就是按照方位将 28 个星座分为东、南、西、北四个部分，每方各有七宿。白虎就是西方七宿的总称。如果将西方的七个星宿用线条勾勒出来，其形状就像老虎，因此，就有了“西方白虎”之称。在一年四季之中，四象之中会随季节的变化出现不同的星宿，这样又把四象配以春、夏、秋、冬，以观星宿的方位变化。东方苍龙配春，南方朱雀配夏，西方白虎配秋，北方玄武配冬。白虎司秋令，秋天意味着由热转凉，因此，白虎汤一方就是一副清热剂。这样就应该将其翻译成：Decoction for Removing Pathogenic Heat。

2. 二妙散

二妙散由黄柏、苍术两种药组成，属于清热药。方中的苍术，辛苦而温，芳香而燥，其作用是燥湿强脾；黄柏苦寒下降，其作用是清下焦湿热。这两种药相配，阴阳相济，标本兼治，中下两宣，是相得益彰的绝妙配伍，因此，被命名为二妙散。这里的“妙”字是指这两种药搭配起来所产生的绝妙效果，并不是指这两种药本身有多么妙，因此，用 wonderful 一词就不大合适，而应该将其翻译成：Powder (Pill) of Two Well-matched Drugs。

3. 小青龙汤

根据《中国古方方名考》，小青龙汤中的“青龙”与“白虎汤”中的“白虎”所指一样，并不是“青色的龙”的意思，而是四象之一。这里的“龙”指的是“东方苍龙”。《周易·文言》中说：“云从龙”。也就是说龙兴云就会生，有了云就会有雨，雨能润及万物，天下太平。人如果出现太阳病无汗又兼烦躁的症状，也可以“兴云致雨”，施以汗解。青龙为东方木神，司掌春天。春天之时，万物生长，因此，青龙木神具有生长发散的性能，大、小青龙汤也具有这些作用，所以取名“青龙”。大青龙汤与小青龙汤的区别在于，大青龙汤方中的麻黄用量比麻黄汤中的麻黄用量增加了一倍，其发汗作用更强。小青龙汤能驱除水饮，如龙潜隐在波涛之中。这样，大、小青龙汤就应该分别译成：Decoction for Diaphoresis with Larger Dose of Ephedra 和 Decoction for Diaphoresis with Smaller Dose of Ephedra。

综上所述，在将中医方剂名翻译成英语时，一是要比照拉丁语药品命名法中的制剂类药品命名法的公式，这样可以使译名在格式上规范统一，符合国际标准。二是注意方名的内涵，不要望文生义，翻译出会使外国人产生误解或文化休克的译名来。

[原载《中国中西医结合杂志》，2004，24（8）：751－752.]

第三节　针灸经络英译实践

浅谈“络穴”的英译

田开宇

随着针灸疗法在国际上的广泛应用，其相关术语翻译的规范化在对外培训和学术交流方面的作用愈显重要。虽然 WHO 也发行过一些有关针灸的出版物，但仅涉及了穴位和头皮针的标准名称，对于针灸其他相关术语尚未能进行统一和规范。目前国内出版的中医针灸书籍的英语翻译多停留在约定俗成、相互借鉴的阶段，使得一些术语的英译未能真正体现针灸学的理论内涵。本文以“络穴”的英译为例说明这一问题。

“络穴”是针灸脑穴中特定穴的一类，是指十五络脉从经脉分出处的 15 个穴位。十五络脉是经络系统的一个重要组成部分，是指直接从经脉别出的 15 条大的络脉，总称为“十五络脉”，其名称也是借用十五络穴的名称分别命名的，如手太阴络脉名为列缺。在 WHO 的出版物《标准针灸穴名》（*Standard Acupuncture Nomenclature*，中“络脉”已被翻译为“Collateral"，而“络穴”却无相应英译。由于“络”有“联络”之意，长期以来“络穴”一直被半音半意译为“Luo-Connecting Point”，并被广泛接受。目前使用较广、影响较大的教材也采纳了此英译，如普通高等教育“十五”国家级规划教材——《针灸学》[1]、全国高等中医药院校外国进修生教材——《针灸学》[2]，(英汉对照）新编实用中医文库——《中国针灸》[3]。然而，笔者在国外从事针灸学交流以及在国内讲授留学生课程时，深感外国学者和学生由于两者英译的无关联性而引起对其理解不便，所以本人认为“络穴”的翻译应当体现出络穴与十五络脉两者的关系，即“络穴”是十五络脉从经脉分出处的穴位，在“络脉”译为“Collateral”的情况下，考虑可否将“络穴”译为“Collateral Point”。

由于汉语中“络穴”和“络脉”中的“络”字的音、形、义完全相同，我们从未担心过有人会将“络穴”误以为是“络脉”的穴位，同样，其对应英译“Collateral Point”也不会被外国学者、学生误以为是“Collateral”的“Point”，相反，却能使他们更好地理解“络穴”和“络脉”这两个概念的关联性，同时也体现了中医术语翻译的一致性和回译性原则。

参考文献

[1] 石学敏. 针灸学. 北京：中国中医药出版社，2002：24.
[2] 张吉. 针灸学. 北京：人民卫生出版社，1999：174.
[3] 赵京生. 中国针灸. 上海：上海中医药大学出版社，2002：27.

[原载《中国中西医结合杂志》，2007，27 (3)：269.]

中医针灸学论文标题的英译

田开宇

为了促进中医药学的国际交流与合作，国内中医学、针灸学方面的学术刊物大都附有由论文标题构成的英文目录。一个好的标题可以起到概括全文、吸引读者和便于检索的作用，同时也反映出原作者和刊物的较高学术水平和较强影响力。

1. 标题的语言特点

标题常用不完整的句子，多用名词、名词词组或动名词。例 1：Effective Acupuncture Therapy for Stroke and Cerebrovascular Diseases[1]。例 2：Using the Power of Belief in Acupuncture and Holistic Medicine：Case Studies[2]。标题一般由一个名词或若干并列的名词加上必要的修饰语构成，没有谓语成分。但个别情况因表述的需要也可例外，亦可使用疑问句。例 3：Can the Addition of Moxibustion during Acupuncture Therapy Improve Recovery from Bell's Palsy ?[3]

2. 标题的写作要求

2.1 主题突出，简短明了

标题字数一般在 10 个单词以内，最多以不超过 15 个词或两行为宜。例 4：Conservative Therapy with Acupuncture for Injury to the Sciatic Nerve Resulting from Intramuscular Drug Injection[4]。副标题往往用以突出论文的某一方面，如病例数、研究方法、重点内容或连载论文各分篇等。所以若表述需要导致标题较长，可以副标题的形式处理。例 5：The Demystification of Chinese Pulse Diagnosis：An Overview of the Validations，Holograms and Systematics for Learning the Principles and Techniques[5]。标题首单词为 Observation、Effect、Analysis、Influence、Study、Treatment、Relationship 等时，其前的冠词可以省略。

2.2 避免冗余的谦虚套语

中医论文的标题常带有表示谦虚意味的词，如“初步分析”“初步观察”“初探”“心得体会”“之我见”等。这类句式在国外期刊已不用，甚至连“Study of”“Investigation of”“Report of”等开始的形式也已少见。科技论文应立足于事实材料，非实质性内容皆可省略不译，而并不会影响文章的主题和文献检索。

2.3 尽量避免使用缩略词语

为了使读者准确地了解文章内容，标题中使用缩略词有失恰当，特别是疾病名称，更应避免使用非标准缩略词语。如此缩略词已通用且无歧义，亦可使用。例 6：Determination of Safety Needling Depth via CT-Scan Studies of Tissue Thickness[6]。例 7：Diagnosis and Treatment of Idiopathic Thrombocytopenic Purpura[7]。本标题未使用“ITP”指代“Idiopathic Thrombocytopenic Purpura”。

2.4　标点、大小写要求

标题中虚词（冠词、连词、介词等）除了 4 个字母以内并且不位于句首的以外（例 5、9），每个词的首字母都应大写，末尾一般不用标点符号。例 8：Investigation into Potential Synergism Between Body and Auricular Points for the Treatment of Hypertension[8]。

2.5　病例数的处理

在外文期刊中，因病例数不列入检索题目，为了突出文章主题，又不影响检索，通常不将病例数列入正标题中，必须使用时可置于副标题中。例 9：A New Classification System and Combined Treatment Method for Idiopathic Facial Nerve Paralysis：Report on 718 Cases[9]。

3. 标题中涉及针灸术语的英译

经络、腧穴、针具等术语的翻译应遵从 1991 年由 WHO 马尼拉会议制定的《标准针刺术语命名》（*Standard Acupuncture Nomenclature*）。如：经（Meridian）、络（Collateral）、三焦经（Triple Energizer Meridian）、督脉（Governor Vessel）、足三里［Zusanli（ST 36）］、印堂［Yintang（Ex-H N3）］、三棱针（Three-edged needle）、皮肤针（Dermal needle）、皮内针（Intradermal needle）、头针（Scalp acupuncture）。

参考文献

［1］Effective acupuncture therapy for stroke and cerebrovascular diseases. Am J Acupunt，1993，21（3）：205.

［2］Using the power of belief in acupuncture and holistic medicine：case studies. Am J Acupunt，1993，21（1）：33.

［3］Can the addition of moxibustion during acupuncture therapy improve recovery from bell’s palsy? Am J Acupunt 1998，26（1）：33.

［4］Conservative therapy with acupuncture for injury to the sciatic nerve resulting from intramuscular drug injection. Am J Acupunt，1996，24（4）：241.

［5］The demystification of Chinese pulse diagnosis：an overview of the validations，holograms and systematics for learning the principles and techniques. Am J Acupunt，1993，21（1）：63.

［6］Determination of safety needling depth via CT-scan studies of tissue thickness. 中国中西医结合杂志，1992，12（5）：258.

[7] Diagnosis and treatment of idiopathic thrombocytopenic purpura. 中国中西医结合杂志 1992，12（5）：304-306.

[8] Investigation into potential synergism between body and auricular points for the treatment of hypertension . Am J Acupunt，1995，23（2）：184.

[9] A new classification system and combined treatment method for idiopathic facial nerve paralysis：report on 718 cases. Am J Acupunt，1995，23（3）：205.

[原载《中国中西医结合杂志》，2001，21（11）：871.]

经络学说术语的英译

袁洪仁

经络学说是中医学的重要理论，是古人在长期的医疗实践中，从针灸、推拿、气功等各个方面积累的经验，结合当时的解剖学知识，按阴阳五行、天人合一模式而提出的机体功能调节理论。经络学说术语的英译必须忠实于这个事实。

1. 经络的英译

文献中将“经络”译作“Channels and Collaterals”或“Meridian”，这种意译令人费解。根据《黄帝内经》对经络的论述及现代经络研究的结果，表明经络结构包括血管网络（血行脉中）、神经网络（气行脉外）和感传网络（经气游行），故“经络”应译作“Neurovaso Qiduct”，意为“神经血管性气导管”。这种译法既表达了经络原有神经血管解剖学基础之事实，又表达了经络“内属于脏腑，外络于肢节”之类神经血管必然的网络形态。加上后缀“-Qiduct”又区别于解剖学上的神经血管，表达了中医经络“行气血”的功能特征。可将“Neuro-vaso-Qiduct”缩写为“NVQ”。相应地，“经络学说”译作“NVQology”。

2. 经脉和络脉的英译

“经脉”是经络系统中直行的干线，故译为“Stem of NVQ”，意为“经络之干”，可缩写为“SNVQ”。经脉有正经与奇经之分，前者与脏腑络属，后者与脏腑无络属关系，别道奇行。故“正经”译作“Visceral-SNVQ”，意为“脏腑之经脉”[1]。“奇经”译作“Extra-ordinary SNVQ”，意为“异常经脉”“奇异经脉”。

“络脉”是经脉的分支，故译作“Branch of NVQ”，意为“经络之支”，与“经络之干”（经脉）相对，可缩写为“BNVQ”。相应地，“别络”“孙络”“浮络”分别译为“Bigger BNVQ”（较大的络脉）、“Tiniest BNVQ”（最细小的络脉）、“External BNVQ”（表浅的络脉）。

参考文献

[1] 袁洪仁．谈藏象与脏腑术语的英译．中国中西医结合杂志，2000，20（3）：164.

［原载《中国中西医结合杂志》，2001，21（3）：198.］

腧穴本义与英译

沈雪勇

腧穴，即通常所说的“穴位”和“穴道”，古时又称“气穴”“孔穴”“输”“节”“会”等。在普通英语词典里，腧穴的对应词是 point，但在许多专业词典和专业书刊中多译为 acupuncture point，或简作 acupoint。此种译法有其一定的道理，这是因为 point 一词多义，且“腧穴”又非其常用义项，若无上下文语言环境，当读者看到 point 一词时，首先想到的不大可能是腧穴。若在 point 前加上 acupuncture，读者一看便知这是用来针刺的腧穴。但是，如果我们对腧穴的本义进行比较全面的分析之后，便发现这种译法还是有失偏颇的。

腧穴是针灸治病时用以刺激的部位。腧穴的刺激方法可多种多样，可以用针来刺激，也可用灸的方法。仅艾灸而言，可以用艾直接或间接地灸灼腧穴，也可用艾条在腧穴上面进行熏灼。此外，我们还可采用指压点穴、气功点穴、激光、微波、磁珠、磁片等方法来刺激腧穴。其实，最早用来刺激腧穴的工具是砭石，而非金属针具。从 acupuncture 一词的结构来看，它由 acu 和 puncture 两部分构成。acu 是一个拉丁词头，意为“needle”。可见，acupuncture 意指用针在机体上刺个小孔。这个小孔，当然是腧穴之所在。从这个意义讲，将“腧穴”译成 acupuncture point 是不错的。但是，如上所述，腧穴不只是用针刺激的部位，它还可以通过其他的一些途径接受刺激。如果将腧穴译成 acupuncture point，这会造成对腧穴概念认识得不全面。需要指出的是，我们有时将指压点穴、气功点穴、激光、微波、磁片（或磁珠）、砭石等分别称为指针、气针、激光针、微波针、磁针、砭针等，有时还将艾卷亦称为“针”，如雷火神针等。这里所说的“针”是泛指一种针灸疗法，而不是指用以针刺的针（acupuncture needle）。英语中的 needle 一词不具备这种含义，所以上面讲的这些“针”是不能用 needle 对译的，因此，采用这些方法刺激的腧穴，也就不能译成 acupuncture point，因为被译作 acupuncture point 的腧穴必须是用针在其上面刺扎成孔的部位。如此，读者很容易产生误解，以为腧穴只是用针来刺扎的部位。

我们再从腧穴的性能来看，它具有两方面的意义，除了上面所说的腧穴是针灸治病的刺激点外，腧穴又是疾病症候的反应点。也就是说，腧穴不仅具有治疗意义，还有诊断意义。当人体某一脏腑或器官发生病变时，常可在其相应的部位出现异常反应，可表现为该处皮肤形态、色泽或皮肤温度的改变，或出现皮下结节、压痛等异常变化。这些异常反应部位便是腧穴，所以，腧穴有时还被称为反应点、压痛点等。如果将这一意义上的腧穴也译为 acupuncture point，显然有失原义。

腧穴是针灸学中一个重要、基本的概念，为避免对腧穴概念认识的局限性和片面性，笔者以为，不宜将其译为 acupuncture point，而直接译成 point 为妥。point 前无须加限定词 acupuncture，否则，恐将对腧穴本义亦有"限定"。其实，point 作腧穴解时，大多出现于中医针灸等专业书刊中，读者一看便知其意。有时和其他义项不易分辨时，通过上下文，也不至于混淆。

[原载《中国中西医结合杂志》，1995，15（1）：50－51.]

奇经八脉英译当议

沈雪勇

目前有关“奇经八脉”一词的英译颇不一致，其中最多见的是将其译成 eight extrachannels 或 eight extrameridians，有的作（译）者还译作 extraordinary vessels，等。笔者以为，产生这些不同译法的主要原因在于对“奇经八脉”一词本身的中文含义认识的不同。

奇经八脉中“奇”字的主要含义是奇特、奇异的意思。“奇经”，又称“奇脉”，是奇经八脉的简称，是和“正经”相对而言的；“正经”，又称“常经”，是指十二正经，即十二经脉。可见，“奇”和“正”“常”相对，是“正”和“常”的反义。extra 的常用词义是“外加的，额外的”，如果把“奇”字译作 extra，读者很可能认为奇经八脉是外加于十二经脉的附属部分。虽说奇经八脉是指十二经脉之外的八条经脉，但它绝非十二经脉的隶属部分。事实上，就奇经八脉的作用而言，它不拘于十二经脉，即不受约于十二经脉，恰恰相反，它对十二经脉有统率和主导的作用。此外，从机体原气的产生和发展来看，奇经八脉之气也应先于十二经之气。据此，笔者以为，将“奇”字译作 extraordinary 似更贴切，它反映出了“奇”字的“不同于一般”“奇异”等意思，同时也避免了使读者产生“奇经八脉是十二经脉的隶属部分”的误解。

“奇经”又称奇脉，可见，此处的“经”字和“脉”字义同。再从“奇经八脉”的词语结构来看，其中“经”和“脉”字可互换，均为“经脉”之义，即“奇经八脉”意为八条奇特的经脉。若把“脉”字简单地理解为“脉管”而译成 vessel，这是不全面的。有人将八条奇经名称中的“脉”字，如“督脉”的“脉”字，也译为 vessel，这也是不妥的。也许，采用这种译法的作者是想将“奇脉”的“脉”，字与“十二经”的“经”字相区别。其实这是没有必要的。至于将“经脉”译成 channel 还是 meridian，笔者认为，译为 meridian 为宜。channel 为水道、沟渠之义，而 meridian 作子午线、经线解。channel 一词太具体，容易使读者将经脉误解为一条有形的水沟，而 meridian 一词的含义比较抽象，用来作组织结构尚未明了的经脉的英译显然比 chanenl 一词确切，因此，奇经八脉一词似应译成 eight extraordinary meridians 较为适宜。刍荛之言，还望方家以教之。

[原载《中国中西医结合杂志》，1993，13（10）：627.]

关于针灸学中“寸”的英文译名

张玉娟　张坤杰

具有悠久历史、源于我国的针灸学是中外医学交流的重要内容之一，为便于在学术研究和技术交流中对于针灸学中“寸”的理解更为准确，所以探讨针灸学中“寸”的英文译名的确切性就更为重要了。

在现代汉语中，一般“寸”字为市寸的通称，是中国市制测量单位。在中医经典著作中，事实上对于“寸”这一测量单位有两个比较明确的基本含义。其一是指表示测量的绝对不变的单位（an absolute and constant unit of measure），它的尺度大小由中国特定的历史时期所决定。譬如：在《黄帝内经》中，寸用于量取古代针刺针的长度。其二则表示测量的相对单位（a relative unit of measure），其长度可根据身体和年龄的个体差异而变化。人体各个不同部位的宽度和长度可分别分为一定数目的相等分（equal divisions），把每一等分称为一寸，或称此为“同身寸法”（the measure of individual Cun）。例如：从肘横纹至腕横纹折作 12 寸；下肢部外踝尖至足底折作 3 寸。根据中医学经典著作中“寸”字的两个基本含义，一般在英语中常常译作“Cun”或“individual Cun”。

在临床实践中，遵循腧穴主治作用的基本规律，通过针刺某些腧穴以达到治疗疾病的目的。人体的腧穴很多，且每个腧穴的位置又不同，故这些腧穴定位是否准确直接关系到治疗效果，因此，历代医学家都非常重视腧穴的定位与取法。现代临床常用的腧穴的定位与取穴方法有 3 种，即解剖标志法、骨度分寸法和手指比量法。本文主要论及把寸作为测量单位的取穴方法。骨度分寸定位法古称“骨度法”。这种腧穴定位法始见于我国最早的医学文献《灵枢·骨度》篇，此法将人体的不同部位，依其尺寸，按比例分别规定为一定等分，每一等分称为 1 寸。手指比量法则是以患者手指的长度与宽度为标准，进行测量定位的方法。临床常用的是中指同身寸，即以患者的中指中节屈曲时内侧两端纹头之间作为 1 寸。正如唐代医学家孙思邈在其名著《备急千金要方》中解释“指寸”（fingers Cun），就是怎样用“同身寸”来确定针刺穴位的一个典型范例。在这两种方法中，确定正确的针刺穴位的测量单位“寸”，实际上意指“同身寸”。在某些英语书中翻译为“Cun”并没有表达出“寸”字的真正含义。

从另一方面讲，针刺治疗的效果与行针的深度有关。一般来说，在确定特别的治疗原则之后，理想的进针深度应视下述情况而定：针刺穴位的解剖部位，患者的个体特征，包括年龄、体格、体质和对针刺的敏感性以及治疗情况等，即患者的体型如身高、肌肉发达程度、脂肪堆积和年龄是确定针刺深度的重要因素。明代医学家扬济洲在其医学论著《针灸大成》中，论述了用“同身寸”作为测量针刺深度的标准单位，而且他还从王丙的医著中直接引证了对某些穴位针刺深度的描述。在这本书中，他把“同身寸”缩略为寸。

鉴于此，“同身寸”作为测量技术来确定针灸穴位和进针深度，已在我国针灸医学的临床实践中应用了数千年，其可靠性和实践性在针灸医学的实践和发展中已得到充分的证实。正如明代著名医学家徐春福在他的医学论著《古今医通》中所评述：“同身寸”被古人应用的原因是它可以按照不同的个体情况自动地变化，所以这种测量用于胖、瘦、高、矮都不能产生错误。然而在大多数现代汉语针灸书的英文版的翻译中，对“寸”这一测量单位还没有明确的参数（parameter），如在《针灸穴位解剖图谱》一书的英文版中，表明针刺深度的寸是指我国正在使用的测量单位，即 1 寸等于公制（the metric system）的 3.33cm。在《中国针灸学概要》一书的英文版中，则把“寸”译成“英寸”（inch），并作为每个穴位针刺深度的测量单位。而在《中英日对照实用针灸手册》一书的英文中，表示定位的寸被直接译为“Cun”。由于“寸”的译名没有统一和标准化，致使针灸定位和针刺深度的概念和参数含糊不清，甚至失去了其真正的含义。

美国医学博士伯凯辛先生在对中国针灸针刺深度的测量单位的研究后认为，在针灸学中，把汉语的“寸”视为绝对单位而翻译成市制的寸（Cun）或公制单位（3.33cm），以及英/美制单位（inch）来确定进针的深度都是不正确的。

纵观古今，中外学者在对针灸医学的研究中，认为把表示针刺穴位和深度的“寸”字的真正含义理解为“同身寸”更为准确、更为可靠和合理，因此，与其相对应的英文译名应为 individual Cun。这样才能表达“寸”字的真正内涵，才能更为确切地表达取穴、定位以及确定进针的深度，从而取得比较理想的治疗效果。

［原载《中国中西医结合杂志》，1996，16（7）：443.］

经络和穴位名称的翻译

刘兴华

在翻译经络和穴位名称时常遇到一些问题，现综述如下。

1. “经络”的译法

按国际标准经穴名称方案（WHO 公布，1989）[1]，“经络”一词应译为 Meridians and Collaterals，而我国多年采用的译法为 Channels and Collaterals，这多少引起了一些麻烦。针灸文献分析检索系统（Acupuncture Literature Analysis and Retrievel System，ACULARS）主题词表采用前一种译法，将“经络”译作 Meridians and Collaterals，但在一般情况下，只译作 Meridian（s），如“经络现象”译为 Meridian Phenomenon；“经络学说”译为 Meridian Theory，“经络研究”译为 Meridian Research 等。国内书刊大都采用后一种译法，即 Channels and Collaterals，也有时将“经络”笼统译作 Channels。

2. 经络名称及缩写

国内标准与国际标准有所不同。1989 年 WHO 公布的国际标准经穴名称方案中经络名称和缩写与 1990 年我国国家技术监督局发布的《经穴部位》[2]标准使用的经络名称和缩写不一致，因此，穴位编码亦不一致，涉及 75 个穴位（三焦 23 个，督脉 28 个，任脉 24 个）。如三焦经：国际标准为 Triple Energizer Meridian（TE），国内标准为 Sanjiao Meridian（SJ）；督脉的国际标准为 Governor Vessel Meridian（GV），国内标准为 Du Meridian（DU）；任脉的国际标准为 Conception Vessel Meridian（CV），国内标准为 Ren Meridian（RN）。

3. 新旧穴位编码的不同

WHO 1984 年公布的西太区标准穴位名称方案与 1989 年总部批准的方案不完全相同，在穴位编码，主要是经络缩写方面有区别。目前有些书刊或工具书还沿用旧编码是不妥的。新、旧编码经络缩写的区别见表 1，新缩写均为两个字母。

表 1　新旧编码经络缩写

经络名称	旧缩写	新缩写
Lung Meridian	L	Lu
Large Intestine Meridian	LI	LI
Stomach Meridian	S	ST
Spleen Meridian	Sp	SP
Heart Meridian	H	HT
Small Intestine Meridian	SI	SI
Bladder Meridian	B	BL
Kidney Meridian	K	KI
Pericardium Meridian	P	PC
Triple Energizer Meridian	TE	TE
Gallbladder Meridian	G	GB
Liver Meridian	Liv	LR
Governor Vessel Meridian	GV	GV
Conception Vessel Meridian	CV	CV

4. 穴位的读音和别名

因汉字读音不同，对穴位的音译中出现的问题常见的有：①攒竹（BL 2）：Cuanzhu 和 Zanzhu，国际标准用 Cuanzhu 或 Zanzhu，国内标准用 Cuanzhu。②膻中（CV 17）：Shanzhong、Tanzhong、Danzhong，国际标准用 Tanzhong 或 Shanzhong，国内标准用 Danzhong。③曲差（BL 4）：Qucha 和 Quchai，国际标准用 Qucha 或 Quchai，国内标准用 Qucha。④仆参（BL 61）：Pucan 和 Pushen，国际标准用 Pucan 或 Pushen，国内标准用 Pucan。看来，攒竹用 Cuanzhu、曲差用 Qucha、仆参用 Pucan 都已不成问题。膻中的拼法不一致，但仍以拼作 Danzhong 为宜。还有同一穴位有两个名称的情况，如悬钟（Xuanzhong，GB 39）与绝骨（Juegu），人中（Renzhong，GV 16）与水沟（Shuigou，GV 26），长强（Changqiang，GV 1）与龟尾（Guiwei）（注：以上所说国际标准用 Guan zhu 或 Zan zhu，指将前一拼法为主放在前面，而将后者用括号放在后面）。

5. 国外常用缩写及代号

以往国外常用代号有日、法、德、英、美等体系（1964 年我国《中国针灸学概要》也有非正式的代号），法国又分莫兰特（Soulie De Morant）和富耶（Roger De La Fuye）两种。日本经络经穴委员会制定了日本的代号。对经穴名称，大都采用本国语言或中文罗马拼音。美国《美洲中医杂志》（*American Journal of Chinese Medicine*）在20世纪70年代初出版时，曾试图意译穴位名称，如将“合谷”译为 connecting the valleys，“足三里”译为 walking three miles，“内关”译为 inner pass 等，但未能推广使用。目前因已有国际标准穴位名称，穴位编码已趋向于统一。

在翻译国外文献时，对新提出的穴位，注意不要翻译错，如 Tianmee（腕部戒烟穴），应译“甜味”（按广东读音），而不应译“甜蜜”。

6. “穴位”一词的翻译

尽管有的国外学者，如德国的满晰驳（Mansfred Pokert）等反对，目前已普遍把“穴位”译作 point，而随着 acupuncture 一词进入词典和医学主题词表，acupoint 一词也开始广泛使用。《美洲中医杂志》自创刊以来，一直将“穴位”译作 Locus（Loci）。

在中医的词汇里，穴位又称经穴、俞穴、腧穴、输穴（俞、腧、输同意）。国外文献有时将俞误读作 Yu。我国文献翻译常把俞穴、腧穴、输穴一律译为 Shupoint，当然是错误的。俞穴、腧穴、输穴一般都是指穴位，即 point 或 acupoint。作为特定穴位，“五输穴”应译为 Five Shu Points，五输穴之一的“输穴”译为 Shu Stream Point。以上所述仅限于体针，耳针、头针的穴位更为复杂，在国际上尚难取得统一。

（注：国际标准见《国外医学·中医中药分册》，1990，12（5）：52－64. 国家标准见《经穴部位》国家技术监督局 . GB12346－90. 1990）

［原载《中国中西医结合杂志》，1997，17（6）：370－371.］

也谈针灸穴位名称的翻译

李经蕴　李永安

20世纪70年代，随着中国针灸麻醉术的研究成功，这种古老针刺疗法很快得到了西方世界的认识。目前，针灸疗法已传播到世界上许多国家和地区，已被许多国家政府认可，并成为这些国家的合法疗法。

由于针灸穴位名称古奥玄秘、含义丰富，长期以来，对其翻译是一个非常棘手的问题。随着全世界对中国针灸的重视和认可，WHO在20世纪80年代委托西太平洋地区研究制定国际标准化针灸穴位名称。

1991年，经过近10年的努力，WHO最终出台了针灸穴位名称的国际标准化方案。该方案规定，针灸穴位名称统一采用汉语拼音，并附加国际代码。例如，“涌泉”翻译为Yongquan（Kid. 1）。其中，“Kid.”为肾经“肾”的英文kidney的缩写，“1”表示该穴位为肾经的第一号穴位。这种简明易记而实用的翻译穴位方法受到了广泛的欢迎，从此以后一直被用在国际针灸界，为针灸的对外传播起到了非常积极和重要的作用，从而也结束了针灸穴位名称翻译的混乱局面。

然而，近两年来，不时有国内外专家学者，特别是中医专家学者，著书立说，发表论文，提倡意译中医针灸穴位名称。他们认为，音译的穴位名词有以下弊端：首先，读者无法根据穴位的名称了解相关穴位的位置特点、主治内容和用法要求等信息。这些学者认为代码译法使得穴位名称的文化、生理和诊治意义丧失殆尽。例如，“睛明”穴的名称含义为此穴位主治眼部疾病，确保眼睛明亮。按照这些学者的意见，“睛明”穴应该意译为Bright Eyes[1]。另外，西方著名的中医翻译专家魏迺杰（Nigel Wiseman）也是意译穴位名称的积极倡导者。在他编写的《实用英文中医辞典》（*A Practical Dictionary of Chinese Medicine*）中，对所有的针灸穴位名称都作了意译。

其次，这些学者认为，由于汉语穴位名称存在着较多同音字，也使得有些穴位名称的音译有些混乱不清。他们列举了3组例子为证：“伏兔”与“扶突”，“腕骨”与“完骨”，以及“中渚”与“中注”。

以上是主张意译针灸穴位名称学者的主要观点。我们如何看待这些观点呢？

首先，让我们看一组这些学者意译的穴位名称：日月——Sun and Moon，承山——Mountain Supporter，太渊——Great Abyss，风市——Wind Market，库房——Storehouse，云门——Cloud Door，等。其中，“风市”为胆经穴位，是疏散风邪的主要穴位。将其意译为Wind Market会使外国读者不知所云，怎么还有

"风的市场"？太渊为肺经穴位，因此处脉气旺盛如深渊，故名"太渊"。将其意译为 Great Abyss（大深渊），外国读者能明白其深刻含义吗？"云门"为肺经穴位，位于胸上部，如肺气出入的门户，故名"云门"。"云"实际指肺气。将"云门"意译为 Cloud Door 显然也无法揭示出其真正含义。从以上意译的穴位名称可以看出，意译针灸穴位名称并不能向读者传递穴位名词的真正生理、解剖和主治等意义，更无法说明穴位名称中深邃的中医文化内涵。相反，这些意译的名称反而使外国读者无法理解，如读天书，甚至有滑稽可笑之感。与 WHO 出台的简洁、明了、实用的方案比较，有着很大的差距。

由于针灸穴位的命名体现着典型的中国文化特色，穴位名称含义丰富，命名规则非常复杂。有以星象命名，以示直观；有以天象命名，以表曲折漫回；有以山脉走势命名，以喻主治；有以沟壑谷渎命名，以明形位；有以道路冲市命名，以明出入；有以宫府殿堂命名，各有所喻；有以庭廊房屋命名，寓意别异；有以户门牖窗命名，类比形象等[1]。

面对如此复杂的穴位名称，就是国内的中医专业人士也未必知晓多少，更不说是外国人，因此，在意译穴位名称的过程中，出现翻译错误屡见不鲜。在国内外的出版物中，可以看到，"人中"被译成 Middle of Man（人的中间），"缺盆"被译成 Empty Basin（空脸盆），"少商"被译成 Young Merchant（年轻的商人），等。其实，这里的"少商"中的"商"跟"商人"没有任何关系。它是中医五行学说里的五行"金、木、水、火、土"配中国古代音乐中的五音"宫、商、角、徵、羽"的配属关系。"商"在五行中属金，属肺经（肺在五行中属金）。少商为肺经的最后一个穴位，其气少而不冲，故名"少商"。如此复杂和深刻的含义要用几个英语单词翻译成一个名词几乎不可能。

至于提倡穴位名称意译的第二个原因，这些专家认为，由于汉语存在着较多同音字，使得有些穴位名称的音译有些混乱不清。虽然汉语中存在大量的同音词，但在 361 个针灸穴位名称中，同音的也只有以上意译穴位名称的倡导者用来支持自己观点的 3 组例子。而且，虽然这几组穴位汉语拼音相同，由于分属不同的经脉，在用国际化标准方案标记时，根本就不存在所谓的混乱不清。例如，"伏兔"属胃经第 32 号穴位，标记为 Futu（ST 32），而"扶突"属大肠经第 18 号穴位，标记为 Futu（LI 18）；"腕骨"属小肠经第 4 号穴位，标记为 Wangu（SI 4），而"完骨"属胆经第 12 号穴位，标记为 Wangu（GB 12）；"中渚"为三交经的第三个穴位，标记为 Zhongzhu（TE 3），而"中注"属肾经第 15 号穴位，标记为 Zhongzhu（Kid. 15）。

对于外国中医针灸专家来说，他们所关心的是哪个穴位治什么病，就像什么药治何种病一样，掌握这些信息就足够了。穴位名称只是一个符号而已。这就好比家长给孩子起名时也许在姓名中寄予一定的含义，但对于周围其他人来说，姓名只是孩子的代号而已，其作用仅仅是用以和其他孩子相区别而已。如果将穴位名称的文化含义翻译出来，反而误导影响了读者对信息的接收。毕竟，中医是一门自然科学，是一门医学科学。尽管中医学是建立在中国古代文化的基础上的，但在翻译时，我们一定要强调医学信息的传递，并且淡化，甚至放弃其文化含义[2]。

1991 年 WHO 制定的针灸穴位名称标准化方案简洁、实用、易记、科学。经过 10 多年的使用，该方案已被海内外广大中医界人士接受。作为一个世界性的卫生管理和学术组织，WHO 能为一门传统的医学——中医制定标准化针灸名称方案，这是我们应该感到十分荣幸而拥护的一件事。我们应积极推广使用这个标准化方案，不应该否定它而倡导意译针灸穴位名称。

参考文献

[1] 李照国．中医基本名词术语英译国际标准化研究．上海：上海科学技术出版社，2008：40-47.

[2] 李永安，李经蕴．奈达的翻译理论在中医翻译中的应用．中国中西医结合杂志，2006，26(9)：857-859.

［原载《中国中西医结合杂志》，2009，29（12）：1133-1134.］

针灸穴位翻译与中医文化传承

朱函亭　李亚平　郑芳子

笔者在中医临床一线从事中医的口译、笔译工作多年，期间亲眼目睹了中医，特别是针灸在世界范围内得到迅速的发展，深感欣慰。笔者认为，这不仅是我国中医学在西方国家的传播，更是我国古老中医文化的传承和传播。

应该看到，东西方的文化背景差异很大，思维方式也不尽相同，这对跨文化的交流必将带来一定的影响，针灸穴位名称的翻译便是其中一例。

WHO 于 1989 年统一了 361 个穴位的名称，对穴位名称引用了由英文字母和数字相结合的命名方法。诚然，这个举措对于当时没有规范的针灸穴位命名的现状，以及方便外国学员学习和记忆针灸穴位带来了不可低估的积极作用，对中医特别是针灸在国外的传播和发展做出了有益的努力。然而，1989 年距今已有 18 年之久，期间世界科学技术突飞猛进，特别是医学领域也发生了前所未有的变化，境外针灸从业人员的结构，不管是数量上还是人员的素质上都比 18 年前有了大大的提高。那么，针灸穴位翻译情况又是如何呢?

1. 针灸穴位名称翻译现状

在长期的中医药翻译实践中，笔者发现，境外留学生学习和记忆针灸穴位名称是按照该穴位所属经络走向的先后次序进行学习和记忆的。如，足三里穴是足阳明胃经上一个非常重要的穴位，主治胃肠疾患、下肢瘫痪等疾病，由于它位居“足阳明胃经”第 36，就被称为“St. 36”(St. 即中文“胃”的英文缩写)，这也是笔者从事翻译工作多年唯一能记忆住的针灸穴位号码。再比如，血海穴是足太阴脾经上的一个穴位，主治月经不调、功能性子宫出血等疾病，因为它位于足太阴脾经第 10，就被标记为“Sp. 10”(Sp. 即中文“脾”的英文缩写)。

2. 关于腧穴学的命名原则

归纳起来，中医学腧穴命名的依据及方法大致有以下几种。

2.1　自然类

以天文学上的日月星辰和地理名称结合腧穴的形象而命名的，如日月穴、承山穴、少海穴等。

2.2　物象类

以动物和植物名称，以及建筑物和生活用具来形容某些腧穴的部位，如伏兔穴、攒竹穴、天井穴、缺盆穴等。

2.3　人体类

以人体的解剖部位、生理功能、治疗作用以及人体部位和经脉分属阴阳来命名，如大椎穴、血海穴、三阴交穴等。

唐代医家孙思邈在《千金翼方》中说："凡诸孔穴，名不徒设，皆有深意。"由此可知，古人对腧穴的命名，取义十分广泛，可谓上察天文，下观地理，中通人事，远取诸物，近取诸身，结合腧穴的分布特点、作用、主治等内容赋予一定的名称[1]。从我们目前的中医对外交流以及教学来看，虽然针灸穴位极富我国中医文化内涵，但是其教学内容严重缺失。

3. 语言国情说是中医翻译中保持中医特色的指南语言

国情说认为，任何一种语言中都有一些反映该民族特有事物的词，而这些词常常带有一个民族的文化背景，是一个民族有别于其他民族的象征，因而，这类中医特有的文化词汇在翻译时应反映出来。奈达在《翻译的理论和实践》中指出，不能也不该将《圣经》翻译得听起来好像发生在邻近小镇上 10 年前的事一样。因为《圣经》所涉及的历史环境至关重要。《圣经》语言中的历史遗迹使得《圣经》有别于其他书籍，因此，在翻译时应予保留[2]。事实上，奈达的理论与语言国情说很相似，两者都可作为中医翻译时保持中医特色的指南。

4. 针灸穴位的翻译

对于目前针灸穴位翻译中存在的问题和不足，应该引起足够的重视，应采取有效措施加以完善，确保中医药文化成分在对外传播过程中尽可能完整地保存。

笔者认为，是否可以在原来针灸穴位名称翻译的基础上增加针灸穴位含义的翻译。具体处理方法大致有以下几类。

4.1　第一类

以天文学上的日月星辰和地理名称结合腧穴的形象而命名的，如主治胆囊炎、胆囊结石、肝炎、呕吐等的日月穴，在原有翻译 Riyue（GB 24）的基础上增加其含义的翻译，翻译成 Riyue（GB 24，sun and moon）。

4.2　第二类

以动物和植物名称，以及建筑物和生活用具来形容某些腧穴的部位，如主治肘关节疾患、偏头痛、颈淋巴结结核等的天井穴，在原有翻译 Tianjing（SJ 10）的基础上增加其含义的翻译，翻译成 Tianjing（SJ 10，courtyard）。

4.3　第三类

以人体解剖部位、生理功能、治疗作用以及人体部位和经脉分属阴阳来命名，如主治月经不调、功能性子宫出血的血海穴，在原有翻译 Xuehai（Sp. 10）

的基础上增加其含义的翻译，翻译成 Xuehai（Sp. 10，sea of blood）。

这样翻译针灸穴位既保留了原有针灸穴位翻译的命名方法，方便境外学员和从事针灸治疗的从业人员的学习和工作，更为主要的是它丰富了针灸穴位翻译的文化内涵，使得针灸穴位这一部分中医文化得以传承。

5. 中医文化传承应贯穿对外中医药交流的全过程

很显然，如果听任目前针灸穴位翻译的现状继续下去，那么十几年乃至几十年后，针灸穴位含义这一富含我国特有中医文化的内容必将随着时间的推移而在境外被慢慢淡忘甚至消失。这肯定不是我们传播中医药学的初衷，结果将是令人痛心的！因此，为了能使我国古老的中医文化尽可能完整地介绍给国外的中医爱好者、同行以及热爱我国博大精深中医文化的外国朋友，从现在开始我们应该积极采取各种有效的措施，以期尽快改变这种现状。笔者对此有以下几点建议。

5.1　规范针灸穴位命名方法

通过我国针灸协会、学会包括政府等组织机构向世界针灸联合会以及 WHO 呼吁，建议组织相关的中医、针灸专家和中医翻译工作者共同商讨，在原有穴位名称由英文字母和数字相结合的命名方法的基础上，增加针灸穴位的含义，以便制定出更为规范、完整的针灸穴位命名方法，使我国古老的针灸穴位这一宝贵的中医文化得以传承。

5.2　重视经典针灸图书的整理和出版

根据《腧穴学》记载：杨上善撰注《黄帝内经明堂》时，曾对经穴名称逐一注释，惜原书散佚，现仅存手太阴肺经一卷。以后张介宾等医家对腧穴含义亦有解释，因此，呼吁我国出版界积极出版针灸穴位含义一类的书籍，使我国的中医文化得以延续。

5.3　重视对外教学

那些从事国外留学生教学的大专院校以及中医研究院、中医院等要加大管理力度，认真履行工作职责，直接负责留学生带教的老师以及译员要热爱留学生带教和翻译工作，为传承祖国中医文化尽力。

笔者认为，中医文化既是民族的，同时又是世界的，我们只有尊重历史才能更好地展望未来，而历史和未来的连接就靠传承，因此，笔者愿与同道一起在中医翻译领域不断探索，为祖国中医文化的传承尽自己一点绵薄之力。

参考文献

[1] 罗永芬．腧穴学．上海：上海科学技术出版社，1994：4－5.
[2] 李永安．如何处理中医翻译中的文化因素．陕西中医学院学报，2002，25（2）：71.

[原载《中国中西医结合杂志》，2008，28（6）：556－557.]

下篇　书评及其他

为谢竹藩教授英译中专著 *On the Standard Nomenclature of Traditional Chinese Medicine* 写的序言

陈可冀

Professor Xie Zhufan, Director Emeritus of Peking University Institute of Integrated Traditional Chinese and Western Medicine, is a renowned internist and integrated traditional Chinese medicine and Western medicine specialist in China.

A distinguished, erudite scholar and a clinician par excellence of forthright character, Professor Xie is a highly respected and close friend of mine for decades. His exemplary works on basic neuroendocrinology studies of Cold & Heat Theories of traditional Chinese medicine have been leading the field with solid progresses. Over the years, Professor Xie has headed several task forces on English standardization of traditional Chinese medicine nomenclatures sponsored by World Health Organization and State Administration of Traditional Chinese Medicine of China with outstanding achievements. With his extensive proficiencies in both traditional Chinese and Western medicines, Professor Xie excels in the adaptation of traditional Chinese medical science into English and has been universally recognized as the best in the field. Amongst his abundant translated works, "On the Standard Nomenclature of Traditional Chinese Medicine" has been the most representative.

An energetic octogenarian of highest professional standards, Professor Xie works ceaselessly and tirelessly to promote academic exchanges and international collaboration in medicine. This book, *Contemporary Introduction to Chinese Medicine in Comparison with Western Medicine* in one of his recent works in collaboration with Dr. Xie Fang. The aim of this work is to provide Western practitioners a systematic approach to study, comprehend and practice traditional Chinese medicine. In spite of the vast and all-encompassing nature of traditional Chinese medicine and considerable difficulty in technical adaptation to English, Professor Xie and Dr. Xie are able, on the one hand, to maintain Chinese cultural characteristics throughout the dissertation, and on the other, stand on the Western readers' perspectives to ensure that the essence of this work is easy to read, study, comprehend and hence, to apply. This book faithfully lays out basic theories of traditional Chinese medicine, and diagnostic and therapeutic principles, with full attention on the most updated treatment of diseases commonly seen in the West, such as allergic, arthritic and gastrointestinal disorders, hypertensive, coronary heart and diabetic diseases, metabolic syndromes and tumors. Fluent in language and style, it is an extremely handy and practical tool, the best of its kind one can find nowadays.

It is indeed most rewarding, and my great pleasure, to preface this work to all.

Prof. Chen Keji, MD
Member,
Chinese Academy of Sciences
Chairman Emeritus,
Chinese Association of Integrated Traditional and Western Medicines
Beijing, July 2009

评杨谦志著《中药与方剂手册》（*Handbook of Chinese Herbs and Formulas*）

陈可冀

由杨谦志医师（Him-che Yeung，CA，Ph. D.）编著的英文版《中药与方剂手册》（*Handbook of Chinese Herbs and Formulas*）一书，分上下二卷，1983 年开始在美国洛杉矶出版。本书共收录中药 402 种，常用方剂 302 种。本书系统全面，既重视传统知识，也注意结合现代药理和方剂的研究进展，故本书在美国颇受欢迎，被不少针灸和中医大学或学院所广泛接受，多年来成为这些学校的基本教材或重要参考书。

1. 尊重中医传统理论和经验

本书关于中药分类及中医方剂分类，均按中医传统功能分类法为主，中药分为 22 类，方剂分为 19 类。中药分为 Diaphoretics（解表药），并分：①For affection due to wind and cold（发散风寒药）；②For affection due to wind and heat（发散风热药）；Antipyretics or Febrifuges（清热药）；Anti-malaria Herbs（抗疟药）；Anti-tussives，Expectorants and Antiasmatics（化痰、止咳、平喘药）；The Digestives（消食药）；The Warming Herbs（温里药）；The Tonics（补益药）；The Carminatives（行气药）；Herbs of Regulation of Blood（活血祛瘀药）；Hemostatics（止血药）；Laxatives（泻下药）；The Diuretics（利水渗湿药）；Herbs with Fragrant Odour for Resolving Dampness（芳香化湿药）；The Anti-rheumatics（祛风湿药）；Anticonvulsants（平肝药）；The Sedatives（安神药）；The Aromatic Stimulant（开窍药）；The Astringents（收涩药）；Anthelmintics（驱虫药）；Herbs for Tumor（抗肿瘤药）；The Analgescs（麻醉止痛药）；Topical Agents（外用药）。中医方剂分为：The Diaphoretics（解表剂）；The Anti-pyretics or Febrifugal Formulas（清热剂）；The Mediating or Regulating Formulas（和解剂）；The Phlegm Expelling（Expectorant）Formulas（祛痰剂）；The Antitussives and Anti-asmatics Formulas（止咳平喘剂）；The Warming Formulas（温里剂）；The Resolving or Discutient Formulas（消导剂）；The Tonifying Formulas（补益剂）；The Carminatives Formulas（理气剂）；The Blood Regulating Formulas（理血剂）；The Purgative Formulas（泻下剂）；The Diuretic Formulas（祛湿剂）；The Anti-convulsant Formulas（治风剂）；The Moisturizing Formulas（治燥剂）；The Sedativeor

Tranquilizing Formulas（安神剂）；The Resuscitating Formulas（开窍剂）；The Astringent Formulas（固涩剂）；The Anti-thelmintic and Anti-parasitic Formulas（驱虫剂）；The Emetic Formulas（涌吐剂）。

在以上这些纲要的分类之下，又以中医理论为主，分为若干不同功用的亚目。以清热药为例，又分为：Herbs for reducing intense internal heat（清热泻火药），其中又分为 Herbs for clearing the heat in the Qi（inner defensive）system（清气分实热药）、Herbs for eliminating heat and dampness（清热燥湿药），以及 Herbs for eliminating pathological heat from blood（清热凉血药），Herbs for clearing the heat caused by Yin deficiency（清虚热药）、Herbs for clearing pathogenic heat and toxin（清热解毒药）等。后者又分为 Herbs for febriles diseases（治温热病的药），carbuncles，boils or abscess（治痈疮肿毒的药）；For dysentery or diarrhea（治泻痢的药）；For sores，For inflammation of the throat（治咽喉肿痛的药）及 eliminating the heat in the eyes（清热明目药）等。这种分类基本符合中医传统理论结构。

方剂方面，如 Anticonvulsant Formulas（治风剂），又分为两大类，即所谓 Dispelling the exogenous wind for mulas（疏散外风方）及 Dispelling the endogenous wind formulas（平熄内风方），又如 The Moisturizing Formulas（治燥剂），又分为两大类，即所谓 Eliminating the external dryness formulas（轻宣外燥方）及 Eliminating the internal dryness formulas（滋润内燥方）均甚合理。

2. 中药和方剂名称的综合引用

为了便于西方学者学习、应用和研究中医药学，该书作者采用综合多种名称的方式介绍中药及方剂名称，每一种药物，例如巴戟天，不仅有现在公布的汉语拼音名称 BaJi Tian，且有过去习用的拼音名称 Pa-chi-tien。此外，有通用名称（common name）Morinda Root，植物学名称 Morinda Officinalis How，药学名称（Pharmaceutical name）Radix Morindaeofficinalis。方剂名称方面，例如普济消毒饮，不仅列有汉语现行拼音名称 Pu Ji Xiao Du Yin，还有以往习用的拼音名称 Pu-Chi-Hsiao-Tu-Yin，还有按其功能译意的名称 Universal Anti-phlogistic Decoction，以及其他著作（包括许鸿源医师所著《常用中药方剂图谱》（*Commonly used Chinese Herb Formulas with Illustrations*），所曾采用的名称 Scute and Cimicifuga Combination（见第 189 页）等，因而，甚为实用、方便。

在索引方面，中药索引计有 4 种：即药学名称索引、拉丁文名称索引、通用名称索引及中文名称索引。方剂索引有三种，即英文名称索引，中文名称索引及中西医诊疗时针对病证和方剂功用的索引。后者最有特点，堪称本书之一大特色。例如在腹痛（Abdominal pain）的项目之下，可按索引查找：Caused by cold

（寒痛），列出 Liang Fu Wan（良附丸）和 Tong Mai Si Ni Tang（通脉四逆汤）；Caused by heat（热痛），列出 Da Cheng Qi Tang（大承气汤）；Caused by asthenia or deficiency（虚痛），列出 Xiao Jian Zhong Tang（小建中汤），Da Jian Zhong Tang（大建中汤）及 Fu Zi Li Zhong Tang（附子理中汤）；Caused by sthenia or excessiveness（实痛），列出 Due to stagnation Qi and bloodstasis（气滞血瘀）及 Due to stagnation of food（饮食积滞）两大类，前者列出 Chai Hu Shu Gan Tang（柴胡疏肝汤）及 Shao Fu Zhu Yu Tang（少腹逐瘀汤），后者列出 Bao He Wan（保和丸）。又如现代医学病名支气管哮喘（Bronchial asthma）项下，列出中医四大证候索引：With cold phlegm（寒痰），列有 Xiao Qing Long Tang（小青龙汤）及 Su Zi Jiang Qi Tang（苏子降气汤）；With heat in the Lung（肺热），列有 Ding Chuan Tang（定喘汤）；With deficiency of Kidney（肾虚），列有 Du Qi Tang（都气汤）；With deficiency of both Lung and Kidney（肺肾虚），列有 Ren Shen Hu Tao Tang（人参胡桃汤）等。

3. 继承发扬兼顾，注重中西医结合

本书在介绍每种药物时，除注意介绍科属（Family）、药用部位（Used part）、中药性味（Property and Taste）、归经（Entering Meridian）及功用（Function）、剂量（Recommended Dosage）和处方（Prescription）举例外，还援古引今，中西结合地介绍适应证（Indication）、禁忌证（Contraindication）和化学成分（Chemical Component）等，所以十分实用，便于掌握和理解。例如介绍了大枣可用于过敏性紫癜，苍耳子可用于过敏性鼻炎及鼻窦炎头痛。厚朴含有厚朴酚（magnolol）、异厚朴酚（isomagnolol）、挥发油（machilol，eudesmol）、生物碱（magnocurarine，magnoflorine salicifoline）等。当然，在各药结合中医理论和经验的传统临床应用上，介绍尤为详细。

在介绍方剂方面，不仅介绍了各方剂的组成及常用剂量，而且介绍了其作用（Action）、适应证（Indication）和临床应用（Clinical application）。例如关于七味都气丸的应用，在介绍传统经验之后，指出其可用于支气管哮喘、肺气肿及肺结核等。尤为可贵的是，在许多方剂之后，还附有如何掌握（Modification）一项，如独活寄生汤之用于慢性风湿性关节炎及风湿性坐骨神经痛，在该项中更列出加减之法度，如指出痛剧者可加川乌头，有瘀血者可加桃仁、红花等。又如在当归六黄汤之后的该项中指出，夜间盗汗剧者（with severe night sweat）加麻黄根、浮小麦、糯稻根须。侧重养阴（to replenish Yin-vital essence）时，加牡蛎、龟板及鳖甲等。再如六一散加西瓜翠衣、丝瓜络治疗夏季热；加海金沙及金钱草用于尿路结石及排尿烧灼感；加青黛而成碧玉散治咽喉痛及火眼等，均符合教科书及临床用药的实用原则。

总之，本书是一部很好的英文版中药及方剂著作，不足之处在于尚应补充各药图片，以及各方剂的新制剂或新品种。当然，如果增加了这些内容，则会增加篇幅，售价可能相应要高些。

注：本书为英文版，本文列出该书对中药、方剂分类的英译名称，供读者参考。

［原载《中国中西医结合杂志》，1989，9（3）：187－188.］

评魏迺杰先生的《实用英文中医辞典》

谢竹藩　刘干中　吕维柏　方廷钰　张庆荣　王　台　王　奎

魏迺杰（Nigel Wiseman）先生是英籍人士，现任台湾长庚大学中医系英语讲师，从事中医翻译工作多年，曾有几部汉英中医词典问世，如1990年由美国标登出版社（Paradigm Publications）出版的《中医及针灸穴位名词词汇》（*Glossary of Chinese Medical Terms and Acupuncture Points*），1995年由湖南科学技术出版社出版的《英汉汉英中医词典》，以及1998年由美国标登出版社出版的《实用英文中医辞典》（*A Practical Dictionary of Chinese Medicine*），后者于2002年由人民卫生出版社影印再版。作为一位外籍人士，对中医学长期不懈地坚持钻研，做出如此大量的贡献，实属难能可贵。其所制定的中医英文名词，有一些确能较好表达中医原义，理应考虑采用；尤其是他重视中国文化，力求在翻译中反映出中国文化精髓的这种努力方向更是值得赞许。

但是，中医学毕竟历史悠久、内容浩瀚、用词古朴，能用英文词语正确地反映中医名词的医学原意已非易事，要想通过中医名词的英译完全融合中西文化上的分歧，则是难上加难。我们认为《实用英文中医辞典》（下文简称《辞典》）中有些原则性和方法学的问题值得商榷。

魏迺杰在《辞典》再版序中十分强调中医词汇英译应以直译为主，通过直译仿造中医英文词汇最能反映中医概念，忠实地呈现中医原貌。他认为“惟有藉仿造为主的翻译方法重新制定一套中医英文词汇，才能有望使西方人对中医的真实面貌一览无余”。本文暂不讨论直译、意译等翻译原则问题，先从《辞典》的具体内容来探讨是否真的忠实呈现了中医原貌，是否确实能让西方人对中医的真实面貌一览无余。

在《辞典》中，大部分词汇是用直译法仿造出来的英文中医名词术语。从这些具体词汇很容易领会魏氏的直译法。其直译和仿造过程如下：首先确定一个中文单字的对应英文词（在《辞典》正文之前列出3638个常用的中文单字及其英文对应词），然后在不同的名词术语中凡遇该汉字时尽量都用规定的英文对应词置换，有语法矛盾时可稍加变化以改变其词性。这样一来，中医名词的英译便成了一项很有规律的工作，甚至是简单的机械性工作，只要对一个个汉字确定相应的英文词，中医词汇的英译问题便可迎刃而解，并创造出一套仿造的中医英文词汇。

下面举一例来说明魏氏的这种做法：他在单字表中规定“神”的英文对应词

是 spirit，“昏”“情”“气”“水”“志”“舌”等字的英文对应词分别是 cloud、affect、Qi、water、mind、tongue，于是一系列有关的英文中医名词便从而产生：神昏 clouded spirit，神情 spirit-affect，神气 spirit Qi，神水 spirit water，神志 spirit-mind，舌神 tongue spirit。其他与“神”有关的中医名词英译也基本上是见“神”就用 spirit，例如：神明 spirit light，神膏 spirit jelly，神疲 fatigued spirit，神犀丹 Spirit-Like Rhinoceros Horn Elixir，神脏 spiritual viscera，神志昏糊 clouded spirit-mind，神志昏乱 confused spirit-mind，神珠 spirit ball，瞳神 pupil spirit，安神 quieting the spirit，精神 essence-spirit，四神丸 Four Spirits Pill，五神汤 Five Spirits Decoction，六神丸 Six Spirits Pill，润神散 Spirit-Moistening Powder，神仙活命汤 Spirit Immortal Life-Giving Decoction，神封 Spirit Seal，神阙 Spirit Gate Tower，四神聪 Alert Spirit Quartet，等。

这些英文对应词只是从字面上与中文对应，其中有不少英文词汇会使西方说英语的人感到十分费解：spirit water 是不是含酒精的饮料，spirit jelly 是不是含酒的果冻，Spirit-Like Rhinoceros Horn 到底是什么样的犀角？

用这种魏氏直译法仿造出来的英文词实际上并不能忠实呈现中医的原貌。仅就这个“神”字的英译而言，还出现了另外一方面的问题。魏氏的中英字词对照表中“灵”字的对应词也是 spirit，于是神明的英译是 spirit light，灵光的英译也是 spirit light，例如磨障灵光膏为 Obstruction-Abrading Spirit Light Paste，但是中医学中的神明和灵光根本不是一回事，英译却把两个不同的概念合二为一了。这种情况还见于“神道”和“灵道”，魏氏大概自己也感到不应把两个不同的穴位都叫做 Spirit Path，于是后者用 Spirit Pathway 来表示。为什么同是“道”，一个为 path，另一个为 pathway，这既违反魏氏自定的原则，也无理可讲。

在这种译法中，魏氏直译法的根本问题在于对中文文字学缺乏正确的认识。他认为单个汉字是意义的单位，与英文的“词（word）”相应[1]。对于字和词的区别，许多中文专家都有过论述，例如吕叔湘、朱德熙明确指出：“字是形体和声音的单位，词是意义的单位。一个字可能也是意义的单位，那个字就同时是一个词；但是许多词是两个字合成的，有些词是三个或四个字合成的。前者我们管它叫单音词，后者我们管它叫多音词”[2]。这个概念对于古今汉语都适用，例如周光庆等在讨论古汉语词汇的构成时指出：“对于古汉语词汇来说，一个重要的问题是区分字和词。字不等于词，词是语言的单位，字是记录词的文字符号。……研究古汉语词汇要以词为单位，而不能以字为单位”[3]。所以，上列各词，两个字的也罢，三个字或四个字的也罢，都是意义的单位，与其中所含的单音词在意义上可以有密切关系，也可以没有密切关系。神明就是神明，不是什么神之明，神情就是神情，也不是什么神加情。瞳神译为 pupil spirit 的问题更是显而易见。瞳神、瞳子、瞳仁是同义词，都指眼球的同一个部位，即现今所说的瞳孔

pupil，如果应该用 pupil spirit 作瞳神的对应词，那么瞳子、瞳仁又该如何按瞳＋子、瞳＋仁来处理？常用的中医名词如瞳神散大和瞳神缩小是不是都该译成 dilated pupil spirit 和 constricted pupil spirit？

魏氏的另一个严重错误是忽略单音词的多义性。许多单音词是多义的，就“神”而言，仅在《黄帝内经》和《难经》中它就有多种不同的含义：“阴阳不测谓之神”（《素问·天元纪大论》），这里的“神”是指玄妙；“望而知之谓之神”（《难经·第六十一难》），这里的“神”是异常高超的意思；“两神相搏，合而成形”（《灵枢·决气》），这里的“两神”即男女两性；“得神者昌，失神者亡”（《素问·移精变气论》），这里的“神”是显露于颜面的气色，即神采之意；“神者，水谷之精气也”（《灵枢·平人绝谷》），这里的“神”是指维系人体脏腑功能活动的神气；“五脏所藏，心藏神”（《灵枢·本神》），这里的“神”是人的意识、思想和精神。像这样一个多义词不可能在英文中找到一个词恰恰也有同样相应的多义性。

中文单字单音词的多义性容易造成误解，其解决办法之一是把由一个单字形成的单音词改变成由两个字组成的双音词或更多的字组成的多音词。仍以上述与“神”有关的词为例，由于“神”字的多义性，为了使其意义明确，产生了一系列的双音词，如神明、神情、神气、神采、神志等。魏氏的译法则反其道而行之，不顾“神”字的多义性，固守 spirit 一词，一律将“神”与 spirit 画等号。这种译法当然无法解决“神”的多义性问题，只会加重由多义性造成的误解。这些与“神”有关的名词，魏氏直译法的问题还只是以偏概全，更严重的问题则是从一开始规定中文单字的英文对应词时就不正确，由此产生的一系列仿造中医英文词汇当然更成问题了。下面也举例说明。

魏氏把“疝”当作了会意字，还在其《辞典》中注明“疝 is composed of 疒，illness，with 山，mountain. ［见《辞典》第 400 页。在 1995 年出版的魏氏《英汉汉英词典》中对此有明确的论述：“‘疝’本字从山，指（邪气）堆积成山之义。如此的比喻，在本书以 mounting 译出，也就是从 mount up，堆起如山（mount，mountain）而来。”见第 22 页］[1]。显然，正是由于这种 illness ＋ mountain 的认识，便产生了 mounting 这个病名作为“疝”的英文对应词，并由此形成若干仿造的中医英文词汇：肺疝 lung mounting，pulmonary mounting，筋疝 sinew mounting，厥疝 reversal mounting，寒疝 cold mounting，狐疝 foxy mounting，vulpine mounting，气疝 Qi mounting，湿热疝 damp-heat mounting，水疝 water mounting，胎疝 fetal mounting，小肠疝 small intestine mounting，心疝 heart mounting，血疝 blood mounting，阴疝 Yin mounting，疝瘕 mounting-conglomeration，疝气 mounting Qi，疝气痛 mounting Qi pain 等。由于魏氏从一开始就没有理解“疝”的意义，规定了不正确的英文对应词，在此基础上产生的仿造中医英文

词汇当然就更令人不知所云了。难道心、肺、筋、小肠等疝就是心、肺、筋、小肠（或其邪气）堆积成山吗？顺便指出，筋疝中的“筋”是指阴茎，不是 sinew。

中文“疒”字旁的单字，除“疒”本身是象形字，表示人有疾病之外，一般都是形声字。“疝”在《说文解字》中就明确注明“从疒，山声，腹痛也”。最初对“疝”做出医学定义的是《黄帝内经》：“病在少腹，腹痛不得大小便，病名曰疝”（《素问·长刺节论》）。无论从《说文解字》还是《黄帝内经》给予的定义，都看不出“疝”与 mounting 有什么关系。后世论“疝”，虽有所发展，提出五疝、七疝等不同名目，但无一能使“疝”与 mounting 发生联系，“疝”的定义也未变，例如《诸病源候论》：“疝者痛也”（第二十卷）。与“疝”类似的还有“痧”字。古代没有“痧”字，甚至在《康熙字典》中尚无收载。虽然后世偶有人将“痧”“沙”并用，但毕竟作为病症的名称以“痧”字比较合理，故现在采用“痧”字。魏氏在其中英文单字对照表中规定“痧”字的英文对应词是 sand，并从而产生了一系列仿造中医英文词，白面痧 white face sand，丹痧 cinnabar sand，风痧 wind sand，刮痧 sand scraping，绞肠痧 intestine-gripping sand，烂喉痧 putrefying throat sand，暑痧 summerheat sand，痧毒 sand toxin，痧筋 sand veins，痧块 sand lump，痧气 sand Qi，痧胀 sand distention 等。对这些仿造的中医英文词，恐怕连魏氏本人都感到难以理解，所以提出“颗粒状疹与以腹部症状为特征的疾病之间的精确病因学联系不明”（The precise etiological connection between a granular eruption and disease characterized by abdominal signs is not clear）[1]。其实，问题出在魏氏的一对一直译法上面。魏氏把“痧”译为 sand，这本身就没有反映“痧”字含有疾病的原意。更重要的问题是魏氏忽略了“痧”作为病症名除了表示“疹”之外还有其他意思，他想把中文的多义单音词改为单义字词，用一个 sand 来表达“痧”的多种含义，而结果却是一个含义也没有表达出来。在这里也许有人会提出质问，把上列中医名词中的“痧”译为 sand 固然不对，译成什么才对呢？我们的答案很简单，译成什么都不对，因为这种考虑问题的方法就错了。丹痧、风痧、绞肠痧都是完整的病名，是独立的意义单位。应该考虑的是“丹痧”译成什么，“风痧”译成什么，“绞肠痧”译成什么，而不是“丹”“风”“绞”“肠”“痧”等单音词分别该译成什么。

以上这些例子虽然都说明魏氏直译法问题影响了一系列的中医英文词的正确制定，但毕竟只限于一定的领域，下面这个例子则影响的范围要大得多。许多中文单音词不仅本身具有多义性，而且即使是同一意义，还可以由于其主体的改变而需要有不同的考虑。“虚”和“实”是一对中医学中极为常用的汉字单音词，虽然具有多种词性，但词义变化不大。不过当主体不同时用同一英文对应词便未必合适了。例如对于脉象，虚脉是举之无力，按之空虚的脉象；实脉是举按均有力的脉象。对于辨证，虚指正气不足，实指邪气盛实。因此，虚脉和虚证，实脉和实证都是有独立意义的词语，没有必要把其中的“虚”和“实”分别都用同一英文对应词来表达。但是，按照魏氏直译法这类情况是必须用同一英文词的，于是规定“虚”的英文对应词是 vacuous 或 vacuity，据此形成的中医英文词数以百计，例如：虚脉 vacuous pulse，虚证 vacuity pattern，虚邪 vacuity evil，虚中 vacuity stroke，虚胀 vacuity distention，虚肿 vacuity swelling，虚里 vacuity Li，以及五脏六腑气血阴阳诸虚。“实”的英文对应词是 replete 或 repletion，据此形成的中医英文词也为数众多，例如：实脉 replete pulse，实证 repletion pattern，实邪 repletion evil，实胀 repletion distention，实肿 repletion swelling，胃实 stomach repletion，胃实呃逆 stomach repletion hiccough，以及其他五脏六腑诸实。

由于“虚”和“实”的英译对中医英文名词的制定至关重要，有必要对这两个单音词的英译本身加以讨论。首先，让我们查阅一下英文词典，无论是《牛津现代高级英汉汉英双解辞典》还是《韦伯斯特大辞典》，对 vacuity 的解释都不外乎：① the state of a vacuum；emptiness；nothingness；② vacant space；a void；③idleness；④lack of intelligence。以上几种注解，只有前两种能勉强用于中医，即空虚、全无。用于脉象，已嫌过重；用于辨证，则难以想象。虚证是正气不足，无论气血阴阳，哪一项皆不可空虚、全无，一旦如此，即使不是死亡，至少也是亡阴、亡阳、亡气、亡血，接近死亡，绝非一般的虚证。中医用词，“虚”与“不足”是通用的，例如李经纬等主编的《中医大辞典》中“肺气不足，即肺气虚，详该条”，“肺气虚，又称肺气不足”。其实，魏氏是完全同意这一点的。对“不足”皆译为 insufficiency，在《辞典》中多处出现与上述《中医大辞典》类似的情况，如“insufficiency of heart Qi 心气不足：see heart Qi vacuity”，“heart Qi vacuity 心气虚：the manifestation of insufficiency of heart Qi...”，“insufficiency of gallbladder Qi 胆气不足：Synonyms：gallbladder vacuity and qi timidity；gallbladder Qi vacuity”[4]。问题在于，vacuity 和 insufficiency 这两个英文词真的是同义的、通用的吗？这个问题只能由魏迺杰先生自己来回答了。

把 replete 或 repletion 规定为“实”的英文对应词，更是望文生义。无论是《牛津现代高级英汉汉英双解辞典》还是韦氏词典，对 replete 的解释都是：①well-fed or gorged；②abundantly supplied or stocked，即“吃饱喝足的”和“充分供应的”。repletion 则是“吃饱喝足的或充分供应的状态”。这样良好的状态与“邪气盛则实”有什么关系？把 repletion pattern 作为“实证”的英文对应词，用一个丝毫没有病态意思的词来表示病证，这种译法是无法让人接受的。至于虚邪 vacuity evil、虚中 vacuity stroke、虚肿 vacuity swelling、虚里 vacuity Li、实邪 repletion evil、胃实 stomach repletion 等令人莫名其妙的中英对应，这类例子很多，在此就不一一评论了。

总之，《辞典》中出现的这些问题无不与魏氏所强调的逐字对应的直译法有关。这种译法错误的根源在于，它混淆了中文的字与词的区别，忽略了中文构词的规律，把中文的字与英文的词等同起来，片面追求字面上的中英文吻合，用简单机械的方法处理像中医名词术语英译这样极其复杂的问题，因而很多仿造的中医英文名词未能真正反映出原有的中医学意义。

生理、病理及疾病的预防、诊断、治疗、康复和保健的综合科学，有其学术内涵的共性。这种差异与共性并存的特点必然反映在中医名词术语的英译上，即一部分能找到相同或相近的西医（现代医学）对应词，另一部分是中医特有的概念，没有西医对应词。我们认为，能否用西医名词翻译某一中医名词术语，关键是要看两者有无学术内涵的对应性；在此问题上我们与魏迺杰先生有较大分歧。

魏迺杰先生在《实用英文中医辞典》（下简称《辞典》）再版序中一再告诫，大量采用西医名词无法准确传达传统中医的精髓。但是，他没有明确指出哪些西医名词可用，哪些不可用。对此魏氏在其《英汉汉英词典》（1995）中曾作过探讨。他把西医词语分为三类：一类是借用普通语言用词所构成的西医词语，例如 fever、chill、cold、influenza、malaria、leprosy、hiccough、headache 等。这些词语是可用的，因为一般人都能够明白。另一类是西医用以描述特定专业概念的词语，例如 conjunctivitis、anemia、hypertension、paranasal sinusitis、trichomoniasis 等，“由于这些名词所反映出的专业知识与一般的认知有很大的距离”，魏氏认为应该绝对避免。第三类介于上述两类词语之间，例如 enuresis、lochia、tumor、fistula、diphtheria 等，这些词语“不需要任何专业知识或设备便能加以了解或确定”，也能够予以使用[5]。从具体中医英文词来看，《辞典》仍然是沿用这种对西医词语的界定方法，如果有什么改变的话，只不过是进一步强调逐字固定直译而增加了一些古怪的英文对应词。例如，1995 年版“发热”的英文对应词是 fever，而 1998 和 2002 年版虽仍用 fever，但增加了一种译法，即 heat effusion，并以后者为主。其他名词变化不大，看来《辞典》对西医名词的使用原则未变。

这种以“一般认知”“不需要任何专业知识或设备便能加以了解或确定”作为能否使用西医名词的界定标准实属别开生面，在科学性、学术性、实用性等方面均存在问题。首先，对什么是一般认知缺少判断标准。比如说《辞典》中“肛漏”的英文对应词是 anal fistula，“肛裂”的英文对应词是 splitting of the anus，而不是 anal fissure，不知是如何判断 fistula 属于一般认知，而 fissure 则超出了一般认知的范围。再举例来说，把“痉”的英文对应词规定为 tetany，从而仿造出一系列带有 tetany 或 tetanic 的中医英文词：风痉 wind tetany，寒痉 cold tetany，刚痉 hard tetany，痉病 tetanic disease，痉厥 tetanic reversal，解痉 resolving tetany，等等。什么是“痉”，让我们从文献上做一考察，《灵枢・热病》指出：“热而痉者死。腰折，瘛，齿噤也。”《金匮要略・痉湿病脉证治》中有一段专门对“痉”的论述：“病者身热足寒，颈项强急，恶寒，时头热，面赤目赤，独头动摇，卒口噤，背反张者，痉病也。”《温病条辨·痉病瘛总论》中说：“痉者强直之谓，后人所谓角弓反张。”李经伟等主编《中医大辞典》说：“痉，病名，以项背强急、口噤、四肢抽搐、角弓反张为主症。”普通高等教育中医药类规划教材《中医内科学》（1997）中对痉病的论述如下：“痉病系指由于筋脉失养所引起的以项背强急，四肢抽搐，甚至角弓反张为主要特征的临床常见病。”由此可见，自古至今，中医对“痉”的认识没有大的变化。现代西医学对 tetany 一词的定义如下：它是由于细胞外钙离子浓度降低引起的神经肌肉兴奋性增高，可见于甲状旁腺功能减退、维生素 D 缺乏和碱中毒，其特征是手足痉挛、肌肉抽搐甚至喉痉挛[6]。由此可见，tetany 与“痉”的临床表现是不同的，tetany 一般只限于手足，特别是两手的屈肌，没有项背强急、角弓反张等现象，故而tetany的相应中文是“手足搐搦”，而不是一般的痉病。令人不可思议的是在诸多与“痉”有关的英文词中为什么偏偏选中 tetany 这样一个有特定含义的西医用语，难道是因为没有医学专业知识的一般人都认识这个词吗？要知道除了医学词典外有些非医学专业的英文词典，例如《牛津高阶英文词典》（*Oxford Advanced Learner's Dictionary of Current English*）根本就没有收载这个词。

对于《辞典》中的有些英文词，魏氏可能认为不是西医专业用词，但实际上并非如此。例如中医学中的“发”是指面积较广、病情较重的体表痈疽，魏氏则从字义考虑，“发”字意为“emit（发散），issue（放出），present an appearance（使之呈现）”（《辞典》第 168 页）。由于 effuse 意为“发出”，与中文字义相符，于是把“发”字的英文对应词定为 effusion，从而仿造出发背 effusion of the back、发脑 effusion of the brain、发乳 effusion of the breast、发颐 jowl effusion、发热 heat effusion、经行发热 menstrual heat effusion、对心发 heart-level effusion、对脐发 umbilical-level effusion 等一系列的英文病症名。其实，effusion 是一个常用的西医名词，意思是向体内某部位或组织内有液体渗出或漏出，也指所渗出或漏出的液体，故中文称渗漏或渗漏液，例如 pleural effusion 指胸膜渗漏或胸腔积液，pericardial effusion 指心包渗漏或心包积液。西医从不把体表的痈疽或其流出的脓液叫做 effusion，所以上面这些与痈疽有关的“发”译为 effusion 是不正确的，它们不可避免地会引起误解。尤其像“发脑”这样的名词用 effusion of the brain 作为对应词，实在可怕，会让人误认为是脑脊液渗漏出来了。即使把 effusion作为一个普通用词对待，也无法让人承认上述各种 effusion 的合理性，人们见到 heat effusion 首先想到的是“热发散”，既然热能够发散出来就不会导致体温升高而发热。我们实在难以理解为什么魏氏在原来列举可用的西医词语中第一个就是 fever，现在却变了，而且还影响其他有关词汇，如“恶寒发热”的英文对应词成为 heat（effusion）and（aversion to）cold，即 heat and cold，这样一来，与八纲的“寒热”cold and heat 就无法区分了。

有些中医名词明明有相应的英文对应词，只因为是西医名词，魏氏便避而不用，宁可使用生搬硬套的中文式英文，或者至少也得在使用西医名词的同时加一条中式的英文词。例如，经闭与 amenorrhea 相应，魏氏是同意这一点的，但又增加 menstrual block 作为同义词，并以后者作为重点。这显然与逐字对应直译法有关，因为在中文单字表中规定“闭”的英文对应词是 block，所以尽管 amenorrhea 与经闭相应，魏氏仍强调用 menstrual block 作为对应词。其实，这种直译并不比用 amenorrhea 更能反映中医原意。“经闭”是女子年逾 18 岁尚无月经来潮或来潮后又中断，amenorrhea 即是此意，而 menstrual block 首先让人想到的是经血被阻塞不能流出，与经闭的含义不同。

中医的鹅口疮与西医的鹅口疮（即 thrush）并无二致，让人疑惑为什么英文对应词非创造出一个 goose-mouth sore 新词不可。尤其令人费解的是《辞典》中注明鹅口疮又名“雪口”snow mouth，尽管 snow 也有“雪白的东西”的含义，但西医英文名词已有非常合适的对应词，即 thrush 又名 white mouth，另外再译出一个新词 snow mouth 实在没有必要。

中文“抽风”是一个很普及的医学名词，一般中国人都知道其含义，与 convulsions 十分相应，魏氏舍此不用，生给搞出个 tugging wind。如果这样的译文出自中国人之手，会有人不客气地称之为洋泾浜，但出自以英语为母语的英文讲师之手，真不知该如何称呼了。是不是魏氏因为 convulsions 是西医名词就舍弃不用呢？并非如此，《辞典》中“抽搐”的对应词就是 convulsions，“搐搦”的对应词也是 convulsions，既然 convulsions 这个词是可以用的，“抽搐”“搐搦”与“抽风”这三个词又是同义，为什么“抽风”就必须译成 tugging wind 不可？究其原因，很有可能是与其所制定的中文单字的英文对应词表有关。表中无“抽”“搐”“搦”三字的英文对应词，只能意译，但对“风”规定其英文对应词是 wind，所以就出现了 tugging wind 这样的英文词。假如真是如此，那么魏氏所制定的西医名词取舍标准实际上是可以随意改变的。坦率地讲，用 convulsions 表达“抽搐”和“搐搦”没有歪曲中医原意，而 tugging wind 实令人不知所云，不但是西方人士，就是懂得英文的中国人也猜不透它说的是什么。

这类情况在《辞典》中非常多，例如“丹”的规定对应词是 cinnabar，并衍生出这样那样的 cinnabar。要知道 cinnabar 也是西医药名词，即硫化汞，人们见到 cinnabar toxin，大概首先会想到硫化汞毒，最多也只能想到朱红色的毒素，不知有谁能想到丹毒。人们见到 cinnabar sand，大概也只会想到丹砂（朱砂）或砂状的硫化汞，怎么也不会想到是丹痧。作为专业名词总应该包含一些反映基本概念或特征的信息，如果丝毫没有这样的信息，而且还能引人误入歧途，那还不如用汉语拼音，汉语拼音最多是令人不知所云，但不至于引起误解。其他如 fire cinnabar、red wandering cinnabar 更是令人难以琢磨的谜语。不知魏氏是否会争辩，cinnabar 与“丹”同义，为什么中文可以称火丹、赤游丹，却不可以照此英译。我们认为“丹”有多义，作为朱砂，译成 cinnabar 当然是可以的，但中文的“丹”又指一种肤红如丹、热如火灼的病症，英文 cinnabar 作为名词的含义十分明确，无论是天然的还是人工合成的都是硫化汞，与皮肤发红的病症没有关系，故魏氏所创造的 cinnabar toxin、cinnabar sand、fire cinnabar、red wandering cinnabar之类的中医英文词皆属误译。又如，子痫为一种中医产科急症，西医有明确的对应词 eclampsia，而魏氏将子痫译作 epilepsy of pregnancy（妊娠癫痫）——一种需与子痫相鉴别的神经科急症。可见，将有对应性的西医专业名词弃之不用，自创逐字固定直译的词语，不仅能产生误译、误解，并有导致临床误诊之可能。

其实，当初西医传入中国时将西医名词译为中文的经验对中医英译如何应用西医名词问题很有参考价值。其中有两点特别值得提及。

其一是如西医与中医所指确是同一事物，西译中时直接应用现有的中医名词，不另觅其他中文词语。例如，在解剖用语方面，tragus 译为耳珠，uterus 译为子宫，glans penis 译为龟头等无不都是原有的中医名词。这些中英文名词完全可以往返互译，经过 100 多年的考验从未出过问题，但在《辞典》中这种相应性被否定了，耳珠不再是 tragus，而是 pearl of the ear，子宫是 infant's palace，龟头是 tortoise's head，也许魏氏可以争辩，这些名词的西医相应词从《辞典》中能够找到。例如从索引查出“guītóu 龟头”在 621 页，在该页可以查到 tortoise's head 的注解是“YIN HEAD”，然后再从 710 页查出“yin head 阴头”的同义词里有 glans penis 一词。通过这样复杂的程序才能明白 tortoise’s head 到底说的是什么。假如手头没有这本《辞典》，要想读懂用魏氏这套英文中医词汇翻译或撰写的中医书籍，那就太难了。如果说像 pearl of the ear 和 tortoise's head 之类的词，对于说英语的西方人来说作为字谜来猜还有可能猜中，但是 infant's palace 就无法猜中了，没有人会想到已经出生的婴幼儿怎么又会回到母亲的腹中居住。有些症状和疾病，中医和西医的名称也是相通的，有不少西医病症名称译为中文时所采用的也就是中医词语，应用多年从未有过异议，例如 opisthotonus 译为角弓反张，edema 译为水肿，wheal 译为风疹块，rubella 译为风疹等。这些中文译名现在为什么不能回译为原来的英文？西医所说的“角弓反张”“水肿”“风疹块”“风疹”与中医所说的“角弓反张”“水肿”“风疹块”“风疹”所指的都是同一事物或现象，当初英译中是贴切的，现在从中文回译为英文也同样贴切。如果说必须按照魏氏的翻译方法把“角弓反张”译为 arched-back rigidity 才能反映“中医原貌”，那么当初把 opisthotonus 译为角弓反张就有问题了，因为它没有反映“西医原貌”。英文 opisthotonus 源自希腊文 ππθεγ（向后）和（搜紧），这里没有角弓的字样。就连 edema 当初也译错了，因为它源自希腊文 αβγδ（swelling，肿），不含水字。由此可见，魏氏所谓的“中医原貌”并不是中医作为一门医学所具有的原貌和精髓，而只不过是中医在文字表达上的某些习惯和方式而已。《辞典》中“水肿”的英文词是 water swelling，“风疹块”是 papular wind lumps，“风疹”是 wind papules，我们怀疑这种译法的实际效果究竟是能让西方人了解中医的原貌和精髓，还是教西方人认几个汉字。语言文字的隔阂是中医向西方传播的主要障碍之一，要消除这种隔阂绝不是教西方人学会几百个中文单字或创造一些中文式的中医英文词所能解决的。相反，这种中文式的中医英文词越多，越使西方人感到中医玄妙莫测，难以理解。

其二是如何处理同一事物的不同名称问题。西医名词也有不少“又称”“别称”，例如 felon、whitlow、panaris 和 panaritium[3]，它们虽各有出处，有的本来就是英文，有的源自拉丁文，但全都指的是化脓性指头炎。当初把西医名词译成中文时没有考虑要反映这种用词不一的情况，一律译为“瘭疽”。假如把这 4 个词分别译为不同的中文，这对于西医传入中国只会制造混乱，不会起到什么有益的作用。现在的问题是：把瘭疽译为英文该怎么办。《辞典》中出现 4 个同义词 Biao-ju，tip-abscess，flare-tip abscess 和 whitlow。这样，一个化脓性指头炎的英文名至少有了 7 个。原来的英文名已有多种，在英译过程中还要再人为地增加几个，这样做确实让人难以理解。中医由于历史悠久，中国地域广阔，不同的时代、不同的地区出现了不同的命名，这不足为奇，但是否有必要通过文字上的直译来显示中医学的这种“原貌”值得商榷。像鼻根这个部位，中医有“山根”“下极”等不同说法，这只不过是汉语修辞学中的不同比喻，作为文学辞藻的研究有其价值，作为医学名词分别仿造出 mountain root 和 lower extreme，完全没有必要。说《辞典》中收载这些词是为翻译古籍之用，这不无道理，但在注释中注明汉字原义就足够了，作为医学专业名词对待，实在无法令人接受。

魏氏自诩为向西方传播传统中医的精髓，所以反对大量使用西医名词，但是他自己在这个问题上却是矛盾的，不仅有意无意地使用了许多西医名词，而且《辞典》中竟然还出现了中文西医词汇。《辞典》中既有“阑尾”“菌痢”之类的西医名词，还收载了“先兆流产”“经前期紧张综合征”等中文西医病名。对于“经前期紧张综合征”一词，魏氏用了超过一整栏的篇幅加以注释，可见其重视的程度。

魏氏对中医英文词中的西医名词使用问题还反映出究竟要向西方什么样的人士传播中医，为什么选择西医名词要以一般的认知为准？为什么“不需要任何专业知识或设备便能加以了解或确定的西医名词”就可以使用，“所反映出的专业知识与一般的认知有很大的距离”的西医名词便应该绝对避免？按照常理，选择用词应该根据中英文对应的程度来考虑，而不是根据一般的认知程度；如果确实对应，越是专业性强的西医名词越应优先考虑，因为中西医学都是医学，其名词术语都是专业用语。既然是专业用语，就不可能要求无专业知识的人全都能懂。即使在中国，也不是只要有一般的认知水平就都能读懂中医的中文用词。我们不反对向西方的普通群众传播中医知识，但中医是一门医学，首先须考虑向西方的医学界传播。针灸之所以能够在西方流传，正是因为西方的医学界肯定了针灸的疗效。魏氏为什么那么强调向普通群众传播而不重视对西方医学界传播，这个问题值得深思。

总之，在西医名词的运用上，《辞典》存在着许多严重的问题，每个不妥的用词固然各有其原因，但根本的原因在于魏氏规定以“一般认知”“不需要任何专业知识便能了解”作为能否使用西医名词的界定标准。这种标准所反映的观点实际上就是中医不是真正的医学，只不过是一种通俗的东方文化。这恰恰也是我们与魏氏在对待英文中医名词的根本分歧所在。

参考文献

[1] 魏迺杰. 实用英文中医辞典. New York：Paradigm Publication，1998：18，22，309，512，954.

[2] 吕叔湘，朱德熙. 语法修辞讲话. 上海：开明书店，1952：8.

[3] 周光庆，杨合鸣主编. 古代汉语教程. 武汉：华中师范大学出版社，2001：90.

[4] 李经维. 中医大辞典. 北京：人民卫生出版社，2005：309，952，954.

[5] 魏迺杰 . 英汉 . 汉英中医词典 . 长沙：湖南科学技术出版社，1995：25.

[6] Dorland's illustrated medical dictionary. 29th edition. 2000：1818.

[7] 北京协和医院世界卫生组织疾病分类合作中心 . 疾病和有关健康问题的国际统计分类第十次修订本（ICD-10）. 北京：人民卫生出版社，1998：71.

[原载《中国中西医结合杂志》，2005，25（10）：937－940，
《中国中西医结合杂志》，2005，25（9）：1046－1049.]

评《英汉·汉英中医词典》出版

1. 王一方　（湖南科学技术出版社）

第一部大型中医英汉双语工具书《英汉·汉英中医词典》最近由湖南科学技术出版社出版。该词典收词 14 200 余条，是目前收词最多的一部工具书，编者魏迺杰（Nigel Wiseman）是一位英籍汉学家、语言学家，他潜心研究中医翻译十几年，先后在美国、台湾编纂并出版了数部中医英文教科书及辞书。该书的另一个特点是词条翻译贴近中医词汇源于生活感受、取类比象的建构原则，反映了中医诸多词汇的多义性。该词典的学术水准受到陈可冀院士及文树德（Paul Unschuld，德国）教授的推崇。

2. 魏迺杰（Nigel Wiseman，台湾中国医药学院）

2.1　本书采用的方法

本书所主张的中医英文词汇择定目标就是要在源自于中医整体概念系统的译文中将中医的概念忠实地反映出来。鉴于中医词汇与普通语言极为近似的事实，系统、组织化地选用英文普通语言的对应用词应该是中医翻译的优先选择。至于西医学的术语名词，只有当其含义不至于扭曲中医概念的认知时，如前文中详加说明，方得资以对应施用。而汉语拼音音译词或是新造字则应当尽量避免使用。以下便以一些实例详细说明。

2.2　普通语言对应词

本书尽可能采用自然对应词，譬如脏腑以及身体部位的翻译名称都是以一般说英文的人所使用的名称译出。

而若英文的自然对应词缺乏时，则尽量择取等化性对应词，尤其是将比喻的含义尽可能保留。例如“牛皮癣”“鹅掌风”“鹤膝风”与“白虎历节”，本书分别译之为 oxhide lichen、goose-foot wind、crane's knee wind 及 white tiger joint running。然而，为了顺应一些早已被接纳而成为惯例的翻译，本书仍以 bowels and viscera 来翻译“脏腑”，而更勉强的是纳入以 point 来翻译“穴”的既成事实。至于笔者将痰饮的“饮”译为 rheum，不采用根据字义翻译的 drink，主要是为了避免误导西方读者。

2.3 西医学名称

本书中所择用的西医学名称限制于使用那些字面上的含义并不会表达出任何西医专业认知者，因此，目前已很少被西医使用的名称如 strangury（意指疼痛性尿淋沥）用以翻译“淋”（证），而 diphtheria（字源是指“皮革”之义，原来藉以形容其蔓延于咽后的假膜）则用来翻译“白喉”。至于开始使用的年代可以溯源至西方现代医学发展之前的一些疾病名称，如 measles、malaria 等，是由于其原始的含义并非现代的西医定义，对于西医而言也算是延用性的名词，因此，本书将之视为自然对应词，而不是西医专业用语。一些根据前述判断标准可被接受的西医学诊断用词本书也予以收录，但是笔者在自己的翻译作品当中，尽量以足以令读者望文生义的一般用语来取代这些字。这些西医学诊断用词（其后的括号中列入较适当的一般用语对应词）包括了 hemorrhage（bleeding）出血，hemafecia（bloody stool）便血，hematospermia（blood in the semen）血精，hematuria（bloody urine）尿血，oliguria（scant urine）尿少，polyuria（copious urine）尿多，oligomenorrhea（scant menstruation）月经过少，menorrhagia（profuse menstruation）月经过多，dysmenorrhea（menstrual pain）痛经，oligogalactia（scant breast milk）乳少，galactorrhea（loss of breast milk）乳汁自出，analactia（breast milk stoppage）乳汁不行。而笔者将“经闭”这个名词翻译为 menstrual block（闭）以取代 amenorrhea，就是为了反映出中医对如是现象的认知。

2.4 新造字词

英文多字的复合词就是为了配合中医的复合性词语所制造（如 blood vacuity dizziness，血虚眩晕）。但在某种情况下，英文多字复合词被用以表达出单一的中医用字（如 flat abscess，疽）。

本书尽可能避免使用造新字的方式，不过还是有一些例外的情形存在。比如“利”字被翻译成 disinhibit，这个英文词是组合出 s（解），于 inhibit（抑制，束缚）而来（不过英文原本就有 disinhibition 与 disinhibitory，应该在规模比较大的英文词典中可以查得到）。“升”“降”分别以 upbear、downbear 译出，因为英文并没有任何单一用字足以分别表达出这两个中文字原指的“使之上升”“使之下降”的含义，至于 upbear、downbear 本身则分别是由 bear upward、bear downward 所缩合成的新单字。将中医所指的“暑”翻译成 summerheat，就是把 summer heat 写成单一个字，而从之更可以把“暑热”“暑湿”“暑温”等复合词分别翻译成 summerheat-heat、summerheat-dampness 与 summerheat-warmth，清楚地将这些中医复合词的区分显现出来。至于中医的“胁”，因为常用的译称

hypochondrium 并不符合中医“由腋下至肋骨尽处之总称名”之定义，因此，本书的翻译是 ribside（“肋侧”）。出现于气逆、逆冷的“逆”字以 counterflow 来翻译，亦是新造的词。虽然面对这些新造词时，读者必须熟悉它们的中医专业术语含义（正如中国学生面对中医术语时也必须熟悉这些中文字在中医的特殊意义），但是根据笔者的母语直觉（native speaker intuition），西方读者应该会觉得这些新造词在语境里面传达中医概念的表达力很高，甚至很可能根本不会想到它们是新造的词。

2.5 拉丁文

本书拒绝使用未被英文接纳的纯拉丁文名词，而唯一的例外是由学名变化而来的拉丁文中药名。值得指出的是，中药的拉丁文学名至今仍然尚未完全规范化。本书所收入的近 1730 个拉丁文药名是以尽量简约的方式加以采纳，但并不会因此而发生名词（或中药）之间有重复混淆的情形。这些名称来自笔者一个收集有 5000 多个药物的资料库，而本书所采用的命名方式即足以将这 5000 多种药物在名称上作明确的区分。

本书虽然收录了拉丁文药物名称，但是笔者个人认为英文药名由于好拼好读，沟通性、传达力较高，而且西方临床医师的使用也比较方便，因此，应该远比拉丁文名称理想。而在 1730 多种药当中，其中 733 种具有在规模较大的英文词典里可以查到的现成英文名称（本书以·标明）；842 种具有曾经在植物学用书或中医临床用书出现过的名称（⊙），而只有 285 种是经过笔者以一定的原则所创造出的（○）。

2.6 汉语拼音音译

在本书中，在万不得已时才使用音译的方式。比如“疳”音译为 gan，因为这个字在中医同时可指营养不良与糜烂两种病，而这两种同名病称之间的关系并不十分明确。将“癞”音译为 lai，也是因为其指的麻风与以掉发为病征的头皮疾病之间的关系亦不清楚。而“便毒”译为 Bian toxin，是因为“便”字的含义不明之故。对于外国读者所不熟悉的名词，笔者在其后加上汉语拼音以资参考，如 clove sore（ding）。至于“阴阳”与“气”，仍分别译之为 Yin-yang 与 Qi，因为这样的译词早已被英文所接纳。

2.7 简缩与符号

本书为了遵从已广为接受的惯例（应该说是极其勉强地），采用了常用穴名代号的命名方式，不过也附加了各个穴名的英文译名。而“天干地支”在本书中也是以代号的方式来翻译的，因为这些中文名称的字义并不明确。至于“君、臣、佐、使”及“卫气营血”，除了将全名翻出来之外（sovereign，minister，assistant and courier；defense，Qi，construction and blood），也附加了这两个词的简明译称 drug roles 和 four aspects。

2.8　尚未解决的问题

鉴于语言本身的性质，翻译者并不可能对于其所择定的每一个译语名称尽皆满意。在此谨探讨笔者个人认为的在本书中的未尽完备之处。

翻译者有时必须被迫去遵从习以为常的翻译惯例，如此虽然会与其原则相违背，但却不得不接受。“穴”在本书中以 point 来翻译全然是因为英文语系国家的每一个针灸师都习惯使用这个字。如此的译称仍不免令人抱憾，因为“穴”的本意是指是“洞”或“洞穴”，指出进针之处乃位于人体外在解剖形势上呈现裂缝或开洞之处，而英文 point 的含义不过是指一个抽象几何性定位的“点”，并不能完全地表达出中文“穴”的意思。

而本书把“证”按照“证候、征候”（如呕吐、恶寒等）和“证型”（如热证、表证等）这两种不同的用法分别翻译成 sign 和 pattern。“证”的本义是为证词或证据（testimony，evidence），而病人所表现的“证”（征候），正是医者所观察到的“证据”，但是“证型”的用法却是一种引申出来的含义。欲在英文之中寻得一个名词足以充分地同时表达出“证”的原意、“证候”以及其引申出的“证型”含义，并不容易。大概具有这两种意思的英文词有 display（显示）、manifestation（表现）及 presentation（呈现）三个。但是后两者使用在复合词，如 manifestation identification（辨证）时便显得非常地笨拙。

“证”字所造成的翻译问题因为同音字“症”的存在而显得更复杂。对于这两个字，虽然不同作者主张的用法不同，但常常被混用。在现今的中国大陆，虽然两者的使用一样普遍，但是有人认为“症”应该专指病人的主观症状，恐怕这是受到现代医学影响所致。而在台湾和日本的中医界，“证”字的使用比“症”较为普遍。不过在一般翻译作品上，常见这两个字以同一个翻译名词被译出。

处理“证”“症”问题的同时，其他的相关名词也应该试图一起考虑，如“疾”和“病”。前者常出现在某一个“病种”的复合词，如“痢疾”“疟疾”等。而“病”则是指一种与“健康”相对的生病状态，并常特别指如是状态的一个事例，如“久病”。不过“病”与“疾”相同，也有病种的意思。而英文的 disease 通常具有“不健康”的意思，但是最常用的含义却是指“病种”而言。在现代医学中，disease 倾向于导致身体组织病变的疾病，而与表示功能失调的 disorder 对称。另外，illness 与 sickness 亦可用指病种而言，但这样的用法较少。如此的问题无论是中文或英文都有待进一步的研究，方能建立出确定的翻译原则。

有的中医关键性用词如“证”一般，在本书中根据不同的定义、语境使用双重翻译方式。如“精”译为 essence 和 semen，“气”译为 Qi 和 breathing，“热”译为 heat 和 fever。虽然双重翻译方式并不是十分理想，但以英文清楚地进行定义，还是可以让西方读者意识到存在于这些成对英文翻译用词之间的同一性。而且该当选用 essence 或 semen，Qi 或 breathing，由中文的上下文便很容易作出决定，但是 heat 和 fever 的区分就比较容易造成困扰，因为“热”在中医中尚包括了一些自我感觉的热感（如五心烦热），如此的感觉就并不属于英文 fever 所指的含义。

在本书上，“痈”和“疽”分别被翻译为 welling abscess（“涌出来的脓肿”）和 flat abscess（“扁平的脓肿”）。无奈的是，这两个新造复合词其英文字面上的含义比中文的“痈、疽”较为明确。

最后，“寒”与“冷”虽然在中医的含义上有所差别，但二者皆译为 cold。虽然后者所指有比较属于感官性的“冰冰冷冷”的含义，可以用英文 frigid 来加以表达，但是 frigid 并不能符合“冷”在每一种语境的需求。而更令人不满意的是，frigid 在现代英文的普通语言用法上还特指“性冷感”一义。而“干”与“燥”之间也存在着类似的差别，不过将两者皆译为 dry。

2.9 结论

有关如何翻译中医的讨论常常被以下的错误观念所蒙蔽，一是主张中医的概念必须移植到一个西方人所熟悉的参考体系结构上，而另一个先入为主的错误想法就是认为英文原来的词汇不足以满足翻译中医的新需求。但是，无数的实例告诉我们，唯有使用精准的英文去对应翻译中医词汇才不至于混淆西方人对于中医的认知。

如果一篇为了西方的中医初学者翻译的英文译文是用西方人“熟悉”的语言去翻译的（如应用西医的用词、概念或不尊重中医原文的恣意意译），所带来的影响将会让读者产生他已经对中医有所了解的印象，事实则不然。如果他花了 5 年的时间继续去研读以这种所谓“容易了解”的语言形态所翻译出来的书，他所获得的知识将会只是一个花同样时间研读中文中医典籍的中国人所获得的十分之一。但是，这并非是因为西方人的才智不足以了解一种不同文化的产物。相对的，一种以反映出原始含义的英文词汇来表达中医概念的翻译方式，对于外国读者而言起初可能比较难以阅读。如此的用书无疑地将包含许多用以解释这些词汇含义的注解，或是甚至集结成词汇学用书。但是，使用 5 年的时间去研读这类书籍，读者对于中医学的认知层次即使不能相当于以同样的模式去学习西医的中国人对西医的了解程度，至少也不至于差距太远。

忠实地传达原文信息的翻译书籍必须经由一个与原文词汇紧密配合的词汇来表达。为了加速读者对于术语名词与概念的认知，额外的解释必须以谨慎的注解提供给读者。术语名词的精确翻译对于学生而言起初可能不是那么容易了解，但是只有这样的翻译才能经得起时间的考验，并提供唯一深入学习的途径。

在西传的过程中，中医并不能为了配合西方人的需求而有所改变。而西方意欲学习中医的人也绝对无法经由一种“以其本身较为熟悉的知识系统将中医学加以过滤”的学习方式获得成功，他们必须真正地进入中医的世界。只有当翻译者遵循中医原来被接受的传统方式去看待中医学，并将中医忠实地翻译出来才得以为西方真正想要学习中医的人士开通一条迈入中医的大道。

3. 陈可冀 （中国中医研究院西苑医院）

以下为对本书所写的序言。

20世纪中国医学的一个显著特点是在东西方文化碰撞与交流中发展、更新，并逐步跨越地缘分隔的栅栏，不断地国际化。针灸学在世界范围内的传播就是一个众人知晓的例证。毫无疑问，要推进中国医学的国际化，首先必须致力于中医语汇学的跨文化理解、沟通，在辞书编纂与翻译规范方面做大量筚路蓝缕、开启山林式的工作，以期不断有新的建树。

在中国，兵农医艺被称之为“四大国粹”。与当今各种自然科学相比，中国医学有着更鲜明的东方文化特质与丰富的华夏民族个性以及淳厚的传统积淀，因此，中医译事之难在形神俱合，信达雅兼备；而译者之难在融合东西文化精髓，通晓古今知识流变。魏迺杰先生便是一位迎难而进的学人。他原籍英国，早年专攻语言学，曾主修德文、法文与西班牙文，对中国语言情有独钟，倾注了极大的热情。尔后，由中文研究步入神奇的中医殿堂。他潜心中医翻译十几年，先后在美国、中国台湾编译、出版了数部中医的英文教科书及词汇用书，这部《英汉·汉英中医词典》就是他首次在大陆出版的一部大型工具书。

论特点，该书主要有二，一是能把握中国医学特有的人文精神，摆脱了一味迁就现代医学职业化词汇及译法规则所建立的翻译体系，大量使用日常词语，更符合中医词汇源于生活感受、取类比象的建构原则。二是译出了中医诸多词汇的多义性，揭示出中医词汇与语境规定性之间的微妙关系以及多层次、多风格的适度变化。很显然，魏先生的翻译是在追求一种至高的境界，即基于深入的背景挖掘与丝丝入扣理解的“原味式诠释”，力图把异质文化骨子里的东西吃透、吃准，然后译解、表达出来。

以匹夫之力完成这样一部大的辞书，不可能每一词条都无懈可击，但作为一项中医学术事业，魏先生无疑是成功的。为此他甘于淡泊与寂寞、执着而坚定，付出了百倍的艰辛与劳顿，这一切都值得我和我的中国同行报以诚挚的敬意。

［原载《中国中西医结合杂志》，1996，16（2）：122－125.］

《补注洗冤录集证》第一个英译本简评

邱　功

在中国南宋时期（1247），出现了一部世界上公认的最早的法医学专著——《洗冤集录》，这本书的作者就是被誉为“大宋提刑官”的宋慈。此后，《洗冤集录》不仅出现了众多的衍生本，在实际的司法检验中影响深远，而且，14 世纪以后，《洗冤集录》的衍生本首先传入了朝鲜，随后至日本、越南。18 世纪以后，《洗冤集录》在欧美国家备受关注，衍生本被译成了法语、英语、荷兰语、德语等多国文字。

1873 年，剑桥大学东方文化学教授，英国汉学家翟理斯（H. A. Giles，1845—1935）将《洗冤集录》在清道光年间（1843）童濂所刊的衍生本《补注洗冤录集证》进行了全文的翻译，题为 *The Hsi Yüan Lu*，*or Instructions to Coroners*（《洗冤录或验尸官指南》），这是《洗冤集录》衍生本的第一个英译本。随即翟理斯于 1874 年将译稿投给《中国评论》杂志，然而却与时任《中国评论》的编辑就校对问题发生了不愉快，遂停止向《中国评论》投稿，刊载于《中国评论》的译稿仅为原译稿的一半。1924 年，英国皇家医学会（Royal Society of Medicine）将翟理斯的译稿全文收入该会论文集——《皇家医学会论文集》第 17 卷“医学史”专章（Section of the History of Medicine），同时有单行本问世。这个译本得到了医学界人士的认可，并被誉为“最有影响，最具权威”的英译本[1]。所以翟理斯感慨地说，《洗冤集录》在“那些我从未想到过的地方引起了人们极大的关注”[2]。随后在 1981 年，美国的大学教授麦克奈特（Brain E. McKnight）将《洗冤集录》（岱南阁本）作了全文的翻译，这是《洗冤集录》及其衍生本现存的两个完整的英译本。这里，我们对翟理斯译本做一简单评论。

1. 译本的缺点

在 1924 年的译本首页，翟理斯这样写道：“1873 年我在宁波任职时第一次听说了《洗冤集录》。我发现负责验尸的地方高级官员到达案发现场时总是带着一本我现在翻译的这本书。并且我发现当遇到一个受到严重伤害的生者的时候，要进行查验，对待死者也同样如此。在后一种情形中，任何在验尸官仔细观察和检查之前所进行的诸如搬动或扰乱尸体等的鲁莽干扰行为都将对公正地解释案件发生非常严重的影响。我由此对这一阶段的中国文明产生了浓厚的兴趣，进一步对《洗冤集录》的文本进行了仔细的研究，继而开始翻译”[3]。由此可见，由于翻译的年代较早，且翟理斯翻译的目的是向西方世界介绍中国文化，并非宣传法医学知识，因此，导致其翻译态度较为随意，对有些概念的理解也不够准确。同时，译本中所有的书名、人名、地名所采用的注音方法，乃是翟理斯自己修改并创造的威妥玛——翟理斯注音系统，这是中国清末至 1958 年汉语拼音方案公布前，中国和国际上流行的中文拼音方案。如《洗冤集录》书名的翻译，翟理斯的注音为斜体 *Hsi Yüan Lu*，有别于现代的注音方法。类似之处还有许多，这无疑给现代的阅读带来了一些困难。

1.1　翻译态度较随意

翟理斯在整篇的译文中，没有像麦氏一样采用注释的方法，只是对文章进行了翻译，翻译较为随意和自由。同时，在译文的最后，翟理斯也没有给出参阅的书目以及索引，在内容上显得较为简单。并且译本并非原著的完整本，“《校正本洗冤集录》的尸论、论沿身骨脉、注释，以及王又槐、阮其新等的附记、附考、补注、顶批等均被删除”[4]。“令人遗憾的是，翟理斯将其中他认为不雅的段落译成了拉丁文（如验女尸的章节）或干脆将其删除”[5]，因此，呈现在读者面前的英译本在一定程度上未反映原来的内容。

在翻译卷、节标题时，翟理斯也甚为随意。标题简单，有的仅用一个词表达，光看标题，根本不知是何意，而且出现了正文标题与目录标题译文不相同的情况，通常正文标题译得更为达意。如中文本第一卷第五节标题是“洗罨”，英译本标题将其译为：Preparing Corpse for Examination，意为“检查前的尸体准备”，但正文中的标题却是：Washing and Preparing the Body[3]，意为“洗涤和准备尸体”。无疑正文标题翻译更接近于原文之意。在 1924 年版译本增入的后两卷中，目录没有译出，直接进入正文。1924 年版的译本比 1874 年的译本多了 4 幅相关尸图和解剖图，分别位于第一卷第三节的“尸格、尸图”和第十四节的“论沿身骨脉”处。尸图包括仰面和合面两幅，翟理斯认识到图中的黑白点代表了人体的穴位，并在图下注释道：“人体正面有 16 个致命穴位，背部有 6 个，而非致命的正面有 36 个，背部有 20 个”[3]。至于解剖图，翟理斯只是将原图附上，对于图上详细的部位名称并未翻译，这不得不令人非常遗憾，尤其是给西方读者的阅读造成了一定的困难。这些做法都体现了翟理斯的文人身份以及早期汉学研究的烙印，有着鲜明的个人色彩和时代特征。

1.2　概念理解不够准确

在翟理斯的译文中，对于有些概念的理解并不是十分准确，尤其是对于某些文化负载词的理解造成了偏差，这里仅举一些与中医学有关的概念加以说明。

对于有些中医学概念的翻译，翟理斯很显然借用了西医学的一些概念，由此造成了误译。如“缠喉风”一病，翟理斯将其翻译为白喉“diphtheria”[3]，显然这两种病是完全不同的。缠喉风“指因脏腑积热，邪毒内侵，风痰上壅所致的病证。症见喉部红肿疼痛，红丝缠绕，麻痒连胸，项强如蛇缠绕等”[6]，多指急性的喉科传染，多译为“acute laryngeal infection”。

又如，“气”的翻译，翟理斯尽力在译文中回避，如原文第三卷《疑难杂说》中有一段话，两次涉及“气”的概念，翟理斯均未译出。

原文：“凡因争斗致死而尸上无痕损，此或是被伤人旧有宿患气疾，或是未毆以前先曾饮酒，醉及争斗，时有所触碍，以致气绝而死也”[7]。

翟译文：“Where a man dies in consequence of blows received in a fight but has no wounds visible，it may be that he was suffering from a disease of long standing，or had taken too much to drink before he began to fight，and then from striking against something during the fight，injured himself so that he died”[3]。

而在第三卷的“作过死”一节中，翟理斯没有回避，却将“气绝血凝”中的“气”翻译为“vital liquid”[3]，意为“重要的液体”，这反映了翟理斯对翻译这个中国独有概念的迷惑。

1.3　翻译语言近乎阐释

通读下来，两个译本，语言流畅优美，甚为详备，可读性很强，然而，由于古籍语言所蕴含的信息十分丰富，翟理斯在翻译时，为了能够完整详细地译出，有的时候近乎阐释，正如麦克奈特在他 1981 年的《洗冤集录》译本所指出的：“翟理斯的译文对我帮助非常大……但是，翟理斯在翻译时有时过于自由，甚至变成了阐释，偶尔他也会陷入陷阱之中。对于翻译中国古典文献的西方译者而言，不管他多么小心，都可能陷入这种陷阱。再者，这也是早期汉学研究中难以避免的”[5]。

2. 译本的优点

然而，麦克奈特同样指出：“尽管存在着这些问题，但是，翟理斯的译本还是非常好的译本”[5]。王吉民先生也曾评论道：“运笔畅达”“立意确当”[8]。这些瑕疵并不妨碍翟理斯英译方法的可资借鉴处。这里，我们仅就其中涉及的一些具有文化负载特色的中医学概念的译法作一说明。对于这些文化负载词，翟理斯综合采用了音译、直译和意译的方法，灵活使用，在一定程度上，既保留了文化负载词的文化特色，同时，让翻译更为明白晓畅。

对古籍名称的翻译，翟理斯综合采用了音译和直译相结合的方法。除了译本书名的翻译外，其他如童濂序言一段中《作吏要言》的翻译，采用了音译：“Tso Li Yao Yen”和括号加注直译“Important Counsels to Government Officers”两种英译方法，这不但保存了古籍书名的文化内涵，而且揭示出古籍的内容，这种方法在现代中医古籍英译时也通常被采用。

一些特殊哲学概念的翻译，如“阴阳”，翟理斯综合采用了音译“Yin”

"Yang" 和括号加注意译 "female principle" "male principle" 两种译法。这在当时 "阴阳" 概念为西方人不了解的情况下，意译的方法无疑让翻译更为通达。随着 "阴阳" 概念越来越被西方人所熟知和接受，历史最终保留了音译的方法。"命门" 的翻译，翟理斯采用了 "door of the life" 的直译方法，同样可资借鉴。

一些特殊疾病的翻译，翟理斯多采用音译的方法，如 "重竭" "逆厥"，译成 "Chung Chieh" 和 "Ni Chüeh"[3]，而且，对于这两个概念的解释，翟理斯并不受原文形式的限制。他结合原文及批注，将其意思准确简洁地译出，实现了译文和原文的动态对等，如，原文为："五脏之气已绝于内而用针者反实其外，是谓重竭，重竭必死，其死也静。五脏之气已绝于外，而用针者反实其内，是谓逆厥，逆厥必死，其死也躁。" 批注："脏气已绝于内，阴虚也，反实其外，误益阳，益阳则愈损其阴，是重竭也。阴竭必死，死则静也。脏气已绝于外，阳虚也，反实其内，误补阴也。助阴则阳气愈竭，故至四逆而厥逆，厥必死，死必躁也"[7]。翟译文："If the five viscera are short of the Yin (female principle), and acupuncture is performed (from a faulty diagnosis) with a view to add more Yang (male principle), this is called Chung Chieh. Death is sure to result, the patient dying quietly. The opposite of this is called Ni Chüeh, and is equally fatal, but death is not peaceful."

可见，译文一目了然、简洁生动。当然，纵观翟理斯在翻译时所使用的方法，并非前后完全统一，这同样反映了翟理斯翻译时的随意和自由。

此外，从语言的角度来说，译本句式的灵活多变，用词的明白、简单、丰富，均增加了译本的可读性，这些不失为译本的优点所在。

英国汉学家翟理斯的《补注洗冤录集注》诞生于 19 世纪末，是向西方世界介绍中国文化的早期译作，不可避免地带上了时代的烙印和译者身份的个人色彩，这反映在翻译态度的随意、相关概念理解的不够准确以及近乎阐释的翻译语言。但是，与此同时，对于早期中国文化的外传，翟理斯的贡献功不可没，尤其体现在他在译介中国文化中的相关文化负载词时，灵活使用音译、意译、直译以及释译等各种方法，尊重了中国文化的独特性。这在 19 世纪的西方汉学研究中是难能可贵的。翟理斯在中国文化的早期译介中做出了有益的尝试。

参考文献

[1] 林金水，谢必震．福建对外文化交流史．福州：福建教育出版社，1997：368.

[2] 王绍祥．西方汉学界的 "公敌"——英国汉学家翟理斯研究（1845—1935）．福州：福建师范大学出版社，2004：221.

[3] Giles HA. The "Hsi Yüan Lu" or "Instructions to Coroners". London: John Bale, Sons & Danielsson Ltd, 1924: 1, 2-7, 19, 28, 31.

[4] 贾静涛．中国古代法医学史．北京：群众出版社，1984：217.
[5] McKnight BE. The washing away of wrongs：forensic medicine in the thirteeth century China. Taipei：Reprinted Southern Materials Center，Inc，1982：32.
[6] 原一祥．汉英双解中医大辞典．北京：人民卫生出版社，1997：1042.
[7] 童濂．补注洗冤录集证．清光绪三年丁丑（1877）浙江书局刊本.
[8] 王吉民．西译中医典籍考．中华医学杂志，1928，14（2）：103-105.

[原载《中国中西医结合杂志》，2011，31（4）：555-557.]

中医翻译要追本求源和衷中参西

——评介《中医翻译导论》

李　恩

随着改革开放的深入，中医学已为国际医学界所重视，中医对外翻译日益显得重要了。笔者喜读陕西中医学院李照国所著《中医翻译导论》一书，一是，看到了他对中医翻译有很多独特的见解；二是，现已有人把中医翻译作为一个独立学科而研究，李照国就是邵循道教授培养的一位跨学科的研究中医翻译的硕士。

中医和西医起源和发展是两个完全不同的理论体系。把中医原意译成外语确是一项十分艰难的工作。中医经典著作语义难懂，渗透着古代哲学思想，概念抽象，不易理解。中医术语本身缺乏统一，许多术语在现代医学上又无对应语，使翻译愈为不易。而《中医翻译导论》对上述问题做了有益的探索，把中医翻译提高到了一个理论研究阶段，现就该书的论点，突出围绕中医翻译应追本求源、衷中参西，做一扼要评介。

1. 中医翻译的历史回顾及现状分析

作者首先对中医翻译做了历史性的回顾，这有利于对现有译法进行了解和对存在问题的分析。根据中医翻译的历史，作者对现行中医翻译的特点概括为：仿造法、定义法、多样化、拼音法等。①仿造法：包括词素仿造法（如“肾虚”译为 nephropenia，“得气”译为 acueasthesia）和词语仿造法（如“血厥”译为 blood syncope，“肺热”译为 lung heat）。②定义法：为用外语原语下定义，如“辨证论治”译为以 diagnosis and treatment based on the overall analysis of the symptoms and signs。③多样法：是指由于中医名词术语本身存在一词多义、数词同义及概念交叉现象，如“虚”根据不同的环境，可能有一些不同对应词，如“脾虚”译为 asthenia of spleen，而气血、阴阳之“虚”可译为 deficiency，功能的虚弱也可用 hypofunciton，体虚的“虚”可用 weakness 或 debility 表达。④拼音法：是由于中医理论中特有的概念在英语中很难找到对应语。如“阴阳”“三焦”“命门”等，应用音译法，可避免用意译造成理解和交际上的困难，如把“气”译为 vital energy，“三焦”译为 three warmers，“命门”译为 life-gate 等，即是明显之例。

为了能承担中医翻译的使命，作者对译者提出了一个修养问题，并从两方面做了论述。一是思想修养，要正确看待中医，努力端正译风，勇于创新；二是业务修养，要精通医学外语，对中西医基本知识应有所掌握。如中医的“奔豚”是中医的一个古病名，症见有气从少腹上冲胸咽，伴有腹痛或往来寒热，这与西医的胃肠神经官能症十分接近，因此，在译时不妨对照，把“奔豚”译为 gastroenteoneurosis，而不用现行译名 running-pig syndrome，否则读者很难理解其含义。在业务上译者还应具有一定的翻译学及语言学知识、医古文基础和古典哲学知识，这样才能成为一名杰出的中医翻译工作者。

2. 中医翻译的原则和特色

由于中医为古文，有古典文学和哲学色彩，又无对应语，歧义较多，翻译时多见于直译或意译，缺乏原则做指导。如“五行”有译 five elements、five phase 或音译 Wuxing；将“ 三焦”译成 three warmers，或 triple heaters 或音译为 Sanjiao 等。鉴于目前中医翻译出现的混乱局面，作者提出中医翻译三条原则：

2.1 薄文重医，得“意”忘“形”

中医语言中有浓厚的古典文学及哲学色彩，译者向读者传达的是古老的医学科学知识而不是文学或哲学知识。在大多数情况下对文学过浓的用语，还是得“意”忘“形”为好。有的可用现代医学术语表达，易为外国人所接受。例如《素问·上古天真论》有“上古圣人之教下也，皆谓之虚邪贼风”之语，其中“贼”实为致病的因素，可用现成医学科学术语 pathogen 或 pathogenic factors，而不用 thief wind。

2.2 比照西医，求同存异

中医和西医的差异是显而易见的，但也有相似之处，如心、肝、脾、肺、肾，其含义不尽相同，但又有共同点，相应的译为 heart、liver、spleen、lung、kidney，也有人主张音译为 Xin、Gan、Pi、Fei、Shen。作者认为上述直译也不会使人产生误解。因为中西医早期有不少接近之处，如汉语“伤心”，英语为 heartbreaking，“关心”的英语为 to take to heart，还有一些中西医名异实同病症，如中医病名“痨瘵”，西医病名为 pulmonary tuberculosis（肺结核）、“瘿”的西医为 goitre（甲状腺肥大）等。早期西医传入中国时也采用直译、音译或意译，区别对待，并未引起西医与中医的混乱和影响西医在中国的传播。如 heart 直译为“心”，而没有音译为“哈特”，而 lymph 则音译为“淋巴”等。

2.3 尊重国情，保持特色

语言国情学认为，一种语言中总有一些反映该民族特有的事物，在思想和观念上在别国语言中找不到对应词，中医则有少部分即是。如“失笑散”译为“powder for lost smile”，实际上这里的“失”不是“失去”，而是“得到”，因此，应该音译为“ShiXiao powder”。在文章首次出现时可加一些注解，要少而精，可译为“A powder dissipating blood stasis ”。

3. 中医翻译的基本方法

作者对目前的翻译采用直译、意译和音译，根据中医语言的特点及翻译的具体意境，把中医翻译的基本方法分为深化、浅化、轻化、淡化和等化五个类型。

3.1 深化

对原文理解及表达透彻、入理，而不是表层信息的转述，如“土不制水”现行英译为 earth fails to control water，在表层上对应，但在深层上就值得研究了。“土不制水”是指脾虚弱不能运化水湿，引起机体水液代谢障碍的病理，如译为 fluid metabolism disorder due to hyposplenofunction，此种深化译语，完全可再现源语的信息。

3.2 浅化

指把特殊的东西一般化的一种译法。对有特殊含义的中医术语，如脏象、骨之余、血之余、髓海，可分别译为 viscera、tooth、hair、brain，达到语义对应。

3.3 轻化

用通俗易懂的语言来翻译理论性强又难懂的话语，如“邪之所凑，其气必虚”。首先把其转变成浅显易懂的汉语，为“体弱易病”，然后把轻化了的原文译成英语 Weak physique is liable to illness。

3.4 淡化

对于不完全适合用译入语表达的中文和对不符合外国人欣赏习惯的描写，进行必要删节或改写，主要用于文章摘要及药物说明书的翻译。

3.5 等化

使译语和源语在语义上趋于相等，主要用于借用西医术语和音译两个方面。

4. 中医名词术语翻译及标准化

中医对外交流所反映出的问题很多都与名词术语翻译上的混乱有关。作者从中医名词术语的结构区分，对中医的不同翻译法进行举例说明。如：

4.1 主谓结构

用深化法而不用浅化法，应尽量译成名词术语或词组性术语，而不译成句子。如：“土喜温”不要译为 Earth is fit for warmth。

4.2 动宾结构

可以直译，尽量比照西医用语。如“下利清谷”常被译为 watery diarrhea with indigested food in stool，译语冗长，且概念重复，可译成 diarrhea 或 diarrhea with indigested food。

4.3 联合结构

结构各组成部分平等，可以直译采用深化法。如“金寒水冷”，可译为：pulmonocryosis and nephrocryosis。

4.4　前偏后正结构

前一部分对后一部分有修饰和限制作用。如“肾虚不孕”和“气结腰痛”，可分别译为 nephropenic sterility 和 Qi-stagnated lumbago。

4.5　前正后偏结构

后一部分对前一部分有补充说明的作用，翻译时应尽量从英语医学词汇中寻找对应语，而不要随意直译或意译。如“听力不佳”即西医的 dysacousis（听力不良），不要译为 lowering of auditory acuity。

4.6　连动结构

第一个动词表示治疗手段，第二动词表示治疗目的。如“ 固肾涩精”，应译为 strengthen the kidney and stop nocturnal emission。

4.7　A 则 B 型结构

前一部分表示原因，后一部分表示结果。如“阳盛则热”，常被译成独立的句子 An excess of Yang may bring about heart syndrome，失去了作为术语交流中的作用，且冗长，似应译为 hyperoyang generating heat。

4.8　“取类比象”型结构

这类术语是中医语言文学化的一种表现，如“增水行舟”忌照字面直译，宜采用深化法。

关于针灸经穴标准化问题，在 1984 年召开的国际性针灸经穴名称国际标准化会议上，讨论通过了针灸经穴名称应包括三方面的内容：①英语字母数字编号；②汉语拼音穴名；③汉语名称。此次所定标准为国际合作标准化中医名词术语英译形式之先河，具有重要的现实意义。

5. 中医方剂名称的翻译原则

由于方剂名称命名方式比较复杂，给翻译带来了很大困难。作者首先根据方剂名称构成分类，确定翻译原则，提出规律性的翻译方法。

5.1　方剂名称翻译原则

作者提出三个原则。

5.1.1　简洁性原则

采用音译或中医方剂缩合形式方法，简化目前译法，如“胶艾汤”现译作 Decoction of Colla Corlii（Asini and Folium Artemisiae ），非常冗长。

5.1.2　信息性原则

方剂除指代功能外，都承载有一定的信息，译时要反映这一特点，但又要简洁。如“碧玉散”译为 Jasper Powder。有的则不能二者得兼。

5.1.3　回译性原则

英译的方剂名称在形式上能尽量与其中文形式相近，以有利于国际交流，有利于再现原文所含信息，有利于提高翻译质量。以君药命名的方剂名称都具有回译性。

5.2　方剂名称翻译方法

根据上述三性原则，应以直译和音译为主，并视不同类型而异。

5.2.1　直译法

适合于以主药命名（如桂枝汤 Ramulus Cinnamomi Decoction）、以动物命名（如白虎汤 White Tiger Decoction）、借喻法（如再造散 Recreation Powder）、功效（如温脾汤 Spleen-warming Decoction）以及以数目加主药（如六味地黄丸 Six-Rehmanniae Praeparata Pill）。译时注意不能译成句子，不能有冠词，剂型名排在主药或病症之后。

5.2.2　音译法

音译方剂名称有：组成方药太多（如麻黄杏仁甘草石膏汤，如直译则太长），以及以比喻、传说或以五行配设相关的方剂（如真武汤）。音译时应注意要以词译而不能字译，不能直译音译参半。

5.2.3　方剂剂型翻译

翻译的方式有汤剂（decoction）、散剂（powder）、丸剂（大丸 bolus，小丸 pellet 或 pill）、膏剂［（pate）为煎膏，有软膏、硬膏（plaster），还有浸膏（extract）等］、丹剂（同丸剂）、糖浆剂（syrup）、片剂（tablet）、冲服剂（granula）、油剂（salve）、胶囊剂（capsule）等。

6. 中医典籍名称翻译的新探索

作者有鉴于目前对中医名词术语特别是典籍名翻译的混乱局面，甚至于对一些已经约定俗成的术语，提出一些新看法。如：

6.1　古籍的名称翻译要追源

如对《黄帝内经》一词的理解，如何选词？首先是“黄帝”而不是“皇帝”，译成 Yellow Empeor 或 Empeor 是不大妥当的，当音译为 Huangdi 才对。“内经”不是内科，也不能译成 Internal Medicine。此处“内”的实质为书目编次中的“甲或上卷”。“经”字是梵文 sutra 的意译，即“贯穿”，应该用 sutra 翻译《内经》中的“经”字，均值得讨论，此种直译不如音译为佳。

6.2　创造新词汇

根据词素层仿造法简化出目前的直译或音译，如阴阳、气、命门、三焦、针灸等。

6.2.1　“阴阳”

“阴阳”的音译形式业已统一。作者提出对翻译形式做功能性调整，使其能承载更多信息量，一是将 Yin Yang 动词化；二是将其转化为构词成分，改变单一名词使用。这样就把滋养肾阴 Nourishing the kidney 译为 Yining kidney，把“肾阴虚” the deficiency of kidney Yin 译为 nephroyinpenia，“肝阳上亢” the sthenia of liver-Yang 译为 hyperhepatoyang。

6.2.2 “气”

音译 Qi 已逐步取代 viatal energy。作者认为也可仿阴阳译法一样将 Qi 动词化和转化为构词成分，这样就可以把“胃气虚” the deficiency of stomach-energy 译为 hypogastroqi。

6.2.3 “命门”

认为可采用词素层仿造法将其译为 vitaport（vita-意为“生命”，port 意为“门”），代替目前的 the gate of live。这样，既保持了中医语言特色，又合乎英语构词法则。

6.2.4 “三焦”

目前译法最为混乱，译为 three warmers 或 three heaterd 或 Sanjiao。可根据素层仿造法译为 tripyrogen（tir-“三”，pyro-“热”，gen-“原”）易为国外读者所理解，亦符合现代科技英语构词法的科学译语。

6.2.5 针灸

其译语 acupuncture moxibustion 已国际标准化。为了简便起见，作者提出将这两个术语掐头去尾组合成 acumoxi，此种改法有广泛的语言学基础，也符合现代科技英语的发展趋势。

以上重点概括地介绍了该书有关中医翻译的特点和看法。该书从 1993 年出版以来，很少引起中医翻译者的讨论。笔者认为，《中医翻译导论》是一本有关中医翻译理论体系探讨的书，或者可以称为“中医翻译学”。尽管可能为一家之言，但毕竟把问题提出来了，提出一个问题有时比解决一个问题还难。作为抛砖引玉，欢迎引起大家的讨论，以促使我国中医翻译走向一个新阶段，为中医走向世界，开展对外学术交流，更好地发挥桥梁作用。

[原载《中国中西医结合杂志》，1997，17（8）：508－510.]

对《中医药常用名词术语英译》的一些意见

魏迺杰　冯　晔

2004年由中国中医药出版社出版的《中医药常用名词术语英译》（谢竹藩主编）的英文名词，相对于过去许多汉英中医名词词表所提出的中医英文名词呈现大幅的进步，主要是因为它肯定了名词术语常规的翻译方法，也就是直译（仿造），并避免冗长意译的翻译方式。书中谢教授采用笔者著作中所出现的许多英文名词，笔者觉得很高兴。不过，《中医药常用名词术语英译》仍有许多尚待商榷之处。

1. 选词不当

选词不当就是说所选定的英文对应词与中文名词意义不相同。如，五行 five elements（第2页，为《中医药常用名词术语英译》中的页码，下同）：element是“元素”的意思，five elements似乎类似古希腊的四元素。“行”是运行的意思，与元素无关。大部分英语国家的翻译家早就改用 five phases 并习用多年。现在推行 five elements 是枉费精力。君火 monarch fire（第3页）：在英语国家最普遍的翻译是 sovereign fire。营 nutrient（第4页）：“营”字的原意是军营，当动词有“供应、输运、管理、建设”之义。“营”与“卫”相对，两者为军事性比喻。“营”原与“营养”无关，因为“营养”的“营”也就是供应的意思。92—93页亦有此问题。涎（thin）saliva、唾、（thick）saliva（第5页）：英文有 drool 和 spittle，与涎、唾颇为相近，何必用 saliva？三焦 triple energizer（第6页）：energizer 从 energy，即“气”的不恰当的翻译（谢教授也已不取用 energy 为“气”的对应词）。三焦与气有关，也与水有关，因此，triple energizer 不能完全地反映其义涵；另外，triple energizer 为 WHO 早前所提出，但没有任何英语国家的翻译家采用此名词。宣散 dispersion（第8页）：“宣散”是发散而发挥作用的意思，而 dispersion 是散而消的意思。肌 musele（第11页）：在古文中，“肌”就是“肉”的意思，包括了现代医学所指的脂肪和肌肉，因此，“肌”译成 muscle 是错误的，应该翻译成 flesh。筋 tendon（第11页）：中医的“筋”是指肉中可以摸得到的条状物，以现代解剖学来分析，它应包括肌腱（tendon），也包括肌肉（muscle）。谢教授有时译之为 muscle（见“3. 一词多译”）。脱 prostration/collapse（第28、29页）：“脱”是离去的意思（古人认为气能往外泄），而 prostration 的本义是倒下，医学上表示严重疲劳；collapse 则指昏倒，两者皆无法用来翻译“阳气外脱”。笔者采用 desertion 来翻译（如“外脱”可译为 outward desertion）。

2. 不良英语语法和修辞

热入血分 entering of heat into the blood system（第 24 页）：句型太复杂。笔者用 heat entering the blood aspect。痰蒙心包 clouding of the pericardium by phlegm（第 31 页）：phlegm clouding the pericardium 较恰当。这一类的问题很多。肺失清肃 failure of lung in purification（第 38 页）：in purification 不是英文的习惯用法。寒热错杂 cold-heat in complexity（第 25 页）：in complexity 不是英文的习惯用法。芒刺舌 prickled tongue（第 48 页）：应该是 prickly 才对。目痒 eye itching（第 55 页）：itchy eyes、itching of the eyes 都可以，但 eye itching 违背英文习惯用法。143 页亦如此。朝食暮吐 evening vomiting of that eaten in previous morning（第 57 页）：“eaten in previous morning” 文法明显错误，整句修词不雅，应该是 vomiting in the evening of food eaten in the morning（或 eaten the previous morning）。

3. 一词多译

一个名词如有两种以上的含义，当然可选定两种以上的英文对应词（如“滑脉”和“滑脱”的“滑”）；而一个名词，如有两种以上的合理对应词，难以择其一，则可以在名词表上系统化地采用两种不同对应词（如谢教授使用 pattern 和 syndrome 来翻译“证”）。然而，若一个名词仅具有一种意义，就不应该在不同语境中随便采用不同的对应词。在《中医药常用名词术语英译》中，如此的错误并不少见，本书中一词多译的问题常常出现在病机和证候的名词所使用的动词上。笔者相信，这些动词不是古人任意选定的，所以应该尽可能寻求一对一的固定翻译。如“结”一字，在中医词汇中，是指严重的郁滞、凝固、硬化的现象，是一种特别的概念，因此，应该有一个固定单一的对应词（笔者用 bind，与“结”相同，原意是“绑”，但也具有“凝结”的意思）。如果“结”字有数种不同的对应翻译，那么“结”的概念在译成的文献中就会丧失殆尽。而且，尽可能寻求一对一的固定翻译还有另外一个重要的理由，那就是方便文本翻译人员的使用。如果“结”在不同的名词中有数种不同的译法，那么当翻译人员遇到一个含有“结”字的名词时，就必须要查阅词表。反之，如果“结”字只有一个概念正确的单一对应译词，反复寻查的烦恼就会减少许多。

现举例说明。宣 dispersion/ventilation：宣发 dispersion（第 8 页），宣肺 ventilate lung（第 166 页）。还有将“不宣”翻译为 obstruction：肺气不宣 obstruction of lung Qi（第 39 页）。（另见“1. 选词不当”）。脱 prostration/collapse

（第 28、29 页）：病理上的脱只有一种意思，就是离去。没有必要采用两种对应词。参见“1. 选词不当”。脏 viscus/Zang organ，在水火之脏 viscus of fire and water 中，“脏”翻译为 viscus，其他处则译成 Zang organ。筋 tendon/muscle/sinew/soft tissue（第 11 页）：筋 tendon（第 11 页），经筋 muscle region（第 11 页），筋 ①tendon；sinew ②soft tissue（第 159 页）。参见“1. 选词不当”（第 11 页）。逆 reverse/adverse/counter-flow：气逆 reversed flow of Qi（第 24 页），肺气上逆 adverse rising of lung Qi（第 39 页），Qi counter-flow syndrome/pattern（第 74 页）。笔者都使用 counter-flow。瘀 stasis、stagnant：瘀血 stagnant blood（第 19 页），血瘀 blood stasis（第 28 页）。笔者使用 static blood 和 blood stasis。痹 impediment、arthralgia 等：痹病 impediment disease 或 arthralgia。痹的意思为：①是指风寒湿侵袭经络，痹阻气血，引起以关节、肌肉疼痛、拘急为主症的一类疾病；②泛指病邪闭阻肢体、经络、脏腑所致的各种疾病，包括前义所指的病症（《中医大辞典》，1627 页）。狭义的痹并非仅指 arthralgia（关节疼痛），后文还会说明。谢教授把风寒湿所致的各种痹证译成 arthralgia（第 111 页），“胸痹”译成 chest impediment（第 105 页），“胸痹心痛”译成 angina pectoris（第 105 页），“皮痹”译成 scleroderma。笔者一律用 impediment，动词用 impede。

4. 多词一译

“结”“停”“蓄”“阻”均译成 retention。如：大肠寒结 cold retention in the large intestine（第 39 页），气滞水停 syndrome/pattern of Qi stagnation and water retention（第 77 页），蓄血 retention of blood（第 91 页），湿阻 retention of dampness（第 101 页）。电子版还有“热积膀胱”的“积”和“脾虚湿困”的“困”也都翻译成 retention。“癃闭”和“饮”的英译也出现 retention 一字于其中。“结”“滞”“郁”“积”均译成 stagnancy。如：结阴/阳 stagnation in Yin/Yang（第 22 页），气滞 Qi stagnation（第 28 页），六郁 six kinds of stagnancy（第 42 页），食积证 syndrome/pattern of food stagnancy（第 70 页），胆郁痰扰证 syndrome of gallbladder stagnancy with phlegm disturbance（第 86 页），肝着 liver stagnancy。“宣”“疏”均译为 disperse，如：宣发 dispersion（第 8 页），疏风 disperse wind（第 166 页）。“痞”“塞”均译为 stuffiness，如，痞 stuffiness（第 55 页），塞因塞用 treat stuffiness with tonic（第 165 页）。“纳呆”（第 56 页）“厌食”（第 133 页）译成 anorexia。“纳呆”是胃主受纳功能减弱引起的消化不良、不思饮食，而“厌食”是虽饥亦不欲食，概念上应加以区别。“泻”“泄”“下”“泻下”“攻”译成 purge，如：实则泻之 treat excess by purging（第 165 页），清气泄热 clear Qi (system) and purge heat（第 167 页），下法 purgation（第 169 页）、泻下攻积 remove accumulation with purgative，缓攻 mild purgation（第 169

页)。“遏”“阻”“不宣”译为 obstruction/retention，如：卫阳被遏 obstruction of defensive Yang（第 24 页），痰浊阻肺 obstruction of the lung by phlegm turbidity（第 38 页），肺气不宣 obstruction of lung Qi（第 39 页）。

5. 过度使用汉语拼音

谢教授采用汉语拼音来翻译经络名称和方剂名称。在国外，经络、中药和方剂也使用汉语拼音名词，但许多外国文献翻译者，对于穴位名称、中药名称、方剂名称和书名都采用双语表达法（英译加上汉语拼音），如“麻黄汤”翻译成 Ephedra Decoction（Ma Huang Tang），“伤寒论”译为“On Cold Damage”（Shang Han Lun）。仅用汉语拼音并不理想，因为对于不会讲汉语的外国人而言，汉语拼音是不具有任何意义的。任何汉英中医词表，应该提出经络和方剂名称的英文翻译。谢教授对于方剂名称所采用的半音译半直译的处理方式，如 Guizhi Decoction，恐无太大意义，因为懂 Guizhi 的读者也知道 tang 是什么。既然谢教授把书名翻译成英文，他也应该提出经络和方剂名称的英文翻译。

6. 过度使用现代医学名词术语

谢教授过多地采用现代医学名词来翻译传统中医名词，最常出现的地方是在对病名的翻译。可否采用现代医学名词来翻译传统中医名词，要看其“所指”与中医传统名词是否相同，也要看“概念”是否一致。若“所指”不相同，则现代医学名词绝对不能用，如“痹”译为 arthralgia，但两词所指并不相同，因为“痹”所指包括非关节疾病，如西医的坐骨神经痛，而 arthralgia 专指关节痛。若所指相同而概念不同，则现代医学名词也不宜用，如“瘿痈”译为 acute thyroiditis（第 117 页），如此的译法不仅完全隐没了中医原来病名“瘿”和“痈”的概念，更在翻译的过程中强加入中医原本没有的概念：“急性”“甲状腺”和“炎症”。尤其是翻译古代中医文献时，若将非中医的现代医学概念引入译文中，就会造成所谓“时代错乱”的错误现象。另外，用现代医学名词来翻译传统中医概念，也会造成中医概念系统的破坏，例如，“疔”根据所发生的不同部位，用不同的现代医学名词译解，如 deep-rooted boil、pustule、whitlow/felon、-itis、Gangrene、anthrax（第 114 页）、boil（第 146 页），就会导致英文读者完全无法知道这些依英译名词彼此不同的病变其实在中医传统概念系统中皆属于同类，也就是不同部位的“疔”。

采用现代医学名词来翻译传统中医名词，从现代术语学和历史文献学的角度来看，都有问题。现代术语学强调名词应该反映出其所代表的概念。举例来说，疔叫作“疔”（亦称“丁疮”），“因为其形小，根深，坚硬如钉而得名”。在中医中，属于这种类型的疮疡都叫做“疔”，而谢教授采用的 boil、pustule、 whitlow、-itis 等不同的现代医学病名皆未能反映出中医“疔”的基本特征，因此，从术语学的角度来看，为不理想的翻译。而从历史文献学的角度来看，翻译带有文化特色的专业领域术语时，应该反映出“为何原来选择该名词”（Unschuld，1989），而通常得以反映出“为何原来选择该名词”最好的方法就是直译，因此，笔者和同事将“疔”翻译成 clove sore（clove 为丁香，从拉丁文 clavus，即“钉”的意思；不用 nail sore，是因为英文的 nail 也有“指甲”的意思）。

用现代医学名词替代传统中医名词将使英文读者完全无法了解传统中医概念，因此，对中医传统医学的传播是毫无帮助的。这种“以西代中”的翻译方法能否符合中西医结合的需求，也是有待商榷的。因为中医疾病缺乏客观的定义，所以一般难以作为临床研究的题目。而且，中医现代化不等于废除传统中医，新中医与旧中医仍然需要沟通的桥梁。譬如，过敏性鼻炎的中医疗效研究报告的前言就需要说明，古病名是“鼻鼽”，而若依照谢教授的翻译方法，古病名的英文翻译即等同于现代医学名称，根本就断绝了现代医学与中医学沟通的途径。中西医病名对照当然很重要，但是这应该是中西结合专业戮力的标的，不应该与翻译工作混淆。中医病名应该采用以直译（仿造）为主的翻译方法，而其与现代医学疾病名称的对应应该列在定义中详述。

在现代医学中，以希腊文字根组成的症状名称，如 dyschezia、menostaxis、polymenorrhea，越来越少用，大概是因为患者所告知的症状日益不受现代医学重视所致。但在中医学领域中，症状仍然较为重要，而且分得比较细，只有应用英文词汇译解才得以清楚地表达原本就颇为繁复的诸多概念（如 difficult defecation、prolonged menstruation 等），类如希腊文字根组成的症状名称根本难以望其项背。

在《中医药常用名词术语英译》“各科疾病”的章节中，“以西代中”的现象颇为普遍，以下即提出几个例子。

五官 five sense organs（第 13 页）：五官包括唇，但唇非属 sense organ（感官）。在古代文献中，官是“活的比喻”（官员），并没有现代汉语的“器官”的意思。目飞血 hyperemia of bulbar conjunctiva（第 59 页）：此名词出于《诸病源候论》，那时候没有“球结膜”的概念，若翻译《诸病源候论》时，把“目飞血”翻译成 hyperemia of bulbar conjunctiva，英文读者会误以为《诸病源候沦》的作者巢元方在隋朝就知道“球结膜”为何，这就会产生所谓“时代错乱”的现象。痈 abscess/-itis/phlegmon（第 115 页）：痈 abscess（第 115 页），乳痈 acute mastitis（第 117 页），锁喉痈 throat-blocking phlegmon。译法隐没了中医“痈”的概念。疽 carbuncle/deep abscess（第 115 页）：“有头疽”翻译成 carbuncle，“无头疽”翻译成 deep abscess。英文读者无法了解二者在中医学概念上的关联。

瘤（第 117、118 页）：气瘤 Qi tumor；subcutaneous neurofibroma，血瘤 angioma 和 hemangioma，筋瘤 varix 和 varicosity，肉瘤 lipoma，脂瘤 sebaceous cyst，骨瘤 bone tumor 和 osteoma。说理同前。解颅 hydrocephalus（第 135 页）：解颅为囟开不合，hydrocephalus（脑积水）则是颅内脑脊液增多的意思，两者概念上不相同，所指亦不见得相同。笔者译为 uninited skull。流金凌木 pseudopterygium（第 139 页）：在中医的概念系统中，金与木有重大意义，不只是病名的层次，更与治疗相关。翻译成 pseudopterygium，则中医的概念就完全不见了。神昏 coma（第 113 页）：神昏"即神志昏迷不清，或全然不知"[2]，不完全等同于现代医学的 coma。笔者用 clouded spirit。皮痹 scleroderma（第 120 页）：皮痹是风寒湿邪外袭皮毛所致的痹证，证见瘾疹风疮，搔之不痛，初起皮中如虫行状（《中医大辞典》，475 页），而 scleroderma 则为硬皮病，概念应难等同。骨痿 bone atrophy（第 112 页）：现代医学的 bone atrophy 与 osteoporosis 等同，即骨质疏松症，而中医的骨痿是肾热内盛或邪热伤肾引起的痿证（《中医大辞典》，1090 页），并不等同于骨质疏松症。笔者译为 bone wilting[3]。鹅掌风 tinea manuum（第 119 页）：按照现代研究，鹅掌风在概念上包括现代医学的手癣（tinea manuum）及裂隙性湿疹（fissured eczema）。直接译为 tinea manuum，一则丧失了中医的概念，二则并不完全合理。笔者译为 goose-foot wind[4]。

7. 结论

"选词不当"及"不良英语语法和修辞"两个问题所显示的重点是"母语优势的英文能力"（native speaker competence in English）的缺乏。词句不通的汉英中医词表将不会在英语国家获得认同，而继续采用已逐渐被废弃的译名如 meridian和 five elements，更表现出未能跟进西方的中医西传和中医翻译发展的趋势。"一词多译"的现象并不符合名词翻译的一般原则，显现出名词翻译的工作人员未能充分协调的窘境。实际执行时，"一词多译"和"多词一译"的错误皆会导致文献翻译人员面临难以背记的困扰。至于方剂名称一律采用音译，如此的译法犯下的"过用汉语拼音"的错谬，只会造成对不懂中文的英文读者而言，译文如佛经一般拗口难懂。一套经过文献翻译实际执行考验而渐趋成熟的词汇不应该出现这样的缺点。

"采用现代医学名词"翻译传统中医名词的结果，就是彻底破坏了中医的概念（如"瘿痈"翻译成 acute thyroiditis），而因此所导致"一词多译"四处可见的局面，甚至还会造成名不符实的弊端丛生（如"痹"可翻译成 arthralgia、impediment等）。虽然一般认为中西医结合与中医现代化是当务之急，但传统中医才是中医的"根本"。在中医西传的过程中，将中医传统知识原封不动地传达给西方人应该仍是不二法门，而且只有传统文献学和现代知识领域所采用的"以直译为主的翻译方法”方可达成此目标。制定英译的标准时，对于中医的传统概念若不采用“翻译”，而以“以西代中”的方法取代，将会引致英文读者永远看不到中医原貌的危厄，破坏中医西传的初衷。中西结合的目标应该是建立中医和西医沟通的桥梁，例如中西病名或概念的对照研究自是中西结合领域的专家重要的课题，但绝对不该在翻译的这个层次上，直接以西方医学的名词代表译解中医的病名或概念，因为此举僭越了“翻译者的天职”，徒然毁坏中医学理论的完整性，甚至影响中医西传使其走上歧途。或许谢教授主张“以西代中”的翻译方法的目标是要让落后的中医脱胎换骨，借由西医名词的使用一举让中医得以登上21世纪的医学大雅之堂，但实际上这样做只会抽离中医的灵魂，对中医西传有害无益。

中国大陆中医界普遍的看法认为中医的原始概念是外国人无法了解、无法接受的，因此，翻译时最好是采用“以西代中”的方法。但多年的实践证明，如此的认知是绝对错误的。西方读者绝对不等于西医界人士，如果给西方读者机会，他们一样也能清楚领会中医的奥妙。今日西方医学能够成为医学主流，不也是因为其放诸四海皆准吗？而且其他知识领域所采用的以直译为主的常规翻译模式已然在英语国家的中医翻译界实质地掌握了绝对优势。

参考文献

[1] 李经纬．中医大词典．北京：人民卫生出版社，1995.
[2] 张伯萸等．中医大辞典．知音出版社，1989：1182.
[3] Wiseman N. 英汉汉英中医词典．长沙：湖南科学技术出版社，1995.
[4] Wiseman N. 实用英文中医词典．北京：人民卫生出版社，2002.

[原载《中国中西医结合杂志》，2006，26（10）：953－955.]

关于《汉英医学大辞典》中某些中医药词条的商榷

樊　蓥　龙明照　周仲瑛

人民卫生出版社1987年10月出版的第1版《汉英医学大辞典》是国家权威出版机构会同全国30余所医药院校与研究院的80多位海内外知名学者、专家、教授编辑而成，中国医科大学为其主编单位。该书是国内迄今为止同类辞书中最大型、也是最具权威性的一部辞典，在近10年里已对我国医疗的各个方面以及国际文化交流起到过十分重要的作用。由于国内外对于基础医学、临床医学、预防医学、康复医学等方面的内容理解比较一致，故由英译汉转而汉译英也就比较贴切，但在中医药名词术语由汉语（特别是古汉语）英译方面显得问题较多。兹就初步翻检所及的一些有可能误译的词条提出来商榷，恳请同道批评指正。

1. 不同疾病译成了同一名称　如“疰（注）夏”译为 Summer fever，“暑温”也译为 Summer fever。该译词实际意义是“夏季热”，似乎与“疰（注）夏”对译为好，因为这已是约定俗成的译法（按：“疰夏”比较贴切的意义是 Summer feoricula，即“夏季轻度发热”）；“暑温”一则“暑”为 Summer-heat，二则专指乙脑之类疾病，所以译为 epidemic Summer-heat febricity（流行性暑热病）可能更恰当些。

2. 温病类病名译法　“温病”是 epidemic febrile disease，“瘟（温）疫”则是 pestilence，或译作 infectious epidemic disease。实际上，“温病”和“瘟疫”是同类疾病，只是“瘟疫”是“温病”中之烈性者。该书“春温”译为 Spring-warm syndrome，“冬温”译成 Winter-warm syndrome，按字面义似乎不错，中医书里有时也可能有“春温证”“冬温证”之说。但实际上“春温”“冬温”都是病名，而不是 Syndrome（证），用 warm 一词也体现不出“传染、流行”的意义，译为 epidemic Spring —febricity、epidemic Winter-febricity 可能较妥，因为是病名，故宜略去 febricity 后 disease 一词。同理，上述“暑温”一词不宜改译为 Summer-heat-warm syndrome。该书“伏暑”译为 disease due to latent Summer-heat，若按作为病名要求可按字面译为 latent Summer-heat，但要更贴切些，还是以直译、意译相结合，译为 latent epidemic Summer-heat febricity 较好。

3. “八纲辨证”　译为 analyzing and differentiating pathological conditions in accordance with the eight principal syndromes。其中“八纲” the eight principal syndromes（八个主要证型）译法不妥。“八纲”实际上是中医辨证的四维坐标系

统（four-dimension-axis system），表、里、寒、热、虚、实、阴、阳是该坐标系中的八个“极”（pole，参照系），而不是一般意义上的 syndrome，此处误译乃因中医“证”字多歧义而然。“八纲辨证”宜译为 analyzing and differentiating pathological conditions in accordance with the four-dimension-axis system，在 four-dimension-axis system 后可对其具体内容作注释。

4. “哑”　译为 alalia，但其实际意义是“失语”。中医时常用“哑”的含义并非是“失语”而是“嘶哑”hoarseness，因此，译“声哑”宜用 hoarseness，“失音”则为 aphonia，而不应为“哑”alalia 所惑。该书“暴喑（瘖）”译为 suddenloss of voice，作为注释词尚可，作为病名则过俗，宜用 acute aphonia（急性失音症）或 acute alalia（中枢性急性失语症），译时根据上下文以作选择应用。同理，“暴盲”和“暴聋”译为 sudden loss of vision、sudden loss of hearing 也不妥，而宜分别译作 acute ablepsia/acute blindness 和 acute anacusia/acute deafness.

5. “鼻疖”　译为 nose-boil 或 nasal boil 较妥，不宜用 boil of nose，因为这种构词法造的词组作为病名不宜。同理，“鼻肿”译为 nose-swelling 而不译为 swelling of the nose。采用“名词+名词”的合成法而不用 of 所有格。

6. “和肝”　宜译为 mediating the liver，不宜译作 regulating the liver-Qi（调肝气）。因为“和肝”通常是“柔肝、疏肝”同用的一种方法，不仅针对 liver-Qi，也针对 liver 体。

7. 谚语的译法　“大实有羸状”书中译成 appearance of deficiency in extreme excess，还原成汉语则是“大实证中虚证的外观”；“至虚有盛候”书中译为 symptoms of excess in extreme deficiency，还原成汉语则是“至虚证中实的症状”，显然离原意已远。并且这两句谚语译成了词组，但是这个词组缺少了动词成分。改译成句子则语义较全：extreme excess syndromes are prone to be identified as deficiency syndromes，and upmost deficiency syndromes are subject to be recognized as excess syndromes，两句句式一样，但同义词选择了不同的措辞，是出于修辞的需要。值得一提的是，该书同一词条下注释中有 pseudo-deficiency symptoms 和 pseudo-excess symptoms 等字样，是照搬中医传统的“假虚”“假实”说法而来。仔细推敲，symptoms 绝不会是 pseudo-的，关键问题是：大实确可能有羸状、至虚确可能有盛候，羸状、盛候都是临床表现的一个方面，本身不是假象。该谚语的意思是，在生死攸关之时，根据次要信息施治，而耽误了治疗关键性病理，往往会使患者横夭莫救。用“假象”这种说法来强调“羸状”“盛候”（次要信息）只是修辞的手段，而不是真的 pseudo-，这在概念上要搞清，不宜望文生义式地对译。

8. “扶正祛邪”　译为 strenthening the body resistance to eliminate patho-

genic factor，还原成汉语则是“增强机体的抵抗力以去除病理因素”。姑且不论“扶正”是否仅限于 strengthening the body resistance，就这个词组来讲，一般情况下尚可译成两个并列的动宾结构组成的词组，即 strengthening the body resistance and eliminating pathogenic factors，但此处的“正”似译为笼统的 vital Qi 为好。

9.“对症下药”　译为 prescribing specific medicine for an illness，该词似乎过于直译；一般译为 giving a proper treatment（治疗、处置），意译为好。“对症治疗”译为 expectant treatment，变成了“期待疗法”“自然疗法”的意思，不如直接用 symptom-treatment 贴切。

10.“疔疮走黄”　译为 carbuncle complicated by septicemia，即“由败血症合并疔疮”，显得本末倒置。该词组可直译为 carbuncle running yellow（“走黄”指黄色的脓毒走散全身），或意译为 septicemia from carbuncle。

11.“儿科四大要证”　译为 four chief diseases in pediatrics 不妥，该词组的实际意义是 four intractable diseases in pediatrics，即“儿科四种难治病”。

12. 关于 due to 句式　如书中“寒痰”译作 phlegm syndrome due to cold，“寒嗽”译作 cough due to cold，在具体行文中该种译法尚可，但该词多数情况下是作为词组、甚至当一个专有名词用，这时用 due to 造词就有不当，应参照汉语的组词方法，用英语的“名词（或形容词）＋名词”构词。如“寒痰”译为 cold-phlegm，“寒嗽”译作 cold-cough。同理，“气郁眩晕” dizziness due to depression of Qi 宜改译为 Qi-stagnancy dizziness，之所以“气郁”不译作 depression of Qi，是因为 depression 有“消沉、抑郁、压低、凹洼”等多种含义，与中医“郁”字有过大距离。

13.“动静结合”　译作 association of activity and inertia，词组中少译了动词意味，同时 activity（活动）似不如 exercise（锻炼、练功）符合“动”的实际意义，故改译成动宾词组 combining exercise with inertia 似较传神。

14.“急黄”　译成 acute febrile，jaundice，infectious hepatitis，即“急性发热的黄疸性、传染性肝炎”，离原意过远。“急黄”实指 fulminant hepatitis (-like syndrome)即，“暴发性肝炎（或那样的综合征）”，或者说 severe hepatitis “重症肝炎”之类病死率极高而发病急暴的黄疸性肝炎。

15.“邪气盛则实”　译为 The excess syndrome results when the invading pathogens is exuberant（while the body defensing Qi is not too weak）。姑且不论其具体译词是否贴切，就句法而言，这是个判断句，或许改译成下面句式更为恰当：That the invading pathogens is exuberant is the excess syndrome（while the body defensive Qi is not too week）。

16.“邪气内陷”　译作 invasion of the interior of the body by pathogen（s），

即“病原向人体内部的侵入”。译文组词方式不妥，且未译出该词组确切含义，可改译为 infectious pathogen（s）invading the interior suddenly and the illness getting to critical stage。

17.“邪害空窍”　译成 affection of the facial orifices by pathogens，“邪恋心包”译作 lingering of pathogenic factor in the pericardium，看上去总觉别扭，其实仍按汉语方式译成“主谓（宾）”词组即可解决问题，如上述两词组可分别译作 pathogen（s）affecting the facial orifices，pathogen（s）lingering in the pericardium。

18. 关于五脏藏神志　该书“心藏神”译为 spirit stored in the heart，“肺藏魄”译作 the lung stores the spirit/soul。另外，“意”“志”都译为 mind，对于“神、魂、魄、意、志”等词相互混译。这五个精神活动相关词在英语中是否能分开是很成问题的，与其无止境地考证，不如将这类词用汉语拼音音译造词，作为 Qi、Yin、Yang 一样处理，译成 Shen、Hun、Po、Yi、Zhi 是否更好。

综上所述，该辞典中许多译词之不当，主要原因当是翻译人员不甚了解中医名词术语的确切含义以及组词方式和应用习惯造成的。有些纯属望文生义，译词浮于表面；作为病名和证名的一些词组，译词过于松散或导致含义倾斜。从译文可以看出，该辞典中医药名词术语英译经过了信息的两次加工，即由中医学者将原文（多为古汉语）译成白话（通常变为注释），再由英语专家英译（译成其他语言也然），这两类学者互不搭界，在许多问题上不可能进行太深入的、具体的沟通，所以出现了原文信息量被丢失和曲解，同时语法关系也被忽略。建议今后编写或修订这类辞书时应请相当比例的精通英译的中医、中西医专家以及精通中医的英语专家加入，至少在审订时严格把关。只有这样，才能提高这类辞书的编译质量，维护其权威性。

［原载《中国中西医结合杂志》，1997，17（2）：109－111.］

评《中医药学名词》中的对应英文名词

谢竹藩 廖家桢 刘干中 张庆荣 李 磊 唐 汉 王 台

任何一门学科都有其专用的名词以表述该学科所特有的概念、理论和实践。一门学科的科技名词的规范统一是关系到这门学科发展的大事，这对于中医药学来说尤其重要。中医药学起源于我国，有数千年的悠久历史，名词浩瀚，亟须规范统一，特别是当前为了促进中医药的对外交流和走向世界，中医药学名词的中英文对应问题更是重中之重。但是，要真正完成这项任务是极其困难的，远非其他学科制定对应英文名词所能比拟。其他科学技术名词大多已有国际名词的基础，甚至有不少名词原本就是从西方引进的，即使是我国创建的名词也不乏原有的命名规律可循。但中医药学，尤其是与理论有关的名词，一般没有现成的西方名词可以借鉴，而中文名词又大多古朴，往往与现代汉语含义有别。《中医药学名词》（以下简称《名词》）于 2005 年由科学出版社出版，确是我们翘首以待的大事。但是在惊喜之余，我们发现这本《名词》并不像前言中所说的那样具有系统性、规范性和权威性。相反地，仅就我们最关心的对应英文名词而言竟然是错误百出，无法遵照使用。

由于在《名词》的“内容提要”中明确提出“本书是全国科学技术名词审定委员会审定公布的中医药学基本名词”，“这些名词是科研、教学、生产、经营以及新闻出版等部门应遵照使用的中医药学规范名词”，因此，此书在全国范围内造成了误导。本文作者之一曾遇到这样一件事，一位答辩委员质问答辩人为什么中医骨伤科中的“骨科”一词的英译不按照《名词》中规定的 osteology 翻译，由此可见该书所引起误导的严重性。为了维护中医药学的正常对外交流，我们认为有必要提出意见，消除《名词》在国内造成的误导。由于书中错误过多，限于篇幅，不可能将所有错误一一列出，只能就各种不同类型的错误分别举例说明。另外，确定中医名词的英文对应词是一项极其复杂的工作，是否贴切，是否实用，难免见仁见智，各执己见，因此，本文所述不涉及这类问题，只限于提出一些无可争辩的错误。

1. 存在英语语法错误

作为名词的英文对应词，在语法方面的要求应该说并不复杂，有些语法问题因涉及意思的表达，虽然明显不妥，本文也不拟讨论，但像名词的单数和复数这样简单的问题竟然也有错误，那就难以令人容忍了。

1.1　中正之官

Fu-viscera with decisive character（03.175，为原书编码，下同）。姑且不论此英文词是否与原文对应，仅就语法而言其错误是绝对的。“中正之官”是胆的别称，人只有一个胆，而 viscera 是复数（单数是 viscus）。

1.2　配穴法

points combination（08.1630）。名词作定语时一般用单数形式，无论用多少穴位配方，都应是 point combination。

1.3　衄血

bleeding from five aperture or subcutaneous tissue（04.134）。这里也不谈英文对应词是否规范，单就五个孔窍用单数 aperture 这一点就无法令人接受。

2. 违反英文用语习惯

既然是英文对应词，那就应该尊重英文的用语习惯。《名词》不论具有多大的“权威性”，也无权更改英文的用语习惯，更不能否定现有的英文习惯用语。

2.1　黑睛

black eye（03.335）。中医所说的黑睛是眼球外壁前部的中央，即角膜部分。英文 black eye 是习惯用语，指被打得眼圈乌青。这样一来，“黑眼珠”译成英文就成了“黑眼圈”。撇开常用的英文习惯用语，black eye 最多也只能说明眼睛的颜色，即虹膜的颜色，与 blue eyes、brown eyes 等并列，不过按英语习惯很少会这样理解，因为即使是黄种人也只是 brown eyes 或 dark-brown eyes。再退一步来说，即使这样解释，black eye 也不能作为黑睛的对应词，因为黑睛是眼球一个部位的名称，不属于黑眼睛、蓝眼睛之类的用语。

2.2　白睛

white eye（03.334）。这个对应英文名词的错误与黑睛 black eye 恰恰相反，后者是乱用英文的习惯用语，而“白睛”则是放着现成的对应词不用，硬要创造新词。白睛是指眼球外壁白色不透明的部分，与此相应的英文是 white of the eye，译成 white eye 则与 blue eyes、brown eyes 属于同类的概念，不过从未闻有谁长着一双白眼睛。

2.3　吐舌

wagging tongue（04.199）。吐舌为“舌常伸出口外，不立即缩回的舌象”。这并不是什么难用英语表达的词语，《名词》却偏偏选中一个与“伸出”“不缩回”不相干的 wag（摇摆）。tongues wag 是英语常用的口语，意为“说闲话”“造谣”。wagging tongue 与中文的“摇唇鼓舌”倒可以相应，与临床症状中的“吐舌”实难联系。

3. 与中医原义根本不对应

3.1 暴风客热

sudden wind and invading fever（14.027）。所谓客热是指外来入侵的热邪，而 fever 是体温不正常升高，即发热。实际上此病并不以体温升高为主要表现，故此热非彼热，无对应可言。

3.2 食鱼蟹类中毒

allergy after eating fish and crab（10.203）。这个名词的定义为："因进食有毒或变质鱼、蟹所致……的中毒类疾病"，既然是中毒，怎么在对应英文词中一下子变成了变态反应。即使在症状中有"以头晕、肤痒、胸闷烦躁，或腹痛呕泻，甚至虚脱为主要表现"的描述，但这并不能说明就是变态反应。如果说是对鱼蟹的变态反应，只进食鱼蟹就能发生，无须进食有毒的或变质的鱼蟹，更不必强调是中毒类疾病。

3.3 但欲寐

analeptic（04.016）。这个对应英文名词更是令人莫名其妙，analeptic 是苏醒剂、兴奋剂，用它来治疗但欲寐也许还算说得过去，怎么会成了"但欲寐"（又称"嗜睡"）的对应英文名词？正文和索引中的"但欲寐"和"嗜睡"三处都是用 analeptic 作对应词，所以不可能是偶然的拼写错误。

4. 随意摘取部分原意

《名词》中有不少对应英文名词是摘取中文中的部分含义而拟就的，其结果不是歪曲原意，就是令人不解。

4.1 本经配穴法

combination of affected channel；association of affected channel；combination of affected meridian；association of affected meridian（08.631）。这里一下子罗列了 4 个英文对应词，但没有一个与原文对应。原文讲的是本经配穴，英文对应词却只有"经"，没有"穴"，到底是什么东西的 combination 或 association，令人不知所云。

4.2 疾医和疡医

general medicine（02.182）和 royal surgeon（02.183）。只要把这两条加以对比，就可以看出《名词》中的对应英文词的拟定是如何地随心所欲。这两条的注释如下："疾医：周代官方卫生机构中的内科或内科医生"。"疡医：周代官方卫生机构中的外科或外科医生"。再来看看这两条对应英文词，第一条中只有医学，医生的概念没有了，而且医学的范围也扩大了，不只限于内科。第二条的对应英文词中只有医生，学科的概念没有了。同样属官方卫生机构，"疡医"的对应词加上了 royal 作定语，对“疾医”则没有这方面的表示。其实，“疡医”这个名词并非只在周代应用，也并非只限于官方卫生机构，例如明代王肯堂的《六科证治准绳》中就有《疡医证治准绳》(1602)，清代顾世澄撰《疡医大全》(1760)。所以疡医的定义是有缺欠的，但这是中文问题，本文不予讨论，仅就对应英文名词而言，其拟定之随意和轻率，缺乏严肃的科学性的程度实令人吃惊。

5. 乱用西医一般名词

有些英文名词既是西医用语，又是日常用语。这类词语实际上比专业性强的西医名词更适用于表达中医的概念。但是，使用这类名词时首先需要认真考虑其作为医学名词的含义，否则会导致严重的误解。

5.1　转归

sequelae (03.773)。《名词》对“转归”的定义如下：“疾病发展的结局，包括痊愈、死亡，或后遗症等各种情况。”但 sequela 在医学上只限于后遗症一种情况。《名词》中中风后遗症 (10.057) 的对应词就是 sequela of apoplexy。把 sequela 变为复数 sequelae 只不过是多种后遗症而已，并不能因此就包括痊愈、死亡等各种情况。

5.2　里急

abdominal pain (04.453)。对于这样一个简单的名词竟然也会出现问题，确实难以想象。按《名词》所作的定义，里急是“自觉腹内拘急，疼痛不舒，便意急迫的表现。”也就是说里急除腹痛外更主要的表现是腹内拘急不舒，便意急迫。把 abdominal pain（腹痛）和里急对应，显然从逻辑上就讲不通，二者的内涵差别太大了。只要把英文回译，问题立即显现。

5.3　喜食异物

addiction to eating foreign bodies (04.441)。喜食异物是指“嗜食生米、泥土、纸张、煤炭、墙皮等各种非食品之异物的表现”。但是，foreign body 并不能表达上述的异物。这个英文词在医学中十分常用，定义也很明确，它所表达的异物是正常生物体内没有的外来的东西，用在这里实在令人莫名其妙。

6. 乱用西医专业名词

如果中医名词的概念确与西医相符，例如人体的某些部位、病人的症状和疾病的名称等如果相符，理应采用西医名词，以免令人误认为中医在这些方面也有许多概念是西医所不了解的。但是西医专业名词一般都有严格的定义，绝不能望文生义，随便应用。《名词》中不乏错用的情况，其错误的严重程度让人感到《名词》应用了西医名词而实际上却根本不懂所用的西医名词的含义。

6.1 孕痈

abdominal carbuncle during pregnancy（12.061）。孕痈为“以妊娠期间合并肠痈为主要表现的疾病”，英文对应名中的 abdominal carbuncle 显然是指肠痈而言，但西医的 carbuncle 是有严格定义的，它是多个相邻毛囊和皮脂腺或汗腺的急性化脓性感染，不可能发生在腹腔内。令人不解的是为什么《名词》把 acute appendicitis（11.087）作为“肠痈”的对应英文名，而妊娠期间的肠痈则成了 abdominal carbuncle。

6.2 白睛青蓝

blue sclera（14.032）。白睛青蓝是中医眼科的一个病名，按中医眼科学的论述，白睛青蓝与西医学之深层巩膜炎及后期的巩膜葡萄肿有相似之处。blue sclera 的中文名是青色巩膜，它是成骨不全（osteogenesis imperfecta）的眼部表现。成骨不全又称脆骨症（oeteopsathyrosis），是一种遗传性疾病，因此，白睛青蓝与 blue sclera 风马牛不相及，这样的对应英文名不仅造成误解、误译，用于临床还可能造成误诊。

6.3 中医骨伤科学

osteology and traumatology of traditional Chinese medicine（01.019）。这里把“骨科”用 osteology 作为对应英文词实为奇闻。首先让我们引证《名词》对中医骨伤科学所下的定义：“研究骨关节伤折，肌肤、筋肉、脏腑、经脉损伤疾病诊治与预防的临床中医学”。我们不在此讨论这样的描述是否规范，至少有一点是十分明确的，它是一门临床医学。什么是 osteology？它是解剖学的一个分支，研究人体的骨骼结构。它根本不是临床医学，不研究骨关节伤折以及其他组织损伤的诊断、治疗和预防。如果有哪家中医医院的骨伤科挂上 Department of Osteology 的牌子，认识这个英文词语的人谁也不敢进去就诊。

7. 违反中医医理

7.1 阴虚外感证

syndrome of exogenous disease due to Yin deficiency（04.588）。注解中明确说明是“阴液亏虚，又感外邪”，对应的英文名却成了“阴虚所致的外感”。阴虚之人可以再感外邪，但阴虚本身不能引起外感证，外感证只能由外邪引起。

7.2 解颅

hydrocephalus due to non-closure of fontanel（13.058）。这个英文对应词不仅冗长，而且颠倒了因果关系。囟门不闭合为什么会引起脑积水？这种医学常识性的错误竟然发生在这样一本“应遵照使用的中医药规范名词”中，不能不令人感到遗憾。

7.3 干脚气

weak foot due to dryness (10.165)。这里不讨论 weak foot 是否与中医的脚气相应，只谈 dryness 问题。在这本《名词》中 dryness 与“燥”相应，指燥邪或燥证，所以对应英文名词所表达的是“由燥引起的脚气”。按中医理论，脚气是因外感湿邪风毒，或饮食厚味所伤，积湿生热，流注腿脚而成。脚气有干脚气、湿脚气之分。所谓干脚气是指脚气之足膝不肿者，湿脚气是指脚气病见脚膝浮肿者。这里的“干湿”不过是症状的描述，英译成为致病的原因，岂非差之毫厘，谬之千里。

8. 不符合中药学概念

中药学名词由于中华人民共和国药典已有英文版出版，大量的中药名和方剂名都有现成的规定，故需要《名词》拟定的名词为数不多，但即使如此，仍有不少错误。

8.1 土炒

fried with earth (06.110)。英文 fry 是用油煎炸，土炒绝非加土拌匀后用油煎炸。

8.2 线剂

thread formula (07.028)。“将丝线或棉线放在药液中先浸后煮，经干燥制成的外用剂型。”其实不用注解，稍有中药学知识的人都知道这是一种剂型，不是配方，不可能与 formula（配方）对应。

8.3 平

calm (06.056)。“寒、热、温、凉界限不明显，药性平和，作用较平缓，调养脾胃、益气生津等功能的药性。”“平”字作为动词用于治则治法，与 calm 相应是可以理解的，但这里指的是药性，也用 calm 显然就难以理解了。这很可能是张冠李戴，把平肝熄风的“平”搬到这里来了。

总之，从以上所举的例子已能充分说明《名词》在对应英文名方面的错误之严重达到令人吃惊的程度。初步统计书中有上述各类错误的至少 240 条。全书共收载 5283 条，其中 1500 多条已有现成的标准对应英文名词（如中药名和方剂名有英文版药典的规定，针灸穴位名和骨科所用的西医病名有世界卫生组织的标准，历代医家姓名无须英译）。换言之，在 3000 多条中竟有 200 多条无可争辩的错误。至于不规范的问题，本文虽未讨论，但像中成药 traditional Chinese patent medicines and simple preparations，针灸学 science of acupuncture and moxibustion of traditional Chinese medicine 之类远离规范的中英对应更是俯拾即是。这样一本错误百出的《名词》竟然以全国科学技术名词审定委员会公布的形式出版，要求各界遵照使用，措辞之严厉颇似法令，在全国引起了严重的误导，我们认为有必要加以讨论，故撰此文提出我们的意见。更为严重的问题是，《名词》的原稿与正式出版物曾先后以中华人民共和国最权威著作的名义和国家标准的名义两次在世界卫生组织召开的制定西太区传统医学国际标准名词术语会议上散发，要求作为制定国际标准的依据，但两次都被会议否决，严重影响了作为中医药发源地的我国在国际上的声誉。但如何消除在国际上造成的恶劣影响，这就不是我们力所能及的了。

［原载《中国中西医结合杂志》，2006，26（2）：169－172.］

中医对外英语交流的经验与体会

贾德贤　李兴广

由于东西方文化背景、东西方教育体系与方法、英语与汉语之间、中医术语与普通汉语之间都存在着很大差异，如何才能将古老的中医理论用简单明了、恰如其分的英语表达清楚，使学习者能全面而深刻地领悟中医的精髓，提高对外英语教学的质量与效果，确实存在许多问题与困难。在经过几年的国外中医英语教学后，笔者愿意谈谈自己的一些经验与体会，抛砖引玉，以期与同道切磋，共同提高中医的英语教学水平。

1. 不仅要有扎实的中医学基础，还要有良好的西医学基础

这里所讲的扎实的中医学基础，不是仅指对中医教材内容相当娴熟，而是指对中医理论和实践在真正意义上的理解，只有充分理解和把握中医学的全部内涵，授课时才能深入浅出，联系实际，能以生活中的普通知识和临床的实际例子，把深奥的中医理论加以通俗地解释，使初学者感到中医学虽然深奥但能摸得着，科学而又符合客观现实，从一开头就牢牢抓住学生学习中医的兴趣。如：如何阐释自然界的“火”与人体“火热证”之间的关系，从而解释“天人相应”这一观点，可从“火”的自然特征讲起。简单地讲，“火”具有红（red）、黄（yellow）、热（hot or burning）以及“火性炎上”等特点，故“火热证”，如扁桃腺炎（tonsilitis）的临床表现为局部发“红”，化脓后则见脓“黄”，自我感觉热痛（burning pain），与自然“火”的特征一一对应，易于理解。

良好的西医学基础非常必要，因为对于西方人来说，他们不具备最基本的中医学背景知识，不像中国人，从很小起就知道“上火”的含义，但他们一般熟知西医病名与相应的症状，尤其是那些“西学中”的西医初学者。在这样的情况下，若单以中医的英语术语来解释中医，往往使初学者有在云里雾里、摸不着边际的感觉，不易理解，从而产生畏难情绪，知难而退，或觉得枯燥而产生厌烦心理。但若以中医理论去分析、解释一些他们的常见病、多发病，如关节炎（arthritis）、抑郁症（depression）、肠激惹症（irritable bowel syndrome）等，如何跟人们生活中的天气、饮食、情绪、环境等息息相关，如何在中医理论指导下分析及治疗这些疾病，常可激发他们的兴趣，收到很好的教学效果。在这一点上，与国内的本科教学略有不同。

2. 要有较好的公共英语基础

在英语的教学与交流过程中，好的教学效果的取得，除了扎实的专业基础外，还取决于清晰的英语表达，正确的语言表述，包括至少简单语法的正确使用，较清晰的发音，和恰当的选词。对于中国学者来说，我们有较好的语法基础，应不存在很大问题，只是要尽量避免使用冗长的句子。我个人认为关键点、难点和容易引起争议的地方是选词。对于非英语国家的授课者来说，光有大量的词汇还不够，关键还要对词汇有确切的理解，选词要恰当，方能很好地表达中医的真正内涵，否则会导致曲解。这一关相对比较困难，但只要授课者耐心细致，认真考究，还是可以做好的。如 anorexia，意为厌食症、食欲缺乏症，它表达的不是一般意义上的食欲不振，而是一种较难治愈的危重征候，可出现在不正确的减肥或其他严重疾病过程中；脾虚之食欲不振是指脾胃功能一般性紊乱所导致的食欲不好，通过理气健脾，通常是可以治愈的，用 poor appetite 或 lose of appetite 等表示即可，若用前者表达后者，则有言过其实之嫌。还有如 sore 和 painful 的区别，都表示“痛”，但前者通常特指感染性或受伤后的疼痛，后者为一般意义上的身体某一部分的疼痛。其他还有如 deficient 和 insufficient，enough 和 sufficient 等，它们的意思均相近，但在程度上有所不同，应注意区别使用。

有些词的使用是有争议的，缘于不同人的不同表达方式。如滑苔，很多人和教材翻译成 slippery coating，但容易产生与 greasy coating（腻苔）相似的感觉，而《中医诊断学》描述滑苔为水分过多，扪之湿而滑利，甚者涎流欲滴，故笔者认为用 watery coating 表示滑苔更为贴切。再如舌诊中的“老舌”，相关教材大多翻译成“rigid（坚硬的）tongue”，《中医诊断学》描述“老舌”为“舌质纹理粗糙，形色坚敛苍老”，使人想到饱经风霜的老人，故笔者认为用“old tongue”直接来表达更为合适。笔者就本翻译曾与英语国家学生讨论，得到认同。诸如此类的问题还有不少，到底应该怎样翻译，有待进一步讨论。

3. 授课力求生动，避免刻板

西方学生在教育方法上更喜欢生动灵活的教学方式，语言要尽量活泼，举例要生动幽默，能用简单词表达的要尽量用简单词，过于专业的词，对于我们来讲难记，对于他们来说也不容易。如鼻出血（epistaxis）可以用极易记忆的 nose bleeding 代替，学生更愿意接受。

4. 课堂讲解与临床实践及时结合

讲课时不宜采取“填鸭式”教学。中医学的内容对初学者来讲较难理解，长时间的课堂教学容易使学生感到厌倦，所学内容容易被忘记，适时的临床实践非常重要。在实践中将所学知识“小试牛刀”，既可帮助学生对课堂所学加深理解，又能激发学生的学习兴趣，还可发现学习中存在的问题，经过临床多次、反复的实践，必定可以提高学习效果。

5. 图文并茂，列表概括，避免长篇累牍的纯文字解释

纵观西方国家的各类教材，皆为图文并茂，西方人已习惯这样的教学方式，加之形象的图画表达，可以省掉语言赘述，确能收到事半功倍的效果。但这样做，就要求授课者尽量将抽象的中医理论用形象思维的方式客观而准确地表达出来。这样的方式一定是基于对中医理论的精髓深刻把握的基础上，否则，会产生误导。另外，阶段总结，提纲挈领，帮助学生理清思路，提高学生的学习效率，非常必要。否则只见树木不见林，最终将一片混乱，收不到预想的效果。

搞好中医的对外交流需要大家的一致努力，在不断切磋的基础上，共同提高我们的英语水平，促进我们的对外教育的成熟，为发展中医做出贡献。英语不是我们的母语，但它也不是不可逾越的，以此与同道共勉。

［原载《中国中西医结合杂志》，2002，22（3）：236－237.］

英译《中医妇科学》的几点体会

曲　凡　周　珏

笔者对导师马宝璋教授主编的国家本科规划教材《中医妇科学》（第 6 版，上海科学技术出版社，1997）进行了英译，同时还与一些学习中医的外国留学生进行了广泛交流。下面就中医妇科学的英译问题谈几点体会。

1. 《中医妇科学》中名词术语的英译

1.1　应以解释性翻译为主，不必刻意追求高信息密度

译者对中医妇科学理论的理解要准确、透彻，这样的译语才能做到“信”“达”。如英译“五不女”时，就要明确其所指为女性先天生理缺陷和畸形所致的不孕，故译为“five types of female sterility due to congenital factors”；再如“经行吐衄”要明晰其具体的含义，故译为“haematemesis and epistaxis within menstruation”；“盛胎”所指的是受孕之初，按月行经而无损于胎儿的，这里的“按月行经”有别于正常情况下的月经，如译作“menstruation”就不能传达其确切含义，译为“menorrhea at the beginning of pregnancy”为佳。中医妇科学名词术语的英译的最大难点就在于准确把握原词的确切内涵，力争真实地再现原文信息。

1.2　准确掌握名词术语的内涵和外延及其相互区别

如中医学的“胞宫”除了包括子宫的实体外，还包括两侧的输卵管和卵巢，虽然它也有“子宫”的别名，但此“子宫”远非彼“子宫”，故将其译为“uterus”就不准确，应音译为“Pao-gong”；再如“崩漏”与西医的“功血”并不完全对应，译为“dysfunctional uterine bleeding”就与原文有一定距离，根据“崩漏”的定义：妇女不在行经期间，阴道突然大量出血，或淋漓下血不断者，同时结合二者间的相互关系：“崩为漏之甚；漏为崩之渐”将其译为“metrostaxis and metrorrhagia”更妥。

1.3　从西医名词术语的英译语中探寻中医妇科名词术语的相关词素

在词素层面翻译中，构成原文词的每一个词素在译入语的对应词中有一定的相应词素。词素层面是分析词汇的基础和依据，是学习和掌握英语词汇的钥匙，还是中医妇科学名词术语词素层面汉英翻译中的有效翻译成分。采用词素翻译法，可使中医妇科名词术语译语信息密度提高、科学性增强。如“肾阳虚型不孕”译为“hyponephroyang sterility”，“脾阳虚型带下”译为“hyposplenoyang leukorrhagia”。根据科技英语的词素构词法原则，可以大胆灵活地进行词素翻译，如“胞宫虚寒”译为“sthenic frigidity in Pao - gong”。

2. “辨证”英译

辨证论治是中医学的特色之一，英译中医妇科学同样也需要“辨证”。众所周知，英文属形合性语言，汉语属意合性语言。中医妇科学语言往往言简意赅，有些词汇具有多层含义。这就决定了同一个中医妇科学词汇，在不同的环境中译语也会有所不同，这并不是因为要避免重复，而是出于准确透彻再现原文信息的需要。如“带下”一词有广义、狭义之分，广义“带下”泛指妇产科疾病而言；而狭义带下又有生理和病理之别，因此，“带下医”中的“带下”应取其广义而译为“gynecologist and obstetrician in ancient times”。《傅青主女科》中的“夫带下俱是湿症”及《素问・骨空论》所说的“任脉为病……女子带下瘕聚”中的“带下”就应取其病理性的狭义带下之意而译，故译为“leukorrhagia”。而《沈氏女科缉要》引王孟英说“带下，女子生而即有，津津常润，本非病也”中的“带下”是指生理性的狭义带下之意，译为“discharge”为妥。

总之，中医妇科学英译的要旨在于向读者传达古老的中医妇科学知识，而不是文学或哲学知识。所以，在将源语言转化为目标语言的英译过程中既要考虑目标语言读者的承受能力，又要强调翻译的科学性、简洁性、标准性和信息性。

[原载《中国中西医结合杂志》，2005，25（5）：448.]

中医药期刊的刊名英译

周庆辉

我国目前出版的中医药期刊共有 110 多种，其中绝大多数以中文出版，只有 4 种以英文出版，即《中国中西医结合杂志（英文版）》《中医杂志（英文版）》《世界针灸杂志》和《针灸推拿医学》。美国科学信息研究所（Institute for Scientific Information，ISI）的《科学引文索引》（Science Citation Index，SCI）没有收录一种我国出版的中医药期刊。美国国立医学图书馆（National Library of Medicine，NLM）的《医学索引》（*MEDLINE/Index Medicus*）2003 年收录的我国出版的中医药期刊只有 4 种，即《中国中西医结合杂志》《中医杂志（英文版）》、《中国中药杂志》和《中药材》[1]。可喜的是，2003 年 5 月创刊的《中西医结合学报》于 2004 年 6 月通过了 NLM 文献选择技术评审委员会的评审，并于 2004 年 9 月 1 日起被收录于 MEDLINE/PubMed 检索系统[2]。

我国中医药期刊的国际化水平以及期刊的国际显示度尚不尽如人意。影响中医药期刊对外交流的因素是多方面的。但不容忽视的因素之一是期刊英文的翻译。期刊内容的英文翻译若不能达到严谨、准确、流畅，甚至存在文法、句法和拼写错误，就不免会令人怀疑作者和编者工作的严谨性，进而怀疑论文的科学性和可靠性，因此，切不可忽视期刊刊名的英译，它是一个值得研究的问题。

笔者收集并分析了我国目前公开出版的 110 多种中医药期刊中英文刊名，多数刊名译名既忠实贴切，又传旨达意，有的则不尽然，主要存在以下问题。

1. 少数英文刊名不能准确反映期刊特定内容

如《现代中药研究与实践》刊名译为 Research and Practice of Chinese Medicines，《中药材》刊名译为 Journal of Chinese Medicinal Materials，两者对“中药”一词的翻译不够准确，宜加上 traditional 一词。《中医文献杂志》和《中医研究》的英文刊名分别为 Journal of Traditional Chinese Medicinal Literature 和 Traditional Chinese Medicinal Research，若其中的 medicinal 一词改为 medical，则更加符合期刊内容。

2. 刊名中的标点及缩写

《中西医结合心脑血管病杂志》刊名译为 Chinese Journal of Integrative Medicine on Cardio-/Cerebrovascular Disease。将斜线号（virgule）与连字符（hyphen）并

用是不妥当的。心脑血管病可译作 cardio- and cerebrovascular disease、cardio-cerebrovascular disease 或 cardio/cerebrovascular disease。斜线号一般表示“或”“和”，连字符表示“和”，故两者不宜并用。

《湖南中医药导报》刊名译成 Hunan Guiding Journal of TCM，虽然在国际上，英文刊名中也有使用缩写的例子，但仍以译出全名为佳，以使其明了。另外，“导报”一词译作 guiding journal 不符合英语表达习惯。根据报刊内容的不同，“导报”一词可有多种译法，如《汽车导报》：Autonews；《申江服务导报》：Shanghai Times；《中国经济导报》：China Economic Herald。以上均为报纸。在期刊中也有应用，如《材料导报》：Materials Review；《欧华导报》：Chinese European Post。《湖南中医药导报》以中医药信息报道为主，故建议译作 Hunan Traditional Chinese Medical News。

3. 刊名中的赘词

期刊的刊名应以简短、明了为宜，在英译时应避免出现赘词。但中医药期刊英文刊名中这种情况比较多见。如《中医药学刊》译作 Chinese Archives of Traditional Chinese Medicine，英文刊名中两次出现 Chinese，显得累赘，可译为 Archives of Traditional Chinese Medicine。又如《云南中医中药杂志》译作Yunnan Journal of Traditional Chinese Medicine and Materia Medica，翻译“中医中药”或“中医药”时，译成 traditional Chinese medicine 即可。刊名英译中这类问题还见于其他一些期刊。

4. 关于英文与拉丁文混用的问题

一般而言，一个外文刊名应使用一种语言，不宜在同一外文刊名中使用一种以上语言的文字。但拉丁词 Materia Medica 已在英文医药文献中广泛使用，其作为一个专用名词也可以在医药期刊的英文名中使用，这是一个特例。而拉丁文 *acta* 一词却不能在英文刊名中使用，只用于拉丁文刊名。如 2004 年的 Index Medicus 收录期刊名单[1]中，使用 *acta* 的期刊共 87 种，刊名均为拉丁文，因此，《中医药学报》的英文刊名译成 Acta Chinese Medicine and Pharmacology 是不妥当的。

5. 中医学院和中医药大学学报刊名的英译

我国公开出版的中医学院和中医药大学学报共有 22 种。其中 21 种将“学报”译为“Journal”，只有《上海中医药大学学报》译为“acta”。

Journal 一词为英文，在汉语中可译为“杂志”“学报”“学刊”“日报（如《华尔街日报》英文名为 The Wall Street Journal）”等。*acta* 为拉丁文，意为

“记录”“学报”“报告”。英文journal和拉丁文*acta*均为较高级的学术期刊。journal和*acta*一般都由国际性或全国性的专业学会主办，不仅有严格的刊期，且每期都有固定的页数。我国各学术团体及各高校的学报大都用journal。笔者对“万方数据——数字化期刊群”收录的125种高等医（药）学院校学报的外文刊名进行了检索和统计，“学报”一词的翻译有以下4种不同形式的表达方法，分别为：journal，105种；acta，12种；academic journal，6种；acta academiae，1种；bulletin，1种。

毛发生[3]对清华大学电子期刊导航系统约11 000种西文电子期刊（包括自然科学、工程、技术和社会科学）进行检索后发现，使用频率最高的为journal，共3892次，占35.4%；而使用acta者仅79次，占0.7%。通过类似方法，对北京大学1427种国外人文社会科学核心期刊（电子期刊）进行检索，结果发现使用频率最高的也是journal，共400次，占28.0%；acta仅使用2次，占0.1%。

英语是世界性第一通用语言，在国际学术交流中，普遍使用的语言也是英语。期刊语种的通用化有利于期刊的国际交流，也有利于全世界读者阅读和国际检索机构收录。目前科技期刊出版用语英文化已成为一种国际趋势。故《上海中医药大学学报》以使用英文刊名为好。如《上海医科大学学报》就曾译为Acta Academiae Medicinae Shanghai，1999年改为英文刊名Journal of Shanghai Medical University，现已更名为《复旦学报（医学版）》，Fudan University Journal of Medical Sciences。

中医学院和中医药大学学报刊名的英译中存在的另一个问题是英文刊名中的院校名与该院校的英文名不一致，如《安徽中医学院学报》等。

6. 中西医结合类杂志刊名的英译

我国公开出版的中西医结合杂志共有16种。刊名中的“中西医结合”一词见有3种译法。多数译为“Integrated Traditional and Western Medicine”，共9种；有的译为“Integrated Traditional Chinese and Western Medicine”，共4种；另有3种杂志译为“Integrative Medicine”。“中西医结合”是指“综合统一中、西医药学知识，创造新医药学”[4]，而刊名中的“中西医结合”一词实际指的是“中西医结合医学”，即“综合统一中、西医药学知识”而形成的新的知识体系，意指中国传统医学与现代医学（又指西方医学）相结合而形成的医学体系，故国内习惯的译法为“Integrated Traditional Chinese and Western Medicine”。9种将“中西医结合”译为“Integrated Traditional and Western Medicine”的期刊其中文刊名中都有“中国”一词，故英译刊名时，都将“Integrated Traditional Chinese and Western Medicine”中的“Chinese”一词放在英文刊名之首，如《中国中西医结合杂志》的英文刊名译作 Chinese Journal of Integrated Traditional and Western Medicine，仍然做到了“达意”。但这种译法的不足是英文刊名太长，不便著录，特别是给编制英文刊名的缩写带来不便。如《中国中西医结合急救杂志》英译为 Chinese Journal of Integrated Traditional and Western Medicine in Intensive and Critical Care，其中实词多达 9 个。相比之下，将“中西医结合”英译作“Integrative Medicine”，则要简洁得多。

近年来，在中医英语翻译实践中，已趋向于将“中西医结合医学”英文译作 Chinese integrative medicine，并已逐渐被人们认可和接受。如 1997 年，首届世界中西医结合大会召开时命名为 World Integrated Medicine Congress，而 2002 年召开的第 2 次世界中西医结合大会即命名为 World Integrative Medicine Congress；中国中西医结合学会的英文名现已译为 Chinese Association of Integrative Medicine（CAIM），而其原英文名为 Chinese Association of the Integration of Traditional and Western Medicine；《中国中西医结合杂志》英文版于 2003 年更名为 Chinese Journal of Integrative Medicine（中文版英文刊名仍使用 Chinese Journal of Integrated Traditional and Western Medicine）；2003 年创刊的《中西医结合学报》，英文刊名译为 Journal of Chinese Integrative Medicine。

Integrative medicine 一词的日益广泛地被使用，是因为近年来在国际上“整合医学”概念的提出。

20 世纪生物医学迅猛发展，正统的西医（主流医学）受到不少非议，于是一些不属于正统西医的医疗方式悄然兴起，如中医、中药、针灸、气功、按摩、骨伤整治、催眠、心理咨询、心身医学等，不一而足，包括几十种治疗方法。这些诊治方法被统称为“补充和替代医学（complementary and alternative medicine，CAM）”。complementary medicine 是指与正统医学平行不悖、相辅相成、协同运作的一些其他治疗方法；alternative medicine 是指除常规西医以外可以有另一种选择。CAM 也被称为“非主流医学”。

包括中医药、针灸在内的这些所谓“非主流医学”日益受到西方世界的重视。英国国会上院于 2000 年对 CAM 的现状进行调研，从 6000 多份材料中总结出若干条战略性意见，认为应积极开展对 CAM 的深入研究，在肯定其效力的基础上，协调其与主流医学的关系，争取形成一个“整合医学”。正是在这一指导思想下，2001 年 1 月英国查尔斯王子发起在伦敦召开了“整合医学”会议，本次会议的名称被定为“整合医学”会议，副题是“替代医学能否被整合入主流医学?”（Integrated Medicine Conference：“Can alternative medicine be integrated into mainstream care?”）

“整合医学”的概念在我国即相当于“中西医结合医学”。“整合医学”的英文原文是 integrated medicine 或 integrative medicine。那么，在英文刊名中应该使用 integrated medicine 还是 integrative medicine 呢?

integrated 和 integrative 均由英语动词 integrate（意为“使结合，使成为整体，使合并”）加形容词后缀而成。两者从英语和汉语翻译的字面上看，对一般读者来说均难以区分。从两词的实际使用情况看，两者在国际上均有使用。在美国，一般用 integrative medicine，而在英国一般用 integrated medicine[7]。如为配合 2001 年 1 月 23—24 日在伦敦召开的“整合医学”会议，《英国医学杂志》（British Medical Journal，BMJ）于 2001 年 1 月 20 日出版了“整合医学”主题专辑，其中多使用 integrated medicine[5-12]。

笔者分别使用 integrative medicine 和 integrated medicine 作为关键词对MEDLINE 光盘数据库进行了检索，结果见表 1。从检索结果可知，含 integrative medicine 和 integrated medicine 一词的文献数自 1991 年以来逐年递增，2001 年以后文献数明显增加；1998 年以前多用 integrated medicine，1999 年以来则多用 integrative medicine；integrative medicine 的使用频率越来越高于 integrated medicine。

表 1　1990 年以来 MEDLINE 光盘数据库中使用 integrative medicine 和 integrated medicine 的文献数

年份	检索所得文献篇数		
	integrative medicine	integrated medicine	合计
2004 年 1—4 月	21	7	28
2003 年	36	6	42
2002 年	39	15	54
2001 年	32	34	66
2000 年	17	9	26
1999 年	19	10	29
1998 年	7	8	15
1997 年	1	10	11
1996 年	0	6	6
1995 年	1	12	13
1994 年	1	5	6
1993 年	0	2	2
1992 年	0	3	3
1991 年	0	1	1
1990 年	0	0	0

中医药等非主流医学正逐渐走向与目前的西方主流医学相汇合，而形成统一的“整合医学”的潮流，因此，中西医结合类杂志在英文刊名中使用 integrative medicine 将更容易被国际医学界所接受。“中西医结合医学”一词的英译不仅仅是期刊刊名英译的问题，规范和统一其英译，对于促进我国中医药学的对外交流也将产生积极的作用。建议今后将“中西医结合医学”译为 Chinese Integrative Medicine。

期刊刊名既能表明期刊的学科属性、专业范围和期刊层次，也能体现期刊的出版频次和读者对象，是人们加工、管理、存贮和利用期刊的重要依据。刊名翻译时应注意以下几个原则：①以直译为主；②要符合英语刊名的命名特点和英语表达习惯；③刊名要能反映刊物内容；④简洁凝练。在英译期刊刊名的时候必须综合考虑期刊的性质、宗旨与报道内容及内涵等方面，结合刊名英译用语本身的含义，准确把握英语刊名的内涵，这是正确英译刊名的关键。中文刊名英译涉及英语、翻译、情报检索等不同学科，是一个值得深入研究的问题，笔者写作此文的目的在于提请相关学科的研究人员对这一问题引起重视。对于大多数刊物来说，刊名及其译名都已经是固定不变的了，但对于新办的杂志或可从中得到启示，选取一个合适的刊名和译名。

参考文献

[1] National Library of Medicine, National Institute of Health. List of journals indexed in Index Medicus, 2004.

[2]《中西医结合学报》杂志社．《中西医结合学报》被国际权威检索系统 MEDLINE/Index Medicus收录．中西医结合学报，2004，2（5）：345.

[3] 毛发生．中文期刊常用刊名词语的英译初探．中国科技期刊研究，2004，15（2）：227-230.

[4] 陈士奎．关于“中西医结合”及“中西医结合医学”定义的讨论．中西医结合学报，2003，1（4）：241-243.

[5] Rees L, Weil A. Integrated medicine. BMJ, 2001, 322（7279）：119-120.

[6] Morrell P. Integrated medicine: orthodox meets alternative. Integrated medicine is not new. BMJ, 2001, 322（7279）：168-169.

[7] Woolfson T. Integrated medicine: orthodox meets alternative. Challenge of making holism work. BMJ, 2001, 322（7279）：168.

[8] Caspi O. Integrated medicine: orthodox meets alternative. Bringing complementary and alternative medicine（CAM）into mainstream is not integration. BMJ, 2001, 322（7279）：168.

[9] Bodeker G. Lessons on integration from the developing world's experience. BMJ, 2001, 322（7279）：164-167.

[10] Owen DK, Lewith G, Stephens CR. Can doctors respond to patients' increasing interest in complementary and alternative medicine? BMJ, 2001, 322（7279）：154-158.

[11] Berman BM. Complementary medicine and medical education. BMJ，2001，322（7279）：121-122.

[12] Reilly D. Enhancing human healing. BMJ，2001，322（7279）：120-121.

[原载《中国中西医结合杂志》，2005，25（4）：368-370.]